Student Workbook to accompany
Connections for Health
Fourth Edition

Mullen McDermott Gold Belcastro

prepared by

Deborah A. Horne, M.S.

Kathleen D. Mullen, Ph.D.

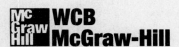
WCB
McGraw-Hill

Boston, Massachusetts Burr Ridge, Illinios Dubuque, Iowa
Madison, Wisconsin New York, New York San Francisco, California St. Louis, Missouri

WCB/McGraw-Hill

A Division of The McGraw-Hill Companies

Contents

Preface

The *Connections for Health Student Workbook* has been prepared to provide you with a framework that will enable you to be the architects of your health through informed decision making. This workbook is designed to provide a clear picture of how your current life-style is shaping your level of wellness both now and in the future. The fourth edition of this workbook reflects the revisions and addition of new material found in the *Connections for Health* textbook.

Wellness is a process that requires hands-on activity and application of concepts. Although self-responsibility is an integral part of wellness, one's social environment is equally important. To that end, an attempt has been made to have you place yourself in social situations where decisons that affect your level of wellness will have to be made.

The chapters of this workbook will guide you through the self-discovery process. Each chapter is divided into four sections. "Where Do You Stand?" provides you with personal assessments to assist in discovering your current level of wellness for each content area. "Review of Important Concepts" acts as a primer to help you clarify the more difficult concepts in each chapter. "Applying What You've Learned" asks you to integrate health information and apply it to real-life situations.

The final section "For Further Study" contains suggestions for pursuing a topic in greater detail outside the classroom. This section is divided into two subsections. "Wellness Activities" suggest experiences that you can explore in your community. These experiences are difficult, if not impossible, to get in a structured classroom setting but add an important dimension to your adventures with wellness. This section has been updated so that you have a list of the most current resources available.

A Wellness Project is included in Appendix A of this workbook. The guides listed under "For Further Study" can be used in conjunction with this project. The project provides a framework for implementing change in some aspect of your life. Although it may not be a requirement in your class, you are urged to make a change in your health behavior. It is the process involved in making the change that is important—not whether you were successful in achieving your wellness goal.

Wellness is an ever-changing process. You are urged to retain this workbook and refer to it in the years to come. Use it to implement change in your life—change that will lead to high-level wellness.

Acknowledgments

A special thank you is extended to William and Rosemary Horne, Patrice Annerino, Julia Lazzara, and all of our friends (you know who you are) for your unending support and encouragement. Appreciation is also extended to Brown & Benchmark Publishers.

1 Wellness: A Quality of Living

Wellness . . . Where Do You Stand?

What does it mean to enjoy high-level wellness? It means feeling really alive, having a gusto for life, a twinkle in your eye, and energy to enjoy it all. In short, it's your capacity to enjoy life to its fullest.

Sound good? Too good to be true? How does one get there? You begin your journey to high-level wellness by taking one step at a time. The Wellness Behavior Inventory is a tool designed to help you. It will help you assess your current level of wellness and at the same time increase your awareness of the elements in your life-style that can be improved.

Wellness Behavior Inventory

After reading each statement choose the response which best describes your *current* life-style.

A = Almost Always
B = Sometimes
C = Almost Never

Personal Habits

1. My appetite is good. _A_
2. I have an up-to-date immunization record. _A_
3. I rarely use medications. _C_
4. I smoke less than one pack of cigarettes per week. _A_
5. I don't smoke at all. (If this statement is true, mark the above statement true as well.) _A_
6. I drink less than two alcoholic drinks per week. _A_
7. I do not drink alcohol. (If this statement is true, mark the above statement true as well.) _B_
8. I minimize extra salt intake. _B_
9. I drink fewer than five soft drinks per week. _B_
10. I do have a monthly self-breast or self-testes examination. _C_
11. I have a yearly breast exam by a physician. _A_

12. I have a Pap test annually. _A_
13. I eat fruits and vegetables fresh and uncooked. _A_
14. I try to eat multiple small meals rather than one or two large meals. _B_
15. I understand that fiber is important in my diet and know sources of fiber. _B_
16. I drink enough water to keep my urine light yellow. _B_
17. I eat a diet that does not require supplements. _A_
18. My weight is within 15 percent of my recommended weight. _B_
19. I minimize refined foods in my diet. _B_ _B_
20. I request that others not smoke around me. _B_
21. I brush and floss my teeth every day. _A_

Feelings and Emotions

22. I enjoy my work. _B_
23. I trust and value my own judgment. _A_

24. I usually admit my mistakes and learn from them. _A_

25. Although I value my own opinion, I can appreciate the views of others. _A_

1

A = Almost Always
B = Sometimes
C = Almost Never

26. I usually know how to create my feelings. _A_
27. I know how to change my feelings. _A_
28. I can recognize and accept my feelings of mad, sad, glad, and frightened. _A_
29. I know feelings are often transient. _A_
30. I know how to deal with my feelings. _A_
31. I can set limits for myself and stick to them. _B_
32. I can say no without feeling guilty. _B_
33. I like being complimented for jobs well done. _A_

34. I think it is OK to cry. _A_
35. I try to accept constructive criticism without reacting defensively. _A_
36. I feel enthusiastic about life. _A_
37. I find it easy to laugh. _A_
38. I would feel comfortable seeking professional help if unable to deal with my feelings. _B_
39. I enjoy my family. _A_
40. I am able to give and receive love. _A_
41. I can accept the responsibility for my actions. _A_
42. I set realistic objectives for myself. _A_
43. I can make and maintain friendships. _A_

Community

44. I do not waste energy. _C_
45. I do not pollute the air. _B_
46. If I see a safety hazard, I will attempt to warn others or correct the problem. _B_
47. I use nonpolluting detergents. _A_
48. I would report a crime I observed. _A_

49. I contribute my time and money to community projects. _B_
50. I try to get to know my neighbors. _B_
51. I belong to a group with other than school or work affiliation. _B_

Automobile Safety

52. I never drink or use drugs while driving. _A_
53. I never ride with drivers who drink or use drugs while driving. _A_
54. I wear safety belts 90 percent or more of the time I am in a vehicle. _A_
55. I wear safety belts and a shoulder harness 90 percent of the time I am in a vehicle. _A_
56. I stay within five (5) mph of the speed limit. _B_

57. I have taken a course in driver education or defensive driving. _A_
58. I stop on yellow if the light is changing. _B_
59. I use radial tires. _____
60. For every ten (10) mph of speed, I maintain one (1) car length distance between cars. _B_

Rest and Relaxation

61. I enjoy my life. _A_
62. I usually have plenty of energy. _B_
63. I fall asleep easily. _A_
64. I can usually go right back to sleep if awakened. _A_
65. I usually meet my need for sleep. _A_
66. I rarely bit or pick my nails or fingers. _A_
67. I have no money problems. _A_
68. I know how to relax my body and mind without using drugs. _A_
69. I recognize and meet my sexual needs. (Note: There are many methods of meeting sexual needs

including art, religion, music, athletics, and sexual activity.) _A_
70. I have made conscious decisions about my sexual activity based on personal/spiritual values. _A_

A = Almost Always
B = Sometimes
C = Almost Never

71. If I were to have sex, I would use a contraceptive method. _A_
72. I feel my job is ethical. _A_

Fitness

73. I know how to measure my pulse. _B_
74. My resting pulse is 60 or less. _____
75. I often avoid using escalators and elevators. _b_
76. I walk briskly two miles or more a day. _C_
77. I bike, or swim, or exercise vigorously at least one hour per day three or more times per week. _b_
78. My daily activities include moderate physical effort (such as rearing young children, gardening, scrubbing floors, or work which involves being on my feet, etc.). _A_
79. My daily activities include vigorous physical effort (such as heavy construction work, farming, moving heavy objects by hand, etc.). _C_
80. I run at least one mile twice a week (or equivalent aerobic exercise). _C_

81. I run at least one mile four times a week or the equivalent. (If this statement is true, mark the previous item true as well.) _C_
82. I regularly walk or ride a bike for exercise. _B_
83. I participate in a strenuous sport at least once a week. _C_
84. I participate in a strenuous sport more than once a week. (If this statement is true, mark the item above true as well.) _C_
85. I do yoga or some type of stretching-limbering exercise for 15 to 20 minutes at least twice per week. _A_
86. I do yoga or a type of stretching exercise for 15 to 20 minutes at least four times a week. (If this statement is true, mark the item above true also.) _B_

The Wellness Inventory is a product of the National Wellness Institute at the University of Wisconsin-Stevens Point. Copyright © 1984. Reprinted by permission.

Selecting a Behavior to Improve

The Wellness Wheel

Directions: In order to get a visual picture of your wellness life-style, complete the following steps for the Wellness Wheel.

1. Refer back to the Wellness Behavior Inventory and assign a point value to each answer using the scale below.
   For each ``almost always'' answer (A), give yourself 2 points.
   For each ``sometimes'' answer (B), give yourself 1 point.
   For each ``almost never'' answer (C), give yourself zero points.
2. Using the Wellness Wheel Rating Key on the next page, figure your numerical score for each wellness area by adding your points for each question listed under the column labeled ``Questions.'' Enter your total points for each wellness area in the blank provided.
3. When you have totaled your points for each area, circle your rating located in the scale column.

Wellness Wheel Rating Key

Wellness Area	Scale			Questions	Total
Self Responsibility					
	Female		Male		
Self-Care Practices	12–16	almost always	11–14	2, 10, 11,	
	5–11	sometimes	5–10	12, 20, 21,	*12*
	0–4	almost never	0–4	41, 73	
	Female and Male				
Minimize Negative Coping Habits	8–10	almost always		4, 5, 6, 7, 66	
	4–7	sometimes			*9*
	0–3	almost never			
Personal Safety	15–20	almost always		46, 52, 54,	
	6–14	sometimes		55, 56, 57,	*14*
	0–5	almost never		58, 59, 60	
Environmental Sensitivity	17–22	almost always		4, 5, 13, 19,	
	7–16	sometimes		20, 44, 45, 46,	*14*
	0–6	almost never		47, 49, 75	
Fitness					
Physical Wellness Life-style	24–32	almost always		18, 61,	
	9–23	sometimes		73–86	*14*
	0–8	almost never			
Vigorous Exercise	15–20	almost always		75–84	
	6–14	sometimes			*5*
	0–5	almost never			
Stretching	3–4	almost always		85, 86	
	2	sometimes			*3*
	0–1	almost never			
Nutrition					
Nutritional Awareness and Habits	6–8	almost always		1, 14, 16,	
	3–5	sometimes		17	*0*
	0–2	almost never			
Reduce Salt	3–4	almost always		8, 19	
	2	sometimes			*2*
	0–1	almost never			

Reduce Sugar	3–4	almost always	almost always	9, 19
	2	sometimes		
	0–1	almost never		
				2
Increased Fiber	3–4	almost always	almost always	13, 15
	2	sometimes		
	0–1	almost never		*3*
Weight Control	12–16	almost always	almost always	14, 18, 19,
	5–11	sometimes		76, 77, 80,
	0–4	almost never		81, 82

Stress

Stress Management	15–20	almost always	almost always	24, 25, 26, 27,
	6–14	sometimes		30, 38, 42,
	0–5	almost never		43, 66, 68
Enjoyment of	8–10	almost always		36, 37, 39,
Leisure Time	4–7	sometimes		43, 61
	0–3	almost never		
Productivity	11–14	almost always	almost always	22, 24, 31,
	5–10	sometimes		32, 33, 35,
	0–4	almost never		42
Rest & Relaxation	12–16	almost always	almost always	61, 62, 63,
	5–11	sometimes		64, 65, 68,
	0–4	almost never		85, 86

Intimacy

Acceptance &	12–16	almost always		26, 27, 28,
Expression of	5–11	sometimes		29, 30, 34,
Emotion	0–4	almost never		37, 40
Feelings about Self	14–18	almost always	almost always	23, 24, 32,
	6–13	sometimes		33, 35, 38,
	0–4	almost never		40, 70, 72
Feelings of	11–14	almost always		39, 43, 46,
Community	5–10	sometimes		48, 49, 50,
	0–4	almost never		51
Sexuality	6–8	almost always	almost always	40, 69, 70,
	3–5	sometimes		71
	0–2	almost never		

4.   Now it's time to complete your Wellness Wheel. The wheel is divided into wellness areas that correspond to the Wellness Wheel Rating Key areas. The inner circle represents ``almost never''; the middle circle represents ``sometimes''; the outer circle represents ``almost always.''

Using your rating for each wellness area, color in the corresponding area of the Wellness Wheel. An example of a partially completed Wellness Wheel is illustrated below.

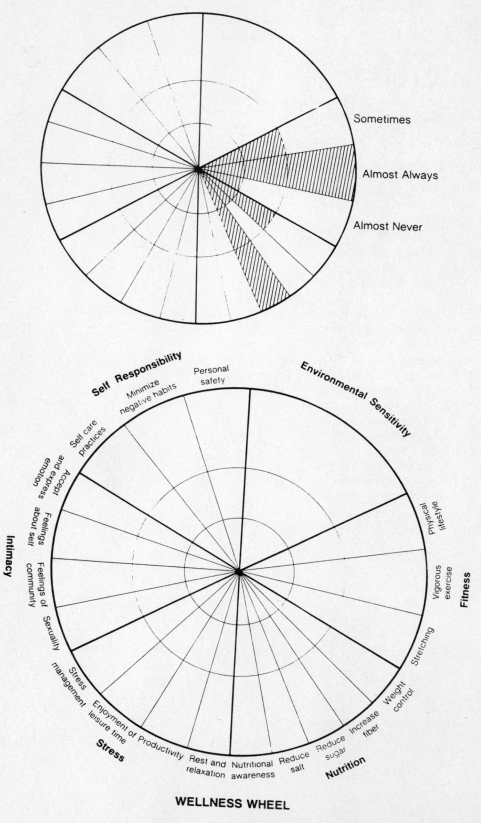

Sometimes

Almost Always

Almost Never

Self Responsibility

Minimize negative habits

Personal safety

Environmental Sensitivity

Self care practices

Accept and express emotion

Feelings about self

Intimacy

Feelings of community

Sexuality

Stress management

Enjoyment of leisure time

Productivity

Stress

Rest and relaxation

Nutritional awareness

Reduce salt

Reduce sugar

Increase fiber

Weight control

Stretching

Vigorous exercise

Physical lifestyle

Fitness

Nutrition

WELLNESS WHEEL

6

Supports and Barriers-to-Action

You've discovered there are areas in your life where you exemplify high-level wellness, and there are areas where you could improve your level of wellness. As part of your activities for this course, you may complete a personalized wellness plan. (Appendix A will help you plan your strategies.)

You can help to insure success with your personalized plan by examining a few behaviors more closely.

List three behaviors you would consider improving. Use Activity for Wellness 1.2 in your textbook and the Wellness Wheel to give you ideas.

1. _Stress_____ (Color Key [X])
2. _nutrition_____ (Color Key [ ])
3. _exercise_____ (Color Key [ ])

There are many reasons why people do or do not practice health and life-style behaviors that lead to high-level wellness. Below is a questionnaire that lists the supports and barriers that play an important role in your decision to engage in positive health and life-style behaviors.

Supports and Barriers-to-Action Questionnaire

Directions:

1. You will need to use three pens each having a different color ink to complete this questionnaire. Use a different color to represent the three different behaviors you would consider improving. (Place an X in the box following each behavior above to identify each color with a behavior.)

    For each item in the questionnaire, circle a number from 1 to 7 that represents the degree to which you think that factor plays a role in your adopting the behaviors listed above. Complete the questionnaire for the first behavior before going on to the next behavior.

2. You now have information concerning the types of supports that you have at your disposal and the types of barriers that will be obstacles for each behavior you have identified.

    Look over your answers for each behavior. Examine the factors for which you scored a 6 or 7. These are your supports (reinforcing and enabling factors)—people, places, and things that will set you up for success in improving your behavior.

3. Examine the factors for which you scored a 1 or 2. These are your barriers—people, places, and things that may impede your wellness planning.

Supports and Barriers-to-Action

Self-Image
Barrier						Support
1	2	3	(4)	5	6	7
I will always be embarrassed		Will have no influence			I will always be proud	

Cost
Barrier						Support
1	2	3	(4)	5	6	7
Will always prevent me		Will have no influence			Will always enable me	

Energy Level
Barrier						Support
1	2	(3)	4	5	6	7
Will always prevent me		Will have no influence			Will enhance my ability	

Convenience
Barrier						Support
1	2	3	(4)	5	6	7
Very inconvenient		Will have no influence			Very convenient	

Family Members
Barrier						Support
1	2	3	4	5	(6)	7
Will always prevent me		Will have no influence			Will always support me	

Comfort Level
Barrier						Support
1	2	3	4	5	(6)	7
Will always be painful		Will have no influence			Will always be pleasurable	

Close Friends

Barrier						Support
1	2	3	4	5	(6)	7

Will always hinder me   Will have no influence   Will always support me

Appropriate Facilities/Equipment

Barrier						Support
1	2	3	(4)	5	6	7

Are not available to me   Will have no influence   Are readily available to me

Other People

Barrier						Support
1	2	3	4	5	6	(7)

Will always hinder me   Will have no influence   Will always support me

Weather

Barrier						Support
1	2	3	(4)	5	6	7

Will always prevent me   Will have no influence   Will always enhance me

Time

Barrier						Support
1	2	(3)	4	5	6	7

Will always prevent me   Will have no influence   Will always enable me

Adequate Transportation

Barrier						Support
1	2	3	(4)	5	6	7

Will never be available   Will have no influence   Will always be available

Ranking My Behaviors: Narrowing the Choices

Ease of improvement, supports, and motivation for improving are three important factors to consider when selecting a behavior to improve. For instance, you might consider cigarette smoking to be a difficult behavior to change. However, if you are highly interested and motivated in this area, then you may want to change your smoking patterns even though you may perceive this as being ``hard.''

To help you determine which behavior to choose for improvement, complete the exercise below.

Directions

1. List the three behaviors you identified in the Supports and Barriers-to-Action section in the blanks below.
2. In the ``Supports'' column, rank each behavior in terms of how much support you believe you have in order to improve the behavior. Number 1 is the behavior you have the most support for.
3. In the ``Ease of Improvement'' column, rank each behavior in terms of how easy you think it would be to change. Number 1 is the behavior you feel would be the easiest to change.
4. In the ``Motivation to Improve'' column, rank each behavior in terms of how motivated you are to change that behavior. Number 1 is the behavior you feel most motivated to change.
5. In the ``Average Ranking'' column, average your rankings for each behavior by adding the 3 scores and dividing by 3.
6. The behavior that has the lowest score is probably the behavior you should consider choosing for your personalized wellness plan. Place an asterisk next to the behavior that scored the lowest.

Behavior	Supports	Ease of Improvement	Motivation to Improve	Average Ranking
1. _____	_____	_____	_____	_____
2. _____	_____	_____	_____	_____
3. _____	_____	_____	_____	_____

Now . . . the choice is yours. After weighing ease of improvement, interest, motivation, supports, and barriers, which behavior do you choose to improve?

Behavior for improvement _____

Reviewing Important Concepts

1. Define *health*.

2. Define *wellness*. Pg. 10 (text)
   * a process of optimal functioning & creative adapting that involves the total person (PM ESS) & strives for an ever increasing quality of life.
   * living life fully and always striving for a better life.

3. What are the major similarities between wellness and health?

4. What are the major differences between the two concepts?

5. Briefly explain the concept of risk.

6. List and describe the six stages of behavior change.

9

Applying What You've Learned

1. Refer to the story of the three cyclers in your textbook (p. 17). What factors do you think play a role in Mike's decision to cycle with the group? List these factors on the chart below.

		Mike	*You*
Predisposing Factors	1.	_____	_____
	2.	_____	_____
	3.	_____	_____
Enabling Factors	1.	_____	_____
	2.	_____	_____
	3.	_____	_____
Reinforcing Factors	1.	_____	_____
	2.	_____	_____
	3.	_____	_____

2. Imagine that Mike, Greg, and Dacia have invited you to join their morning cycling group. What are the reinforcing, enabling, and predisposing factors that would contribute to your decision to join them? List your answers in the column labeled ``You.''
3. Applying Critical Thinking Approaches to Reports of Health News

Applying Critical Thinking Approaches to Reports of Health News

The following is a sample "Critical Thinking Checklist" to help assess media reports about research results. Find an article in a recent newspaper or news magazine that presents new information regarding a health topic. Read the article and then answer the following questions. You will discover that most news reports answer only some of these questions. Analyze what information is given and what information is missing from your news report. How can new health information contribute to your personal health decision making?

1. Credibility of the source
    A. What is the source of the research results?
    B. Who paid for the study? Do the funders have any economic or other stakes in the research results? What is the probability for objectivity or bias?
    C. Has any agency or organization responded to the announcement of research results? Do they have any economic or other stakes in the results? What are the probabilities for objectivity or bias?
    D. Is the reporter known for prior experience in reporting on scientific research?

2. Factors in the study design
    A. What type of research was done? Was the research at the "test-tube" stage, animal-testing stage, or human-testing stage?

B.   Over what period of time did the study take place?

C.   How many subjects were in the study?

D.   Did the subjects have particular characteristics (age range, male or female, past disease history, etc.)?

E.   Was there a control group for the study?

F.   Have all relevant variables been considered?

3.   Interpretation of the results

A.   How are the results being stated? Are there "qualifying" words that limit the applicability of the results (such as "in animals," "some," "may," "probably")?

B.   Do the results depend on a measurement of change? If so, is there an indication of the significance of the change (either statistically or biologically)?

C.   Has the study been repeated by other researchers, with similar results?

D.   Does the article differentiate between "fact" and "opinion"?

E.   Does the study deal with a "risk factor"? If yes, do the results identify actions which will probably enhance health or probably increase the risk of disease?

F.   Are the results part of an ongoing scientific controversy? If so, what side of the controversy has been given added weight by this study?

4.   Application of the news

A.   Does the article make clear what is known and what is not known about the research topic?

B.   Does the article note what questions remain after the study and/or what new questions it generates?

C.   Are the research results reported in this article relevant to one of my personal health decisions? If so, is there enough information in the article to make me consider changing one of my decisions? Do I need to obtain additional information?

For Further Study

Your level of wellness is, in part, determined by what you do to and for yourself. The references and activities that follow will help you begin to explore your level of wellness and show you how to enhance it. Be creative . . . add to this list!

Wellness Activities

1.   What resources are available in your community to help residents achieve higher levels of wellness? You can assess your community wellness resources by looking in the telephone book and campus directory for community wellness resources for each of the areas delineated by the Wellness Behavior Wheel. Once you've done this, go visit the resource and interview an employee about the service they offer the community.

2.   If you have a campus wellness center, talk with a person who works there. What services does the wellness center offer that would enable students to increase their levels of wellness?

3.   Read one of the philosophical articles on wellness that is listed below. What are the major points of the article? How has your philosophy of wellness changed after reading this article?

Ardell, D. B. ``The Nature and Implication of High-Level Wellness, or Why `Normal Health' is a Rather Sorry State of Existence.'' *Health Values: Achieving High Level Wellness* 3(1979):17–24.

Bruhn, J. G., Cordova, F. D., Williams, J. A., and Fuentes, R. G. ``The Wellness Process.'' *Journal of Community Health* 2(1977):209–21.

Dunn, H. L. ``High-Level Wellness for Man and Society.'' *American Journal of Public Health* 49(1959):786–92.

Dunn, H. L. ``What High-Level Wellness Means.'' *Canadian Journal of Public Health* 50(1959):447–57.

Mullen, K., and Gold, R. ``Wellness Construct Delineation: A Delphi Study.'' *Health Education Research* 3.4(1988).

4. What are the barriers and enhancers that affect your level of wellness? Keep a wellness log for two or three days to aid you in discovering these factors.

2 Mental Well-Being and Stress: Coping Positively

Mental Well-Being and Stress . . . Where Do You Stand?

Mental wellness may be the heart of wellness in general. It is important for you to be open to experiences and to be able to try new behavior options if you are to achieve mental wellness. The first two assessments below will help you begin this exciting new journey.

Managing stress for personal growth is one strategy for mental wellness. Am I coping effectively with my life's stressors? Some individuals may not recognize that they are over-stressed. Make the connection between your stressors and how you are reacting to them by completing the third assessment, ``Stress Symptom Inventory.''

How Is Your Mental Health?

Everyone has a combination of emotions, attitudes, and behaviors that create a unique personality. You have considerable control over the items that make up your personality.

Following is a ``test'' that will help you identify several key issues related to mental or emotional health. Circle the answer that best describes you. Be as honest as possible.

My friends would agree that:
1. I am basically a pessimistic person. True False
2. I frequently wish I were somebody else or had another person's qualities. True False
3. I find myself frequently angry at people. True False
4. I tend to blame others for my problems. True False
5. I often assume blame for other people's problems. True False
6. I find it difficult to encourage and support the successes of others. True False
7. It is hard for me to accept encouragement and support from friends or family. True False
8. I do not have many friends. True False
9. I worry constantly about things I cannot change. True False
10. I am frightened about things others do not seem to be concerned about. True False

Scoring: If you answered ``True'' to five or more statements, now is a good time to review your approach to life. The chapter in your textbook and the guides listed at the end of this chapter will help you do that.

From M. F. Raber and G. Dyck, *Mental Fitness: A Guide to Emotional Health.* Copyright © 1987 Crisp Publications, Inc., Los Altos, CA. Reprinted by permission

Starts and Stops in Building Self-Confidence

A deep and confident sense of liking oneself and feeling worthwhile is one of the most universally recognized characteristics of mental wellness. Confidence is not automatic; it must be built and nurtured.

All of us experience failures. These, to a degree, can tend to destroy your confidence. A tendency to make constant comparisons can unintentionally lead to a decrease in self-confidence.

Finding our own uniqueness and then building on it is a key ingredient to insure a good level of self- confidence. Below is a list of ``starts'' and ``stops'' that can help you build self-confidence. Check those you feel need increased personal attention.

[ ] 1. Start liking yourself.
[ ] 2. Stop running yourself down.
[ ] 3. Stop comparing yourself with others.
[ ] 4. Start making full use of your abilities.

[ ] 5. Start viewing mistakes as a way to learn.
[ ] 6. Start remembering past successes.
[ ] 7. Start becoming an ``expert'' at your present job.
[ ] 8. Start finding areas in your life in which you can make positive changes.
[ ] 9. Start initiating a self-improvement program.
[ ] 10. Start *taking* action rather than just *planning* action.

From M. F. Raber and G. Dyck, *Mental Fitness: A Guide to Emotional Health.* Copyright © 1987 Crisp Publications, Inc., Los Altos, CA. Reprinted by permission.

Stress Symptom Inventory

Stress affects us as whole people, so we're likely to experience symptoms of stress exhaustion not only in our bodies—but also in our emotional reactions, our mental state, our relationships with others, and our spiritual life.

Check the symptoms of stress exhaustion you've noticed lately in yourself. (There may be other underlying causes of any of these symptoms that should be checked out by a doctor. However, this list represents common stress-related complaints.)

Mental

_____ forgetfulness
_____ dull senses
✓ poor concentration
_____ low productivity
_____ negative attitude
✓ confusion
_____ lethargy
_____ whirling mind
_____ no new ideas
_____ boredom
✓ spacing out
_____ negative self-talk

Emotional

✓ anxiety
✓ frustration
_____ the "blues"
✓ mood swings
✓ bad temper
_____ nightmares
✓ crying spells
✓ irritability
_____ "no one cares"
_____ depression

_____ nervous laugh
✓ worrying
_____ easily discouraged
_____ little joy

Spiritual

_____ emptiness
_____ loss of meaning
_____ doubt
_____ unforgiving
_____ martyrdom
_____ looking for magic
_____ loss of direction
_____ needing to prove self
_____ cynicism
_____ apathy

Physical

✓ appetite change
✓ headaches
✓ tension
✓ fatigue
_____ insomnia
_____ weight change
_____ colds

_____ muscle aches
_____ digestive upsets
✓ pounding heart
✓ accident prone
_____ teeth grinding
_____ rash
_____ restlessness
_____ foot-tapping
_____ finger-drumming
_____ increased alcohol, drug, tobacco use

Relational

_____ isolation
_____ intolerance
_____ resentment
_____ loneliness
_____ lashing out
_____ hiding
_____ clamming up
_____ nagging
_____ distrust
_____ fewer contacts with friends
_____ lack of intimacy
_____ using people

Reproduced with permission from *Structured Exercises in Stress Management, Volume 1,* copyright 1983, 1994 Donald A. Tubesing. Published by Whole Person Associates Inc., 210 West Michigan, Duluth, MN 55802-1908, 218–727–0500.

Reviewing Important Concepts

1. What are the important characteristics that promote mental wellness? List the ten characteristics and briefly describe each one.

   1. real: honest, say what they feel.
   2. realistic: differentiate real and what ought to be.
   3. satisfy needs: know needs and can satisfy them.
   4. free & responsible: in control of lives.
   5. open to experience: welcome & seek new experiences.
   6. capable of intimate relationships: able to give & recieve love.
   7. tolerant of others: judges others based on merits.
   8. capable of variety of reactions: abilities to react balance out.
   9. joie de vivre: enjoying.
   10. self accepting: like self.

2. Depression is a term widely used to represent a variety of conditions. Explain the difference between mild and severe depression.

3. Stress is a state characterized by distinct physiological changes. List the changes that occur in the body when it is in a state of stress.

4. Hans Selye has said many times that it is not the stressor that is important but ``how you take it.'' One interpretation of ``how you take it'' is how you perceive the event and the kind of meaning you attach to it. Dr. Selye has delineated two ways of perceiving stress: eustress and distress. Briefly describe the differences and similarities of these two concepts and give several examples of each.

eustress   distress
· moving to a   · customers
bigger house   at work.

Applying What You've Learned

1. A role model is someone you admire and respect and who sets an example for you in terms of values and life-style. Using the ten characteristics of mental wellness listed in your textbook, write a description of someone who is your role model. What qualities does this person have that you would like to pattern yourself after?

2. In this competitive world there is often pressure to ``be like somebody else.'' We may have grown up with the feeling we are not acceptable the way we are. If prolonged, these feelings can develop into a poor self-image. Learning to accept oneself as is and making the most of that self are important steps toward good mental health.

    To help you identify your unique qualities, there are three sections that follow. In the first section, list the names of people you see being similar to you, and make a note of the similarities. In the second section, list those you see as being different and state in what ways they are different.

    Finally, identify three characteristics that are uniquely you (third section), and briefly describe how each characteristic is or can be an asset to your future development.

#1 Similar

1. _____

    name   ways similar

2. _____

3. _____

#2 Different

1. _____

    name   ways different

2. _____

3. _____

#3 Uniquely Me

1. _____

    characteristic   why an asset

2. _____

3. _____

In what ways can my uniqueness become an asset?

3. Describe a stressful situation which you are experiencing now. (If you are not experiencing a ``stressful'' situation, use one from your past or create a possible situation that might actually happen.)

   Brainstorm all the possible stress management skills you could try. From this list choose the one you would use in this situation. Why did you choose this option? What was it about the other options that led you to decide against them?

4. Pat has just graduated and landed a new job in Chicago. He doesn't know anyone in town except for a few people at work. The loneliness is starting to get to him. The singles bar scene makes him feel uncomfortable so he spends his evenings at home watching TV or listening to music. Pat finds himself getting depressed and is at a loss as to what to do. List the possible coping options Pat could use.

5. We are all free to choose what to think. However, we have been taught to be critical rather than supportive. Critical, negative thinking is destructive and may keep you in a state of stress.

   One way to reduce the amount of stress in your life is to change the way you think and focus on the positive. You can learn the art of constructive, positive self-talk. It just takes some practice.

   Below are some typically distressing situations. Write a constructive, positive statement for each situation.

   Waiting in a long line to register for classes

   Being stuck in bumper-to-bumper traffic

   Having to make a presentation before a group of people

   Having a relationship break up

From Jerold S. Greenberg, *Comprehensive Stress Management,* 2d edition. Copyright © 1987 Wm. C. Brown Communications, Inc. Reprinted by permission of Times Mirror Higher Education Group, Inc., Dubuque, Iowa. All Rights Reserved.

Stages of Change

Are you stressed out? Complete Activity for Wellness 2.3 on pages 52–53 of your text to find out. If you scored over 347, you may want to consider taking steps to control the amount of stress in your life.

We can never eliminate all the stress in our lives. However, we can learn to deal with it in more productive ways. If you would like to learn to better manage your stress, answer these four questions to assess your current stage of change.

1. I have been in control of my stress level for more than six months.

2. I have taken action to control my stress within the past six months.

3. I am currently preparing to take action to control stress in the next month.

4. I would like to take action to control my stress level within the next six months.

Scoring

No to all statements	Precontemplation
Yes to statement 4	Contemplation
Yes to statement 3	Preparation
Yes to statement 2	Action
Yes to statement 1	Maintenance

Review table 2.8 of *Connections for Health* for tips on moving through the stages of change and taking charge of the way you manage stressors.

For Further Study

You can increase your mental wellness in a variety of ways. Improving your intellectual level, developing spiritual well-being, getting in touch with your emotions, and managing stress are examples of ways you can increase your self-esteem and self-concept. The activities that follow will help you open the door to new pathways—to a higher level of mental wellness.

Wellness Activities

1. Practice a relaxation exercise. While in the relaxed state, imagine yourself in ten years. What do you see? What career path have you taken? Who are the significant others in your life? Where are you living? Let your imagination run freely. In writing, describe what you imagined. How do you feel about your future? Do you feel this future is realistic? What are things you can do now to help you achieve your imagined future?

2. Identify your abilities, talents, and potentials. Make an appointment with a campus career counselor to assist you. There are many vocational inventories you can take to help you do this. What careers match your abilities and interests? Have you ever considered these career paths? Why or why not?

3. Being open to experience and trying something new or ``risky'' is one characteristic of mental wellness. What are three of the most risky things you have ever tried? What were the outcomes? List three times when you did not do something because it seemed too risky, and you later regretted not trying it. Are you pleased with what you see on your lists? How can you begin to experience life to the fullest?

4. With practice, you can develop your creative powers and your imagination. The following exercise will give you an opportunity to practice. Brainstorm at least thirty ways you can use a paper clip. Write quickly, letting the ideas flow without thinking if the ideas are practical, good, or bad. What was this experience like for you?

5. What mental health resources are available where you live? Consult your campus directory and the yellow pages. Call a few of the resources and ask how they could help someone who is depressed or talking about suicide. What credentials do the counselors have? Is there a fee involved? What emergency services do they

offer?

6. To help you begin to control your stress reactions, it is helpful to keep a diary. Be sure to include the following components in your diary: stressors you encounter, your physical and psychological reactions, what coping skill(s) you use, effectiveness of the coping skill, and at least one other method that you could see as a means of coping more effectively.

     Carry a small notebook with you so that you can record this information at any time. Keep your diary for at least two weeks. Periodically review the diary for patterns in life and to understand how you cope with life events.

7. Attend a workshop or lecture on stress management or assertiveness training. Summarize the program. What sort of strategies were discussed? What new techniques or skills did you learn? What did you discover about yourself?

8. Does your campus have a biofeedback laboratory? Make an appointment to interview the biofeedback trainer. What are the benefits claimed? Is biofeedback based upon scientific evidence? Were you able to decrease your muscle tension, heart rate, or skin temperature? What was the experience like for you? Were you able to relax?

3 Nutrition: Eating for Health

Nutrition: Where Do You Stand?

Learning to eat for health can be an exciting adventure. The first step in your adventure is to conduct a dietary recall. The next steps involve analyzing your diet and becoming familiar with your nutritive requirements. Once you have completed these steps, you can compare your nutritive requirements with your current nutritional status.

By completing these steps, you will be ready to determine what changes you may want to make in order to improve your food choices and attain a higher level of wellness.

Step I: What I've Eaten Today

Keep a record of *all* foods eaten for three consecutive days. List the foods and the approximate amounts in the appropriate category. Estimate as closely as possible, using either standard measures or ounces.

The categories listed on each recall worksheet will help you organize your food items so that you can figure your RDAs and nutritional requirements more easily later in this chapter. There is a separate worksheet for each day of your diet recall.

It helps to keep a small note pad with you so that you can write down what you've eaten at the end of each meal or snack. There's a tendency to forget at the end of the day to record everything you've eaten.

If your eating habits change on the weekends, incorporate one weekend day into your three-day diet recall.

Step II: Nutritional Analysis

The nutritional analysis is a summary of your three-day dietary recall. Using the Nutritional Analysis Worksheets on the following pages, combine amounts of similar foods. For example, if two slices of whole wheat bread were eaten each day, list these as six slices rather than using a separate line for each slice. If you ate a variety of foods, you may want to photocopy an extra copy of the nutritional analysis worksheet before beginning. (Note: The worksheets are separated into two types. There are three pages for proteins, carbohydrates, and fats and three pages for vitamins and minerals.)

Refer to the Nutritive Values of Foods and the Nutritive Values of Fast Foods located in Appendices B and C of this workbook. For items not listed in either source, estimate amounts. Enter the nutrient composition of each food.

Total the amounts for each nutrient at the bottom of one of the worksheets.

Step III: Dietary Guidelines Evaluation

The following formulas (pp. 31–33) will help you calculate your percentage of daily calories from protein, fat, carbohydrate, and alcohol. They will also help you calculate the amount of sodium in your diet. Enter the totals from your Nutritional Analysis Worksheet—Protein, Fats, Carbohydrate in the appropriate blanks.

Complete the equations for each nutrient and for alcohol. Next, review the Dietary Recommendations Evaluation Key (Step III-5). Examine your diet and compare it to the dietary recommendations. Then complete the Dietary Recommendations Worksheet.

Record of What I've Eaten Today—Day 1   Tuesday

	Meat, Eggs, Poultry, Fish	Grains, Nuts, Legumes	Milk, Cheese	Fruit	Vegetables, Salad	Bread, Cereal, Pasta, Rice	Fats: Mayonnaise, Butter, Oil, Dressings	Sweets, Desserts, Alcohol	Misc.
Breakfast			2c milk 2%	1 banana		Frosted 1½ c. flakes			
Lunch	2oz. turkey breast		1 slice cheese	1 large fruit		2 slices white bread	2 tsp. red. fat mayo.	1 tbsp. sugar	
Dinner	1 chicken pot pie								
Snacks								1 fudge side	

22

Record of What I've Eaten Today—Day 2   Thursday

	Meat, Eggs, Poultry, Fish	Grains, Nuts, Legumes	Milk, Cheese	Fruit	Vegetables, Salad	Bread, Cereal, Pasta, Rice	Fats: Mayonnaise, Butter, Oil, Dressings	Sweets, Desserts, Alcohol	Misc.
Breakfast		2 eggo waffles	8oz. 2% milk				1tsp. butter	2tbsp. syrup; 1tbsp. hershey syrup (choc. milk)	
Lunch	2 hard boiled eggs					2 slices white bread	1tbsp. low fat mayo.		
Dinner	1 chicken cordon bleu breast				3tbsp. corn; 1 cup fried potatoes		1/2 tsp. butter		2tbsp. ketchup
Snacks									

Record of What I've Eaten Today—Day 3   Sunday

	Meat, Eggs, Poultry, Fish	Grains, Nuts, Legumes	Milk, Cheese	Fruit	Vegetables, Salad	Bread, Cereal, Pasta, Rice	Fats: Mayonnaise, Butter, Oil, Dressings	Sweets, Desserts, Alcohol	Misc.
Breakfast	3 slices bacon	1 pancake = 2	1 (8 oz.) 2% milk				1 tsp. butter	1 tbsp. syrup	
Lunch						2 slices Italian bread →		2 tbsp. Hershey syrup	
Dinner	2 meatballs				spaghetti sauce / 1 sm. bowl tossed salad	2½ cups pasta	2 tbsp. butter		
Snacks								slice of cake / 1 cup vanilla orange ice cream	

24

Nutritional Analysis Worksheet—Protein, Fats, Carbohydrate

Food Eaten	Amount or Weight	Kcal	Protein (gm)	Total Fat (gm)	Saturated Fat (gm)	Mono-unsaturated Fat (gm)	Poly-unsaturated Fat (gm)	Cholesterol (mg)	Carbohydrate (gm)
½ banana	½	53	.5	.5					14
2% milk	2 c.	240	10	10					24
Frosted Flakes	1½ c.	230	2	TR					52
turkey breast 3oz.	3oz.	45	10	3					0
cheese	1 slice	39	4	3					TR
grapefruit	1	80	2	TR					20
white bread 2 slices	2 slices	130	4	2					34
peanut butter	2 tsp.	100	TR	11					12
sugar	1 tbsp.	45	0	0					12
chicken pot pie	1 slice	545	23	31					42

25

Nutritional Analysis Worksheet—Protein, Fats, Carbohydrate

Food Eaten	Amount or Weight	Kcal	Protein (gm)	Total Fat (gm)	Saturated Fat (gm)	Mono-unsaturated Fat (gm)	Poly-unsaturated Fat (gm)	Cholesterol (mg)	Carbohydrate (gm)
Waffles	2								
2% milk	8oz.								
butter	1tsp.								
Maple syrup	2tbsp.								
Hershey syrup	1tbsp.								
lunchmeat	2slices								
cheese	1slice								
hotdogs	2								
bread	2slices								
mayo.	1tbsp.								
cauliflower									
corn	3tbsp.								
green bean	1cup								
butter	1/2 tsp.								
ketchup	2tbsp.								

26

Nutritional Analysis Worksheet—Protein, Fats, Carbohydrate

Food Eaten	Amount or Weight	Kcal	Protein (gm)	Total Fat (gm)	Saturated Fat (gm)	Mono-unsaturated Fat (gm)	Poly-unsaturated Fat (gm)	Cholesterol (mg)	Carbohydrate (gm)
bacon	3 slices								
pancake	3								
2% milk	10 oz								
butter	1 tsp.								
maple syrup	4 tbp.								
	2 tbsp								
meatballs	2								
italian bread	2 slices								
spaghetti sauce	1 cup								
pasta	2 cups								
cake	1 slice								
ice cream	1 cup								
butter	2 tbsp.								

Nutritional Analysis Worksheet—Vitamins and Minerals

Food Eaten	Amount or Weight	Calcium (mg)	Phos-phorus (mg)	Iron (mg)	Potassium (mg)	Sodium (mg)	Vit A (IU)	Thiamin (mg)	Riboflavin (mg)	Niacin (mg)	Vit C (mg)

Nutritional Analysis Worksheet—Vitamins and Minerals

Food Eaten	Amount or Weight	Calcium (mg)	Phos- phorus (mg)	Iron (mg)	Potassium (mg)	Sodium (mg)	Vit A (IU)	Thiamin (mg)	Riboflavin (mg)	Niacin (mg)	Vit C (mg)

Nutritional Analysis Worksheet—Vitamins and Minerals

Food Eaten	Amount or Weight	Calcium (mg)	Phos- phorus (mg)	Iron (mg)	Potassium (mg)	Sodium (mg)	Vit A (IU)	Thiamin (mg)	Riboflavin (mg)	Niacin (mg)	Vit C (mg)

1. Total calories consumed per day (average). Enter the totals from your Nutritional Analysis Worksheets in the appropriate blanks below.

   A. Protein (pro):

   _____ ÷ ___3___ = _____ × ___4___ = _____
   Total gms   Number of   Average   # calories/   Avg. calories
   pro   days in   gms   gram   pro/day
                  recall   [1A]

   B. Total fat:

   _____ ÷ ___3___ = _____ × ___9___ = _____
   Total gms   Number of   Average   # calories/   Avg. calories
   fat   days in   gms   gram   fat/day
                  recall   [1B]

   C. Saturated fat (sat-fat):

   _____ ÷ ___3___ = _____ × ___9___ = _____
   Total gms   Number of   Average   # calories/   Avg. calories
   sat-fat   days in   gms   gram   sat-fat/day
                  recall   [1C]

   D. Monounsaturated fat (mono-fat):

   _____ ÷ _3___ = _____ × _9___ = _____
   Total gms   Number of   Average   # calories/   Avg. calories
   mono-fat   days in   gms   gram   sat-fat/day
                  recall   [1D]

   E. Polyunsaturated fat (poly-fat):

   _____ ÷ ___3___ = _____ × ___9___ = _____
   Total gms   Number of   Average   # calories/   Avg. calories
   poly-fat   days in   gms   gram   poly-fat/day
                  recall   [1E]

   F. Carbohydrates (carbo):

   _____ ÷ ___3___ = _____ × ___4___ = _____
   Total gms   Number of   Average   # calories/   Avg. calories
   carbo   days in   gms   gram   carbo/day
                  recall   [1F]

   G. Summary:

   _____ + _____ + _____ = _____
   [1A]   [1B]   [1F]   Avg. # of calories
                                                   consumed per day
                                                   [1G]

   H. Cholesterol (chol):

   _____ ÷ ___3___ = _____
   Total mgs   Number of days Average mgs
   chol   in recall   per day
                                  [1H]

2. Percent calories from protein, fats, and carbohydrates

A.   Protein:

_____ ÷ _____ × 100 = _____
     Avg. calories   Averge # of   % of daily
       pro [1A]   calories [1G]   calories from pro [2A]

B.   Total fat:

_____ ÷ _____ × 100 = _____
     Avg. calories   Average # of   % of daily
       fat [1B]   calories [1G]   calories from fat [2B]

C.   Saturated fat:

_____ ÷ _____ × 100 = _____
     Avg. calories   Average # of   % of daily
       sat-fat [1C]   calories [1G]   calories from sat-fat [2C]

D.   Monounsaturated fat:

_____ ÷ _____ × 100 = _____
     Avg. calories   Average # of   % of daily
       mono-fat [1D]   calories [1G]   calories from mono-fat [2D]

E.   Polyunsaturated fat:

_____ ÷ _____ × 100 = _____
     Avg. calories   Average # of   % of daily
       poly-fat [1E]   calories [1G]   calories from poly-fat [2E]

F.   Carbohydrates:

_____ ÷ _____ ×100 = _____
     Avg. calories   Average # of   % of daily
       carbo [1F]   calories [1G]   calories from carbo [2F]

G.   Double check your figures to make sure your totals are correct by completing the equation below.
Total number of calories:

_____%   +   _____%   +   _____%   =   _____%
     [2A]   [2B]   [2F]   This number should be 100

3.   Milligrams of sodium consumed per day

_____ ÷ _____3_____ = _____
      Total milligrams   Number of days   Avg. # of milligrams
        sodium   in recall   sodium consumed per day [3A]

4.   Calories from alcohol (may be blank if no alcohol was consumed)
Refer to the Nutritional Analysis Worksheet. Put an asterisk (*) next to all entries pertaining to alcohol (mixed drinks, beer, wines). Total the number of calories for these entries and complete the following equation:

_____ ÷ _____3_____ = _____
      Total calories   Number of days   Average calories
      from alcohol   in recall   from alcohol per day [4A]

If you consume alcohol it is necessary to add ``alcohol'' calories to your calories derived from food in order to get a true picture of your total caloric intake. Complete the following equation:

$$\underline{\hspace{4cm}} + \underline{\hspace{4cm}} = \underline{\hspace{4cm}}$$

| Average calories from alcohol per day [4A] | Avg. # of calories from food consumed per day (1G) | Avg. # of calories consumed per day from food and alcohol |

5. A Dietary Recommendations Evaluation Key is provided below to outline the optimal ranges for the nutrients and calories you examined on the previous pages. Use this key to help you complete the Dietary Recommendations Worksheet. Enter your figures from Step III—items 1–4 under the column ``Your Diet.'' (The numbers following the blank in this column refer to the number you calculated in Step III, items 1–4.) After comparing your diet to the Dietary Recommendations Evaluation Key, rate your diet writing ``Good'' or ``Could Improve'' in the blanks provided.

Adult Dietary Recommendations Evaluation Key

Nutrient	Optimal Range	Rating
Protein	10–15%	good
Fat	30% or less	good
Saturated fat	Less than 10%	good
Polyunsaturated fat	Less than 10%	good
Monounsaturated fat	Remaining % of fat calories 60%	good
Carbohydrate	2,400 mg	good
Sodium	Fewer than 300 mg/day	good
Cholesterol	1 ounce or less pure	good
Alcohol	alcohol/day	good

Dietary Guidelines Worksheet
Where Do I Stand?

	Typical American Diet	Your Diet	Rating: Good or Could Improve
Protein	16%	_____ [2A]	_____
Total Fat	34%	_____ [2B]	_____
Saturated Fat	12%	_____ [2C]	_____
Monounsaturated Fat	14%	_____ [2D]	_____
Polyunsaturated Fat	6%	_____ [2E]	_____
Carbohydrate	50%	_____ [2F]	_____
Sodium	3000–4000 mg	_____ [3A]	_____
Cholesterol	varies	_____ [1H]	_____
Alcohol	varies	_____ [4A]	_____

Remember: The objective of the dietary recommendations is to improve health through informed diet selection: The recommendations are provided to give you direction and incentive for change. These recommendations represent *averages over time,* not per day guidelines!

Step IV: Recommended Daily Allowance Evaluation

The RDA Evaluation Worksheet will help you calculate your percentage of RDAs for selected vitamins and minerals. Enter the totals from your Nutritional Analysis Worksheet—Vitamins and Minerals in the appropriate blanks below.

Next, review the RDA table found in Appendix D. Examine your diet and compare it to the recommended daily allowances. Answer the questions at the end of this section.

1. Calcium:

    _____ ÷ ___3___ = _____ ÷ _____ × 100 = _____
      Total mg   Number of   Average mg   RDA for   % of RDA
                    days in recall   per day   age group

2. Phosphorus:

    _____ ÷ ___3___ = _____ ÷ _____ × 100 = _____
      Total mg   Number of   Average mg   RDA for   % of RDA
                    days in recall   per day   age group

3. Iron:

    _____ ÷ ___3___ = _____ ÷ _____ × 100 = _____
      Total mg   Number of   Average mg   RDA for   % of RDA
                    days in recall   per day   age group

4. Vitamin A:

    _____ ÷ ___3___ = _____ ÷ _____ × 100 = _____
      Total IU   Number of   Average IU   RDA for   % of RDA
                    days in recall   per day   age group

5. Thiamin:

    _____ ÷ ___3___ = _____ ÷ _____ × 100 = _____
      Total mg   Number of   Average mg   RDA for   % of RDA
                    days in recall   per day   age group

6. Riboflavin:

    _____ ÷ ___3___ = _____ ÷ _____ × 100 = _____
      Total mg   Number of   Average mg   RDA for   % of RDA
                    days in recall   per day   age group

7. Niacin:

    _____ ÷ ___3___ = _____ ÷ _____ × 100 = _____
      Total mg   Number of   Average mg   RDA for   % of RDA
                    days in recall   per day   age group

8. Vitamin C:

    _____ ÷ ___3___ = _____ ÷ _____ × 100 = _____
      Total mg   Number of   Average mg   RDA for   % of RDA
                    days in recall   per day   age group

Recommended Daily Allowances Worksheet
Where Do I Stand?

Nutrient	% of RDAs in your daily diet	Your Rating: Good	Could Improve
Calcium	_____	____	_____
Phosphorus	_____	____	_____
Iron	_____	____	_____
Vitamin A	_____	____	_____
Thiamin	_____	____	_____
Riboflavin	_____	____	_____
Niacin	_____	____	_____
Vitamin C	_____	____	_____

Step V: What Does It All Mean?

Directions: Review the results you calculated in Steps I–IV. Then answer the following summary questions. Be specific when comparing your diet!

1. How does your diet compare with a typical American diet?

2. How does your diet compare with the dietary recommendations?

3. How does your diet compare to the *Healthy People 2000* Nutrition Objectives 1–5?

4. How does your diet compare with the RDAs? Be sure to include your caloric intake in your evaluation.

5. Which *foods* are you now eating that contribute to the strengths and weaknesses of your diet?

6. Which *foods* do you need to minimize so that you'll be following an optimal diet for well-being? Would you be willing to make these changes?

7. Identify three foods that you would be willing to try that would enhance your diet (new foods or different preparation).

8. How easy will it be to make the diet changes identified in questions 5 and 6? Consider cost; convenience; and your personal, social, and cultural food preferences.

9. On the average, how many calories did you consume from alcohol? _____ How is this affecting your diet? What changes do you believe you could make (if any) to improve your diet with regard to alcohol?

Reviewing Important Concepts

1. Describe the nine dietary recommendations issued by the National Research Council. How do these guidelines differ from the typical American diet?

   ① reduce fat intake.
   ② eat 5 or more fruit & vegies
   ③ maintain protein.
   ④ Balance food & physical activity
   ⑤ no alcohol
   ⑥ limit salt intake
   ⑦ maintain calcium
   ⑧ no dietary supplements
   ⑨ maintain optimal amount of fluoride.

   * Most people eat what they want or don't know all of these guidelines.

2. What is the difference between dietary cholesterol and blood cholesterol? Which is the risk factor for heart disease?

   dietary us from the food we consume. Blood cholesterol us made in the liver. LDL blood-cholesterol affects the heart.

3. What is the body's preferred form of energy? Why is this nutrient preferred by the body?

4. Some triglycerides are a major source of dietary concern. Describe each of these fats (as discussed in the textbook). List two sources for each type of fat.

Applying What You've Learned

1. If you were determined to switch from a high-fat diet to a low-fat diet, what dietary changes might you make? List four items high in fat that you would cut down on or eliminate from your diet.

   1. butter   3. chocolate

   2. ice cream   4. pizza

2. Suppose you were going to start eating according to the National Research Council's Dietary Recommendations. Plan a dinner that is in keeping with these recommendations. Include the names of all foods and beverages you would consume at this meal. Don't forget to tell how the food is prepared (i.e., broiled, fried, raw, steamed, etc.).

3. How do you apply all the nutrition information in this chapter when eating in a restaurant? The exercise that follows will give you practice. Look over the menu as you would if you were in a restaurant. Select items which would make up a lunch or dinner meal. *Circle your choices.* Directions for completing this exercise follow the menu.

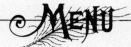

Cocktails

Mixed Drinks
  Your choice
Frozen Strawberry Daiquiri
  House special

Dry Table Wine
  Burgundy and Chablis
Beer
  Bottled and draft

Wine Spritzer
Fruit Juice Cocktail
Sparkling Water
  with a Twist of Lime

Appetizers

Fresh Melon Wedge
  with Lime Slice
Crispy Nachos
  Smothered with melted
  cheddar cheese, served with
  guacamole and sour cream
Fresh Fruit Medley
  Served in a pineapple boat
Fried Wontons
  Served with sweet
  and sour sauce

Chicken Liver Paté
  Served with toasted croutons
Fried Potato Skins
  Served with sour cream
  and chives
Split Pea Soup
  Served with your choice
  of sour cream or sherry

Gazpacho
  A crunchy soup of
  blended tomatoes,
  cucumbers, bell peppers,
  and celery, served chilled
Shrimp Cocktail
  Served with a spicy
  cocktail sauce and
  lemon wedge

Main Course Salads
(Served with rye roll, whole-wheat bread sticks, or croissant)

All-You-Can-Eat Salad Bar
Spinach Salad
  Fresh spinach leaves, crispy bacon bits,
  grated Parmesan, and hard-cooked eggs
  served with a hot vinaigrette dressing
Garden Pasta Salad
  Homemade pasta and fresh vegetables,
  lightly tossed with a dill dressing

Chef's Salad with Choice of Dressing
Seafood Salad
  Tender shrimp, lump crabmeat, and bay
  scallops sprinkled with an herb dressing
  and served on a bed of mixed greens
Fresh Fruit Salad with Yogurt Dressing

For Lunch-Time Appetites

Hot Turkey Sandwich
  Served open face with giblet
  gravy and French fries
Grilled Reuben
  Fresh corned beef, Swiss
  cheese, and sauerkraut
  with tangy Russian dressing
  on thick rye bread
Charbroiled Burger
  Your choice of cheese and
  assorted toppings, served
  with homemade onion rings
  or French fries
Turkey Cordon Bleu
  Slices of ham, turkey,
  and Swiss cheese baked
  in a buttery pastry shell

Pita Pocket Sandwich
  Warm pita bread stuffed
  with a medley of garden
  fresh vegetables and
  chunks of tender cooked
  chicken, tossed with a
  light herb dressing
Tuna Salad
  Served on a fresh-baked
  croissant
Veggie Delight
  Pan pizza smothered with
  mushrooms, green peppers,
  and onions

Pizza Lover's Special
  The ultimate in pizza,
  the crispiest crust in
  town—covered with
  sausage, pepperoni,
  olives, and anchovies
Spinach Quiche
  Filled with fresh chopped
  spinach, onion, and
  Parmesan, baked in a
  flaky crust
Fluffy Western Omelette
  Three fresh eggs mixed
  with minced ham,
  green pepper, and onion

Source: Data from *Home and Garden Bulletin* No. 232-11, U.S. Department of Agriculture, Human Nutrition Service.

Entrees

(Served with your choice of two vegetables and a garden salad)

Pasta Primavera
Ribbons of fettucini and fresh vegetables tossed in a light yogurt sauce, sprinkled with Parmesan

Baked Chicken Breast
Boneless breast of chicken baked in a delicate lemon-basil sauce

Southern-Style Chicken
Fried to a crispy golden brown

Chicken Teriyaki
Grilled strips of chicken marinated in a spicy teriyaki sauce

Beef en Brochette
Skewered cubes of beef round with fresh mushroom caps

London Broil
Delicately marinated and grilled strips of flank steak served in their own juice

Porterhouse Steak (16 ounces)
Charbroiled the way you like it, topped with crispy onion rings

Petite Filet Mignon
Broiled to perfection, topped with mushroom caps

Barbecued Baby Back Ribs
A hefty rack of broiled pork ribs smothered with our own hickory-smoked barbecue sauce

Veal Tenderloins
Plump medallions of veal in a rich cream sauce with mushrooms and capers

Burritos
Your choice of beef, chicken, or bean; served with rice and fresh salsa

Fish and Chips
Fresh filet of sole dipped in a special beer batter and deep-fat fried, served with French-fried potatoes

Crabmeat Au Gratin
Lump backfin crabmeat in a creamy cheese sauce, baked to a delicate brown

Sweet and Sour Shrimp
Batter-fried shrimp coated with a tangy sweet-and-sour sauce

Today's Special

Lemon-Broiled Haddock Filets
Served with steaming brown rice pilaf, green beans almondine, tomato halves broiled with fresh basil, and crusty French bread

Vegetables

French-Fried Potatoes
Herbed New Potatoes
Cheese-Stuffed Baked Potato
Sliced Tomatoes with Basil
Creamy Coleslaw

Broccoli Spears
  with Hollandaise Sauce
Steamed Zucchini-Carrot Medley
Garden Fresh Peas
  with Pearl Onions
Corn-on-the-Cob

Beverages

Fresh Brewed Coffee
Hot Tea
Iced Tea
Assorted Soft Drinks

Milk
  Whole or lowfat
Freshly Squeezed Lemonade
  or Limeade
Chilled Apple Cider

Desserts

Fresh Fruit Sorbet
Assorted flavors

Poached Pears
with Raspberry Glaze

Blueberry Pie A La Mode

New York Style Cheese Cake

Carrot Cake
Topped with a thick cream cheese frosting

Assorted Fresh Pastries
Rich, flaky pastries with assorted fillings

Fresh Strawberries (in season)

Apple Dumpling
Whole apple baked in a flaky cinnamon pastry, topped with whipped cream and chopped pecans

Ice Cream Sundae
A rich French vanilla, topped with fudge sauce, nuts, and whipped cream, served with a cookie

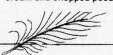

Source: Data from *Home and Garden Bulletin* No. 232-11, U.S. Department of Agriculture, Human Nutrition Service.

In Looking Over the Menu, Did You See . . .

- dishes unfamiliar to you? Ask the waiter to describe how the dish is prepared—and try something new if it fits into the guidelines style.
- preparation terms and ingredients that signal ``low'' or ``high'' fat and ``low'' or ``high'' sodium?
- menu selections that might fit nicely into a guidelines-style meal if you could have dressing, sauces, or toppings on the side?
- selections you might ask to be prepared differently?

Look at the foods you chose for your meal. Did you include a variety of foods from the five food groups shown? Were some foods good sources of starch and fiber? Judging from what you've learned in chapter 3, does your meal appear to be moderate in calories, fat, sugars, sodium, and alcohol? If not, what food selections would you make the rest of the day to provide the balance needed to eat in the guidelines style?

Here are some options within each menu section that tend to be lower in fat, sugars, sodium, or alcohol than others. Generally, they provide fewer calories, too.

Cocktails

Sparkling water with a twist of lime, fruit juice cocktail, or wine spritzer. Dry table wines have about half the calories of sweet table wines.

Appetizers

Melon wedge, fresh fruit medley, split pea soup (sour cream or sherry on the side), gazpacho, or shrimp cocktail (go easy on the sauce).

Main Course Salads

Rye roll or whole-wheat breadsticks to accompany main course salads (watch out for spreads); fresh fruit salad, garden pasta salad, or seafood salad (provided they're light on dressing).

Did You Know?

A typical "diet plate" may be higher in calories and fat than many other selections on the menu. Below is the calorie, fat, and sodium content of a typical "diet plate."

	Calories	Fat (grams)	Sodium (milligrams)
Beef Patty (4 ounces)	325	24	95
Cottage Cheese (1/2 cup)	110	4	425
Hard-Cooked Egg			
Tomato Slices	80	6	70
Rye Crackers (4)	10	Trace	
	110	2	230
Totals	635	36	825

Lunch-Time Appetites

Veggie delight or pita sandwich. If you choose a sandwich such as the tuna salad, lower the fat by having it on a french roll or bagel rather than a croissant. Choose whole-grain bread for additional fiber and nutrients. Watch added cheeses and condiments if you choose the hamburger.

Entrees

Baked chicken breast, beef en brochette, burritos (bean filling for added fiber), pasta primavera (lots of vegetables and the yogurt sauce is lower in fat than traditional cream sauces). If you're ordering a steak, keep in mind that the petite filet is a smaller portion than the porterhouse.

Today's Special

You can't miss here. All the items are foods in the guidelines style.

Vegetables

Herbed new potatoes, sliced tomatoes, zucchini and carrots, peas with pearl onions, or corn-on-the-cob (watch added butter and salt).

Beverages

Lowfat milk, lemonade or limeade, apple cider. If coffee or tea is your choice, drink it plain or limit the sugar and cream you add.

Desserts

Fresh fruit sorbet, poached pears, strawberries (with only a small amount, if any, of whipped cream). Alternative: either fruit item listed under Appetizers.

Getting hungry? The menu clearly shows that eating in the guidelines style need not be dull. It doesn't mean giving up your favorite foods either. If you're really hungry for nachos smothered with cheese, order them. Balance the higher fat and sodium with other menu items that are lower. Or choose lower fat and sodium foods at other meals.

Worth Noting

Sometimes menu names or descriptions send mixed messages. In chicken teriyaki, for example, grilled chicken suggests lower fat, but teriyaki sauce suggests higher sodium. When making choices, you need to consider both the ingredients used and the preparation method. Menu items made with nutritious foods can be quite high in fat and calories—fried potato skins with sour cream, or apple dumpling, for example.

Restaurants are featuring more menu selections that can fit into a nutritious and healthful eating style. Study the foods carefully, however, before you decide. Don't be fooled by the title, ``For Lunch-Time Appetites.'' Some of these selections provide just as much, or more, food (not to mention fat and calories) than the dinner entrees. Also, watch out for menu selections termed ``light fare.'' ``Light'' may or may not mean that a menu item is lower in calories or fat.

Stages of Change

Changing your eating habits is seldom easy, as many of us know from experience. However, eating more healthfully is one of the most important things you can do to maximize your chances of a longer and better life. Complete Activity for Wellness 3.1 on pages 72–74 of your text. If you had a negative score, you may want to consider taking steps to improve your diet.

If you would like to learn to eat more healthfully, pick an aspect of your diet you would like to change and answer these four questions to assess your current stage of change.

1. I have been eating healthfully for more than six months.
2. I have taken action to eat healthfully within the past six months.
3. I am currently preparing to take action to eat a more healthful diet.
4. I would like to take action to eat more healthfully within the next six months.

Scoring

No to all statements	Precontemplation
Yes to statement 4	Contemplation
Yes to statement 3	Preparation
Yes to statement 2	Action
Yes to statement 1	Maintenance

Review table 3.16 of *Connections for Health* for tips on moving through the stages of change and taking charge of your diet.

For Further Study

Increasing your level of wellness through nutrition begins with eating a well-balanced diet that contains a variety of foods. Once you become aware of how to balance your diet, you can incorporate these changes into your meals. The following activities will help you discover new foods, new preparation techniques, and ways to begin eating a more balanced diet.

Wellness Activities

1. Examine the menu at your favorite restaurant. Describe the food items listed. How are these foods prepared? How does the menu compare to the dietary guidelines?
2. On your next trip to the grocery store, examine ten prepared food items (including condiments) for their sodium content. How would the sodium content in these items affect your diet?
3. Invite some of your friends over for an international buffet. Have each friend bring a food from a different country. Discover the tastes of foods you have never tried.
4. What types of fish are available in your local supermarkets? What are the factors (cost, availability, ease of preparation, taste, etc.) that would prevent you from including or enable you to include fish in your diet?
5. Are you brushing and flossing correctly? It's easy to find out. Go to your local drug store and purchase disclosing tablets. Brush and floss your teeth as you normally would. Follow the instructions on the package for using the disclosing tablets. How effective was your cleaning? Look in the mirror; be sure to check your back molars. What areas do you need to concentrate on in the future?
6. Have you ever had your blood cholesterol tested? There are many blood cholesterol screening tests available that can be done while you wait. This test is often available at health fairs. Contact your student health center, local hospital, or county health department to see when and where a screening will be held. Remember, this test is only a screening. Any results should be interpreted with caution. Write a brief paper about your experience. Were your results explained to you? What qualifications did this person have? Explain any dietary advice that was given to you. How are you going to incorporate this advice into your diet? Be sure to hand in a copy of your results.

7. Review the food handling techniques you use in your home. How do you handle eggs, raw meat, and poultry? How do you handle your cooking utensils and cutting boards? Write a brief paper answering these questions. Be sure to include specific ways you will incorporate food safety after your review. If you eat in the dormitory, take a tour through the kitchen and observe the cooks' food handling techniques.

4 Weight Management: A Lifelong Challenge

Weight Management . . . Where Do You Stand?

Weight management is a lifelong process that can be approached in a positive, challenging way. There are many benefits to maintaining optimal body weight and fat. People feel better about themselves emotionally, have more energy, and have a more positive self-image. Discover how you can begin to incorporate weight management into your life-style by completing the following personal assessments.

Do You Know How to Lose Weight?

When it comes to weight control, willpower isn't enough: A sound knowledge of exercise, nutrition and healthy eating behavior is essential. To test your weight-loss know-how, try this quiz, which was developed by Dr. Kelly Brownell, director of the Yale University Center for Eating and Weight Disorders.

INSTRUCTIONS:
In each section, mark the statements
True or **False**

SECTION I: Nutrition
___ **1.** The calorie is a measure of the amount of fat in a food.
___ **2.** If you eat an equal number of servings from each of the five food groups in the Food Guide Pyramid, you'll get a balanced diet.
___ **3.** The recommended daily intake of dietary fat is 30% or less of total calories.
___ **4.** Carbohydrates aren't as important as other nutrients are, and they should make up only about 30% of your daily diet.
___ **5.** One gram of fat contains more than twice the calories of one gram of carbohydrate or protein.

SECTION II: Behavior
___ **1.** Keeping a daily record of what you eat is essential for weight loss.
___ **2.** Ordering à la carte at restaurants is a better idea than ordering package meals.
___ **3.** It's best to take all of what you'll eat in one serving so that you won't need additional helpings.
___ **4.** When you're trying to lose weight, it's a good idea to go food shopping when you're hungry so you can test your willpower.
___ **5.** Controlling how much you eat at a special event is easier if you eat a low-calorie snack before you go.

SECTION III: Exercise
___ **1.** Walking one mile burns almost as many calories as running one mile.
___ **2.** Exercise can help keep you from losing muscle tissue when you're trying to lose weight.
___ **3.** Climbing stairs requires more energy per minute—and therefore burns more calories per minute—than many more popular forms of exercise, such as swimming or jogging.
___ **4.** No exercise can help you lose fat in specific parts of the body.
___ **5.** Exercise must be done in specific amounts—say, at least 30 minutes at a stretch—to help you lose weight.

SECTION IV: Myths
___ **1.** The most important factor in weight reduction is discovering the psychological roots of your weight problem.
___ **2.** There's no such thing as a slow or underactive metabolism.
___ **3.** Since excessive dietary fat has been linked to heart disease and other health problems, it's best to eliminate all fat from your diet.
___ **4.** Eating quickly helps you enjoy food more because your taste buds get more stimulation.
___ **5.** The calorie level necessary to lose weight is the same for all people.

(For answers, see next page.)

Answers
SECTION I: Nutrition

1. False. The calorie is a measure of the energy your body gets from a food. Fat supplies some of the calories in some foods, but so do carbohydrates and protein.

2. False. You should eat the following every day: two to three servings of dairy products; two to three servings of meat, poultry or other high-protein foods (fish, beans, eggs and nuts); two to four servings of fruit; three to five servings of vegetables; and six to 11 servings of breads and cereals (including rice and pasta).

3. True. If you follow the Food Guide Pyramid, you should be able to keep your fat calories under 30%.

4. False. Carbohydrates should make up the largest portion of your daily diet (between 55% and 60% of total calories). It's important, however, to limit high-calorie, carbohydrate-rich foods, such as cookies and pies, and to watch out for hidden calories in sauces for pastas and other high-carbohydrate foods.

5. True. One gram of fat contains nine calories, while one gram of carbohydrate or protein contains only four calories.

SECTION II: Behavior

1. True. People who have lost weight and kept it off generally report that record keeping was one key to their success.

2. True. If you order a package meal—say, a hamburger with french fries and coleslaw—you'll probably end up with more calories than you want or need.

3. False. It's best to take one portion at a time, because it interrupts the tendency to eat without thinking and gives you time to consider whether you really need more food.

4. False. Shopping on an empty stomach is asking for trouble. You'll do less impulse buying if you shop *after* eating.

5. True. Eating a low-calorie food before you go will take the edge off your hunger and help you resist the high-calorie snacks, such as chips and nuts, typically served at parties.

SECTION III: Exercise

1. True. How far you go is more important than how fast you go, so walking helps with weight control.

2. True. Exercise can prevent muscle loss while maximizing fat loss. For weight loss, exercise combined with dieting is preferable to dieting alone.

3. True. Climbing stairs is an excellent way to burn calories.

4. True. You can reduce fat in general, but you cannot dictate where it will come off.

5. False. Any amount of exercise helps, so do what you can.

SECTION IV: Myths

1. False. Psychological problems are at the root of some, but not all, cases of overweight. And there's no evidence that uncovering these causes helps with weight loss.

2. False. There are wide variations in metabolic rate—how fast calories are used by the body for energy—among different people.

3. False. Fat plays an important role in the body, including protecting vital organs and preventing excessive heat loss, so it shouldn't be totally eliminated from your diet.

4. False. Your taste buds catch nothing but a blur if the food shoots past. If you slow down, the food will taste better, and you may feel more satisfied and therefore eat less.

5. False. There are large differences in how much weight people lose when they have the same caloric intake. Some women, for example, lose weight on 2,000 calories a day while others don't lose any on 1,000.

Scoring

Give yourself one point for each correct answer and total the points for each section.

SECTION I: Nutrition

5 You're a nutrition nabob! With so many food facts at your fingertips, controlling your weight should be no heavy task.

3 or 4 Your food choices could use a dash more nutrition know-how if you want to keep your weight at a palatable level.

1 or 2 You need to be en*light*ened on food if you want to scale down. Check out our "Nutrition" department every month, or take a look at books on the topic, such as *Jane Brody's Nutrition Book* (Bantam Books, 1987) by the health columnist for *The New York Times*.

SECTION II: Behavior

5 You ain't misbehavin': Your eating and food-shopping habits are right on target.

3 or 4 You may want to brush up on your p's and q's: Some of your habits may be hindering your efforts.

1 or 2 If you don't break your bad habits, you'll always be fighting the battle of the bulge. You'll find lots of helpful behavior tips in Dr. Kelly Brownell's book *The LEARN Program for Weight Control* (American Health Publishing [no relation to this magazine]; to order, call 800–736–7323).

SECTION III: Exercise

5 You've got a leg up on controlling your weight.

3 or 4 You should work out the kinks in your workout to help keep your weight in check.

1 or 2 Shape up, or you'll never like the shape of things to come! For exercise tips, look at our "Personal Trainer" column and "Fitness" department.

SECTION IV: Myths

5 It's no myth that you know what you're talking about.

3 or 4 Watch out: If you don't separate food fact from food faction, you may be led astray.

1 or 2 When it comes to weight control, don't believe everything you read—unless it's in AMERICAN HEALTH!

From Dr. Kelly Brownell "You Know How to Lose Weight?" *American Health,* November 1994. Reprinted by permission of Dr. Kelly Brownell, Yale University.

Calculating Your Percent Body Fat

You can find out your percent body fat by completing the steps below.

1. Contact your campus wellness center, health education department, or physical education department to have your skinfold measures taken. Note that males have their skinfolds measured in different places than females.

Males		Females	
Chest	_____	Triceps	_____
Abdomen	_____	Thigh	_____
Thigh	_____	Suprailium	_____
Total	_____	Total	_____

2. Sum your three skinfolds. Enter the total in the total column above.
3. Locate the total of your three skinfolds on the nomogram on page 47. Using a straightedge, connect your age to the total. Note the number on the percent body fat scale for your sex where the line intersects. This value represents an estimate of your percent body fat.
4. Use the fatness rating chart below to find out how you rate. Circle your rating. Place an asterisk next to the rating you'd like to achieve.

Rating	Men	Women
Very low fat	7–10%	14–17%
Low fat	10–13%	17–20%
Ideal fat	13–17%	20–24%
Above ideal fat	17–20%	24–27%
Very high fat	20–25%	27–30%
Obese	Above 25%	Above 30%

Norms for female athletes are 13–20%, with an absolute minimum of 10%; for male athletes, norms are 4–12%, with an absolute minimum of 3%.

Used with permission from Procedures for Your Practice: Skinfold Measurements. *Patient Care,* 1987, 21(12):189–196. Copyright 1987 by *Patient Care.*

46

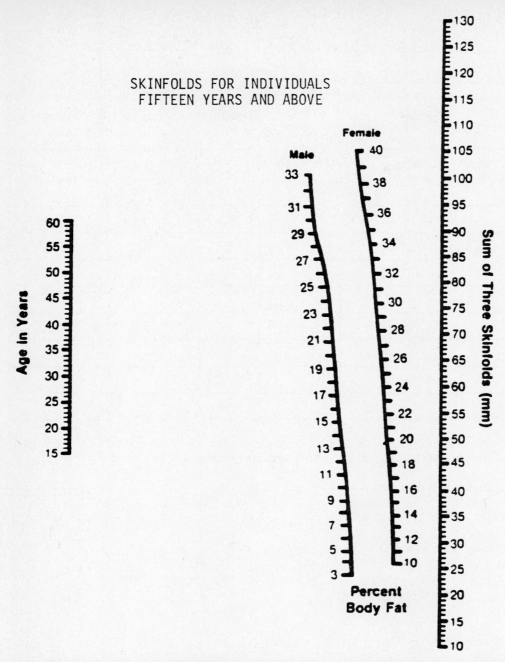

SKINFOLDS FOR INDIVIDUALS
FIFTEEN YEARS AND ABOVE

From W. B. Baum, et al., *Research Quarterly for Exercise and Sport,* Volume 52, August 27, 1985.
Reprinted by permission of the American Alliance for Health, Physical Education, Recreation and Dance,
1900 Association Drive, Reston, VA 22091.

Behavior Modification Tools

1. There are many things that ``cue'' people to eat other than physical hunger. Discover your cues to eating by keeping a diary for a minimum of five days. Be sure to include a weekend in your diary. Whenever you eat any food item, record it in your diary. Use the sample diary on page 46 to help you in the discovery process. IMPORTANT: Complete this step before finishing the rest of the self-analysis!

Day/Time	Quantity and Type of Food	How Do I Feel? (Lonely, Happy)	Where Am I Eating? (By TV, Standing)	How Hungry Am I (Rate Yourself)

2. Review the diary after five days. What patterns do you have regarding your eating behavior? The Mealtime and Eating Behavior Self-Analysis that follows will help you analyze your eating behavior patterns.

   a. Where do you eat most of your meals?
   _____ kitchen table   _____ bedroom   _____ watching TV
   _____ restaurants   other (list): _____

   b. What time do you eat your regular meals?

Breakfast	Lunch	Dinner
6–7 A.M. _____	11–12 P.M. _____	5–6 P.M. _____
7–8 A.M. _____	12–1 P.M. _____	6–7 P.M. _____
8–9 A.M. _____	1–2 P.M. _____	7–8 P.M. _____

   c. How much time does it take you to eat a meal?
   _____ 10 minutes   _____ 30 minutes   _____ 60 minutes
   _____ 15 minutes   _____ 40 minutes   _____ other
   _____ 20 minutes   _____ 50 minutes

   d. How do you feel at the time you normally eat most of your meals?
   _____ tired   _____ fresh   _____ happy
   _____ depressed   _____ starved   _____ lonely

   e. With whom do you ordinarily eat your meals?
   _____ alone   _____ wife/husband
   _____ family   _____ friends
   _____ strangers   _____ acquaintances

   f. Do you eat between-meal snacks? _____ yes   _____ no

48

h.   When you eat between meals, it is because you are:
     _____ hungry   _____ nervous   _____ depressed
     _____ angry   _____ bored   _____ being social
     _____ frightened   _____ for pleasure   other (list): _____

i.   Do you eat second helpings?
     _____ frequently   _____ sometimes   _____ seldom   _____ never

j.   Do you eat sweet desserts such as pie, cake, or ice cream?
     _____ frequently   _____ sometimes   _____ seldom   _____ never

k.   Do you use condiments such as sour cream, butter, catsup, salad dressings, salad spreads, and others?
     _____ frequently   _____ sometimes   _____ seldom   _____ never

l.   Would you classify yourself as a day eater? _____ yes   _____ no

m.   Are you basically a night eater? _____ yes   _____ no

n.   Do you snack as a response to suggestions by advertisements? _____ yes _____ no

o.   Are you a nibbler? _____ yes _____ no

p.   Do you eat on entering your home after work or school? _____ yes _____ no

From G. Carter and S. Wilson, *My Health Status*. Copyright © 1982 Burgess Publishing Company, Minneapolis, MN. Reprinted by permission.

Fat or Fiction?
Take the Nutrition Action Fat Quiz
BY JAYNE HURLEY

Okay. We got the message. We're *trying* to eat less fat. Honest. But does that mean the turkey franks or the "light" beef franks? The tuna salad or the chicken salad? The tortilla chips or the pretzels? That's the tough part. Don't be discouraged if you miss more than you hit. The quiz is tough.

1.   **Which breakfast has the least fat?**
     a.   bagel with cream cheese
     b.   granola with 2% low-fat milk
     c.   McDonald's Egg McMuffin
     d.   Dunkin' Donuts Glazed Yeast Ring

2.   **Which two chicken parts have the most fat? (Assume that you eat equal servings of each.)**
     a.   breast
     b.   thigh
     c.   wing
     d.   drumstick

3.   **Order the following cookies from least to most fat.**
     a.   chocolate chip
     b.   chocolate sandwich (like Oreos)
     c.   oatmeal
     d.   fruit-filled bars (like Fig Newtons)

4.   **Which of these Italian entrees is lowest in fat?**
     a.   fettucini alfredo
     b.   lasagna
     c.   spaghetti with meatballs
     d.   eggplant parmigiana with a side of spaghetti

5.   **2% "low-fat " milk is low in fat.**
     a.   True
     b.   False

6.   **Which of the following Chinese takeout entrees contains almost a day's worth of fat?**
     a.   Szechuan shrimp
     b.   chicken chow mein
     c.   General Tso's chicken (orange chicken)
     d.   shrimp with garlic sauce
     e.   all of the above

7. **Which lunch-counter sandwich has the least fat?**
   a. ham
   b. chicken salad
   c. tuna salad
   d. chicken roll

8. **Which hot dog contains at least seven times more fat than any of the others?**
   a. Hormel Light & Lean 97 Beef Franks
   b. Healthy Choice Beef Franks
   c. Mr. Turkey Bun Size Franks
   d. Oscar Mayer Healthy Favorites

9. **Removing the skin from your roasted chicken breast or drumstick can cut the fat by:**
   a. one-fourth
   b. one-half
   c. three-fourths

10. **Which one of the following Mexican dinners contains less than a day's worth of fat?**
    a. chicken taco platter
    b. chicken burrito platter
    c. taco salad
    d. cheese enchilada platter

11. **"Lite" or "reduced-calorie" salad dressings always have less fat than regular dressings.**
    a. True
    b. False

12. **Which of the following foods has the most fat?**
    a. McDonald's Big Mac
    b. ½ cup of Häagen-Dazs ice cream
    c. McDonald's Chef Salad with a packet of Ranch Dressing
    d. McDonald's Large French Fries

13. **Which of the following is highest in fat? Four ounces of:**
    a. round steak, untrimmed (select)
    b. pork tenderloin, untrimmed
    c. chicken thigh, with skin
    d. sirloin steak, untrimmed (select)

14. **On average, which line of frozen dinners is lowest in fat?**
    a. Healthy Choice
    b. Weight Watchers
    c. Lean Cuisine
    d. Budget Gourmet Light & Healthy

15. **Dry-roasted nuts contain about the same amount of fat as regular (oil-roasted) nuts.**
    a. True
    b. False

16. **Four ounces of Healthy Choice Extra Lean Ground Beef contain four grams of fat. How many grams of fat do four ounces of regular ground turkey contain?**
    a. 5
    b. 10
    c. 15
    d. 20

17. **Order these salty snacks from least to most fat:**
    a. tortilla or vegetable chips
    b. corn chips
    c. "light" potato chips
    d. pretzels
    e. "light" microwave popcorn

18. **Which one of these canned or dried soups has about three times the fat of the others?**
    a. ramen noodle
    b. split pea with ham and bacon
    c. chunky beef
    d. New England clam chowder

19. **Tablespoon for tablespoon, which are the two lowest-fat toppings for baked potatoes?**
    a. "bacon" bits
    b. butter
    c. sour cream
    d. "light" margarine

20. **A Burger King BK Broiler Grilled Chicken Sandwich has more than twice as much fat as a McDonald's McGrilled Chicken Sandwich.**
    a. True
    b. False

Answers

1. **d.** Its 9 grams of fat aren't really low (or healthy), though. Try a bagel with a tablespoon of light or fat-free cream cheese, or a low-fat cereal like Wheaties with skim or 1% fat milk.

2. **b & c.** Dark meat (as long as you're talking drumstick) isn't always fatty. The white meat on wings is, though.

3. **d, c, b, a.** Fat-free cookies by Archway, Entenmann's, and others are your best choice.

4. **c** Spaghetti with red or white clam sauce, tomato sauce, or meat sauce is even lower in fat.

5. **b.** The 5 grams of fat per glass flunks the FDA's limit for "low-fat" (3 grams). Only skim or 1% milk qualify.

6. **c.** The others have half as much or less.

7. **d.** The tuna and chicken salads wouldn't be so fatty if you made them with reduced-fat mayo. The leanest meat for your sandwich is turkey breast or chicken breast.

8. **c.** It's got 11 grams of fat; the others have 1 to 1 ½ grams. In general, though, regular turkey or chicken franks have about a third less fat than regular beef or pork franks. (Unfortunately, all hot dogs are salty.)

9. **b.** If you skin the fattier thigh, you'll cut the fat by about a third.

10. **a.** But that's only because tacos are small and aren't generally served with guacamole and sour cream. Even so, a taco platter uses up two-thirds of your day's fat allowance.

11. **b.** While they usually have less, that's not always the case: 2 Tbs. of Ken's Steak House Lite Honey Mustard, for example, contains 9 grams of fat. Henri's regular Honey Mustard contains just 6 grams.

12. **c.** The 30 grams of fat use up almost half your day's quota. If you get it with the Lite Vinaigrette dressing, the fat plummets to 11 grams (and the sat fat drops from 7 to 4 grams).

13. **c.** Even if you skin the chicken, you'll end up with more than twice the fat of the tenderloin, which is one of the few low-fat cuts of pork.

14. **a.** Healthy Choice dinners average just 14 percent of calories from fat. The others range from 22 to 25 percent. Healthy Choice is also a tad lower in sodium.

15. **a.** Nuts are so fatty that they don't absorb much extra oil when roasted.

16. **c.** Regular ground turkey includes fatty skin. Ground turkey *breast* is as low in fat as the Healthy Choice ground beef.

17. **d, e, c, a, b.** An ounce of pretzels has just 1 gram of fat. Then come "light" microwave popcorn (2–4 grams), "light" potato chips (6 grams), tortilla or vegetable chips (7–9 grams), and corn chips (8–10 grams).

18. **a.** Companies like Campbell, Nissin, and Maruchan fry their ramen noodles in fat—often (saturated) palm oil—before their soups are dehydrated.

19. **a & c.** They've got just a couple of grams of fat. A tablespoon (3 pats) of "light" margarine has 6 grams. Butter has 11 grams.

20. **a.** It wouldn't have been true last year, but sneaky Burger King went and tripled the fat without telling anybody.

WHAT'S YOUR SCORE?

Give yourself one point for each correct answer on this very tough quiz. Your Score _____

If you scored:

17 to 20   **Fantastic!** Even we didn't do *this* well when we proofread the test.
13 to 16   **Hubba Hubba!** Congrats. You're the Fat Champ of your block.
9 to 12   **C-o-o-o-l!** Most people were in this range. You're on the right track.
5 to 8   **Pretty Lean!** *Nutrition Action* is for reading, not for cleaning your windows.
Below 5   **Blubber City!** Keep your cardiologist's beeper number in your wallet.

Reviewing Important Concepts

1. Describe the difference between ``overweight'' and ``obesity."

2. There are currently several important theories which attempt to explain the causes of obesity. Briefly summarize each of the following weight loss theories:

    a. Fat cell theory—

    b. Set point theory—

    c. Insulin theory—

    d. Energy balance equation theory—

    A calorie is a calorie and if the intake doesn't equal the physical weight could be gained.

    e. Dietary fat theory—

    f. Genetic theory—

3. Are scales and height/weight tables good ways to determine how fat you are? Why?

4. Describe Body Mass Index, and explain its relevance as a measure of obesity.

Applying What You've Learned

1. What new behaviors can you practice as alternatives to your current eating behaviors? List five things you can do other than eat. For example, you could take three deep breaths, delay eating for at least five minutes (the urge will go away), water your plants, read a book, write a short note to a friend, or balance your checkbook. The possibilities are endless. Be creative! The next time you find yourself looking for a snack, practice one of these positive substitutes.

2. It is important to reward yourself for practicing the new positive alternative behaviors you are developing. Your rewards should be things other than food. The rewards should also be something you would not have given yourself if you had not achieved your goal. Some examples of rewards include:

do a crossword puzzle	read a new book	go to a movie
play a musical instrument	garden	walk in the park
needlepoint	buy some new cologne	make model planes
discover flower arranging	buy a new album	learn a new hobby

   Identify a reward or rewards for the new positive eating behavior(s) you decide to adopt. Set a time span during which you'll practice the behavior before you give yourself your reward.

3. Your friend Kendall wants to go on a diet. He discovered a new fad diet in the Sunday newspaper. Explain to Kendall why fad diets can be a health hazard. List five questions Kendall can use to determine if a diet is safe and effective.

4. You've convinced Kendall not to go on the fad diet. Kendall asks you for advice. You discover that he weighs 190 pounds and is six feet tall. What is Kendall's body mass index? Using the nomogram in Activity for Wellness 4.1 in your book, determine how much weight Kendall needs to lose to achieve at BMI of 23.

5. Develop a fat-management program for Kendall based on the amount of weight he needs to lose from either the BMI or percent body fat calculations.

Stages of Change

Maintaining optimal body weight is one of the biggest components of wellness—and one of the biggest challenges for many people. Refer to table 4.3 on page 131 and Activity for Wellness 4.1 on page 134 of your text. If your score indicates that you are at increased health risk because of your weight, you may want to consider taking steps to lose or gain weight.

Answer these four questions to assess your current stage of change related to weight management.

1. I have been at a desirable weight for more than six months.
2. I have taken action to lose or gain weight within the past six months.
3. I am currently preparing to take action to lose or gain weight in the next month.
4. I would like to take action to lose or gain weight within the next six months.

Scoring

No to all statements	Precontemplation
Yes to statement 4	Contemplation
Yes to statement 3	Preparation
Yes to statement 2	Action
Yes to statement 1	Maintenance

Review table 4.7 of *Connections for Health* on page 158 for tips on moving through the stages of change and taking charge of your weight.

For Further Study

Optimal body composition and related levels of wellness are a result of your life-style choices. Weight management is a lifelong process involving the development of sound dietary practices and regular activity. The following activities will help you to begin this process. The choice is yours.

Wellness Activities

1. Identify a diet program that is offered in your community. What techniques are used in this program? Do you have to purchase special foods or food supplements? Estimate the cost of going on this diet for one year. Do you feel this is a way of eating that you could continue lifelong?
2. Exercise is the key to weight management. See the activities in chapter 5 ``Fitness Potentials: Discovering Your Play'' to assist you in your weight management goals.
3. Liquid diets are among the most popular diets in recent years. Investigate two or three of these programs. Does a physician supervise the program? What is the liquid supplement made of? Is a behavioral component offered? What is the program length and cost?

4. Interview someone you know who has recently lost weight. How did he or she accomplish his or her goal? What program, if any, did he or she follow? What ``success'' tips can he or she give you?

5. How many times do the characters on your favorite television show eat or drink? Conduct your own study. Be sure to count each eating episode, note the type of food eaten and where the food is consumed (sitting at table, in front of TV, standing). Is it possible to determine the mood of the character while eating? Write a brief report of your findings. Do you eat while watching this particular show? Do you think you are influenced by the eating done on the show?

5 Fitness Potentials: Discovering Your Play

Fitness . . . Where Do You Stand?

In order to begin your new physically active wellness life-style, you need to know how to set up safe and beneficial fitness activities. The following assessments will help you evaluate your feelings concerning physical activity and your level of fitness. Remember, the key to leading a physically active wellness life-style is to find activities that you consider play.

Physical Activity Questionnaire

This quiz will help you evaluate your feelings about physical activity and help you to determine the specific reasons why you do or do not participate in regular physical activity. The term *physical activity* refers to all kinds of activities, including sports, formal exercises, and informal activities, such as jogging and cycling.

Read each of the statements below. In the blank labeled ``Rating,'' rate your response as follows:

> Strongly Agree (SA)
> Agree (A)
> Undecided (U)
> Disagree (D)
> Strongly Disagree (SD)

		Rating	*Score*
1.	Doing regular physical activity can be as harmful to health as it is helpful.	_____	_____
2.	One of the main reasons I do regular physical activity is because it is fun.	_____	_____
3.	Participating in physical activities makes me tense and nervous.	_____	_____
4.	The challenge of physical training is one reason I participate in physical activity.	_____	_____
5.	One of the things I like about physical activity is the participation with other people.	_____	_____
6.	Doing regular physical activity does little to make me more physically attractive.	_____	_____
7.	Competition is a good way to keep a game from being fun.	_____	_____
8.	I should exercise regularly for my own good health and physical fitness.	_____	_____
9.	Doing exercise and playing sports is boring.	_____	_____
10.	I enjoy taking part in physical activity because it helps me to relax and get away from the pressures of daily living.	_____	_____
11.	Most sports and physical activities are too difficult for me to enjoy.	_____	_____
12.	I do not enjoy physical activities that require the participation of other people.	_____	_____

13. Regular exercise helps me look my best. _____ _____

14. Competing against others in physical activities makes them enjoyable. _____ _____

Scoring:

1. For items 1, 3, 6, 7, 9, 11, and 12, give one point for strongly agree, two for agree, three for undecided, four for disagree, and five for strongly disagree. Put the correct number in the blank to the right of the statements under the column ``Score.''
2. For items 2, 4, 5, 8, 10, 13, and 14, give five points for strongly agree, four for agree, three for undecided, two for disagree, and one for strongly disagree. Put the correct number in the blank to the right of the statements under the column ``Score.''
3. Enter your score next to each corresponding question. Determine each of the following seven scores by adding your points together.

Health and fitness score	Question #1 _____ + Question #8 _____	= _____
Fun and enjoyment score	Question #2 _____ + Question #9 _____	= _____
Relaxation and enjoyment score	Question #3 _____ + Question #10 _____	= _____
Challenge and achievement score	Question #4 _____ + Question #11 _____	= _____
Social score	Question #5 _____ + Question #12 _____	= _____
Appearance score	Question #6 _____ + Question #13 _____	= _____
Competition score	Question #7 _____ + Question #14 _____	= _____

Total score _____

4. Determine your total score by adding the seven scores together. Write your total score in the bottom blank.
5. Use the chart below to determine your rating on each score.

Physical Activity Questionnaire Rating Scale

Classification	Each of Seven Scores	Total Score
Excellent	9–10	63–70
Good	7–8	50–62
Fair	6	42–49
Poor	4–5	30–41
Very Poor	3 or fewer	29 or fewer

6. Check your rating for each of the seven reasons for exercising in the box on page 58. Also include your total score rating. These seven scores should reflect your reasons for participating in physical activity. Answer the questions that follow to provide you with more insight to your current exercising behavior.

	Ex	Good	Fair	Poor	VP
Health and fitness	☐	☐	☐	☐	☐
Fun and enjoyment	☐	☐	☐	☐	☐
Relaxation and enjoyment	☐	☐	☐	☐	☐
Challenge and achievement	☐	☐	☐	☐	☐
Social	☐	☐	☐	☐	☐
Appearance	☐	☐	☐	☐	☐
Competition	☐	☐	☐	☐	☐
Total	☐	☐	☐	☐	☐

Do you think the scores on which you were rated ``excellent'' or ``good''' accurately reflect the reasons you might do regular exercise? Explain.

Do you think that the scores on which you were rated ``poor'' or ``very poor'' might be reasons why you would avoid physical activity? Explain.

Those who are physically active should score high on the total score. Is your total score a good reflection of your overall attitude about physical activity? Explain.

Cardiovascular Fitness

A variety of methods can be used to determine your cardiovascular fitness. The 1-mile walk test is one method described in your textbook. Another way to access cardiovascular fitness is the step test. Directions for taking the step test are described below.

1. Step up and down on a twelve-inch bench for three minutes at a rate of twenty-four steps per minute. One step consists of four beats, that is, ``up with the left foot, up with the right foot, down with the left foot, down with the right foot.''
2. Immediately after the exercise, sit down on the bench and relax. Don't talk.
3. Locate your pulse or have another person locate it for you.

4. Five seconds after the exercise ends, begin counting your pulse. Count the pulse for sixty seconds.
5. Your score is your sixty-second heart rate. Locate your score and your rating on the following chart.

Step Test Rating Chart

Classification	60-Second Heart Rate
High Performance Zone	84 or less
Good Fitness Zone	85–95
Marginal Zone	96–119
Low Zone	120 and above

From F. W. Kasch and J. L. Boyer, *Adult Fitness: Principles and Practices,* 1968. Mayfield Publishers, Palo Alto, CA. Reprinted by permission of the author.

In order to make a final assessment of your cardiovascular fitness, take more than one type of fitness test. Use the charts in chapter 5 of your textbook and the step test rating chart above to compare your results. Fill in the box below. How do your results compare?

Step Test	Your 60-second heart rate: _____	Fitness Rating: _____
1-mile walk	Your time:	Fitness Rating: _____

Directions: Within each group of exercises, start with the one that you believe is the most difficult one that you can perform. If you can pass it, try the next most difficult one. You receive points for the most difficult exercise that you can perform. Note: M = point values for males and F = point values for females.

Muscular Fitness Norms (Push-Ups)

Evaluating Isotonic Strength

I. **Push-Up:** Tests pectorals, triceps, abdominals, and other muscles.
   (It is a failure if the hips pike or sag.)

2. One straight-leg push-up, keeping your body rigid.

Point values
M = 3
F = 6

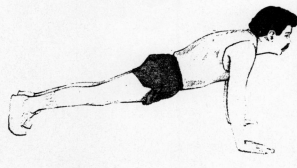

Tests

1. One bent-knee push-up, keeping your body straight and rigid.

Point values
M = 0
F = 3

3. One straight-leg push-up, keeping your body rigid and your feet on the bench.

Point values
M = 6
F = 8

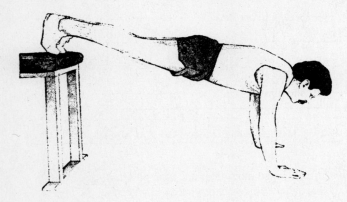

5. Same as no. 2, except use only one arm.

Point values
M = 10
F = 12

4. Same as no. 2, except have partner do a push-up on back of your shoulders at the same time.

Point values
M = 8
F = 10

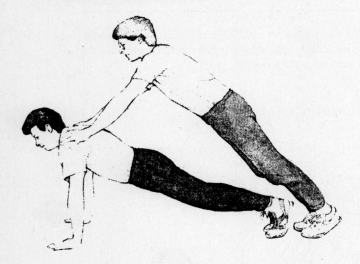

Isotonic Strength *Rating Scale* (Men and Women)					
	Age				
Classification	17–26	27–39	40–49	50–59	60+
High performance zone	31+	28+	28+	26+	24+
Good fitness zone	24–30	22–27	22–27	20–25	19–23
Marginal zone	19–23	17–21	15–21	14–19	12–18
Low zone	<19	<17	<15	<14	<12

Flexibility Tests

Because it is impractical to test the flexibility of all joints, perform these tests for joints used frequently. Follow instructions carefully.

Test

1. *Modified Sit-and-Reach*
   (Flexibility Test of Hamstrings)
   a. Remove shoes and assume the position for the "backsaver toe touch" , except place the sole of the foot of the extended leg flat against the box or bench seat, and place the head, back, and hips against a wall; 90 degree angle at the hips.
   b. Place one hand over the other and slowly reach forward as far as you can with arms fully extended; head and back remain in contact with the wall. A partner will slide the measuring stick on the bench until it touches the fingertips.
   c. With the measuring stick fixed in the new position, reach forward as far as possible, three times, holding the position on the third reach for at least two seconds while the partner reads the distance on the ruler. Keep the knee of the extended leg straight (see illustration).
   d. Repeat the test a second time and average the scores of the two trials.

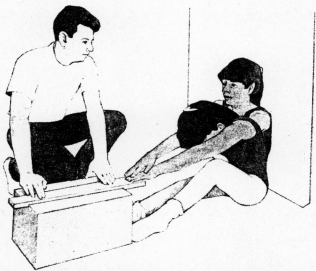

Flexibility *Rating Scale* for Test 1*		
	Men	Women
Classification	Test 1	Test 1
High performance zone	16+	17+
Good fitness zone	13–15	14–16
Marginal zone	10–12	11–13
Low zone	<9	<10

Reviewing Important Concepts

1. When designing an aerobic-exercise program, it is important to consider frequency, intensity, and time. Compare the recommended frequency, intensity and duration of physical activity to gain health promotion benefits with physical activity to gain physical fitness.

2. There are four principles of fitness which apply to cardiovascular endurance as well as to the flexibility and muscular strength/endurance activities. These principles are overload, specificity, individual differences, and reversibility. Describe each one of these concepts. Use bicycling as an example to illustrate your descriptions.

3. Distinguish between resting heart rate, target heart rate, and maximum heart rate as they relate to aerobic exercise.

Applying What You've Learned

1. Your roommate Ken would like to start exercising regularly. Ken decides to join a group of friends who jog every morning. After three weeks you ask Ken how he's doing with his exercise program. He explains that he's only jogged three times because he really doesn't like jogging. What other aerobic activity could you suggest that Ken might enjoy?

2. Develop an exercise program for physical fitness benefits for Ken using the activity you suggested. Remember that Ken is just beginning an exercise program. Develop your plan so that he begins at the initial conditioning stage. Be sure to follow the F.I.T. guidelines.

3.   What changes will Ken need to make to move into the improvement conditioning stage and then on to the maintenance stage? Develop a program for each of these stages.

4.   You are going to an open house at a new health club with a friend. The health club owner tries to make you immediately sign a contract to become a member for a three-year period. How do you assess whether you should join this health club? List the pros and cons of joining on the first visit.

5.   When it comes to physical activity, you may say that you just can't seem to find the time for it. What you need to do is to examine how you spend your time and then determine how you can ``make'' the time.

   To help you find out how you're spending your time, keep a diary of what you do each day for one week. Be sure to include the following: time you get up, time you spend eating each meal, time spent with friends, time spent studying, time spent watching TV, time spent on other activities.

   Look for patterns in your diary. Where can you make time for your fitness program? Is there time in the morning, afternoon, early evening, or late evening? Look for a 10–15 minute block of time to begin with. Can't find 10–15 minutes? Find 5 minutes. Anyone can take 5 minutes to walk around the block. As you get more comfortable with your fitness program, you'll gradually be able to make more time for it! Write some of your observations below.

6.   Keep a daily exercise log. The example below will help you see how you're improving with your fitness program.

Frequency	*Intensity*	*Duration*
Date:	My activity today felt:	Time spent:
Comments*	easy _____	1–20 min. _____
_____	average _____	21–30 min. _____
_____	difficult _____	31–40 min. _____
_____	My breathing:	41–60 min. _____
Mood	came easily _____	61+ min. _____
_____	was labored _____	Distance covered: _____
_____	was labored throughout _____	
_____	Heart rate: _____	

*Comments can include time of day, weather conditions, location, companions.

Reprinted from *Running as Therapy: An Integrated Approach*, edited by M. L. Sachs and G. W. Buffone, by permission of University of Nebraska Press. Copyright 1984 by the University of Nebraska Press.

7.   It is important to reward yourself for practicing the new positive activities you are practicing. The rewards should be something you would not have given yourself if you had not achieved your goal. See chapter 4, ``Applying What You've Learned'' for reward suggestions. List three rewards you will use when you practice your new fitness activity.

Stages of Change

How physically fit are you? Complete the One-Mile Walking Test on pages 176–177 of your text to find out. If your score is in the low fitness range, you may want to consider taking steps to improve your cardiovascular fitness.

Answer these four questions to assess your current stage of change related to cardiovascular fitness, or any aspect of fitness.

1.   I have maintained a high level of fitness for more than six months.

2.   I have taken action to start and maintain a fitness program within the past six months.

3.   I am currently preparing to start a fitness program in the next month.

4.   I would like to take action to become more physically fit within the next six months.

Scoring

No to all statements	Precontemplation
Yes to statement 4	Contemplation
Yes to statement 3	Preparation
Yes to statement 2	Action
Yes to statement 1	Maintenance

Review table 5.9 on page 193 of *Connections for Health* for tips on moving through the stages of change and taking charge of the way you manage stressors.

For Further Study

Now you're ready to begin your exercise program. The following activities will help you discover your ``play.'' Be open to trying new activities—variety is the spice of life. Remember to START SLOWLY and proceed gradually to your fitness goals.

Wellness Activities

1.   Enter a fun run or a bike race that's held in your community. How did you feel mentally and physically before, during, and after the run/race? What was it like to participate in an activity with many other people?
2.   Observe the activity level on your college campus. Do people tend to drive, walk, ride bikes, roller skate? Do people participate in aerobic activities? What types? Do they partake in these activities outdoors or indoors? What kinds of recreational activities are popular with students?
3.   Kenneth Cooper has also developed a 1.5-Mile Walk/Run Test and a 3-Mile Walk Test. If you are currently physically active, try one of these aerobic tests. The book, *The Aerobic Program for Total Well-Being* by Kenneth H. Cooper, M.D., New York: M. Evans and Co., 1982 describes both tests.

4. According to a recent Gallup Poll, the surge in the number of people exercising is due to the ``walking boom.'' For many people, walking is boring and they don't feel they get a good workout. Walking tapes are one way to help you turn a casual stroll into a real workout.

5. Use Activity for Wellness 5.6 ``How fit is your health club?'' to investigate a fitness center that interests you. Write a brief report of your findings.

6. There are a number of exciting new trends in fitness—step, water walking and exercise, strength training, indoor rock climbing to name a few. Choose one activity that you've never tried before. Try the activity at least twice. Write a brief paper describing what you did, how you liked it, why you would or would not continue this form of exercise.

6 Human Sexuality: Behavior and Relationship Options

Human Sexuality . . . Where Do You Stand?

There has been a recent challenge to gender role stereotypes causing many people to reexamine their own sex roles. There are many life-style options available for us to choose from. The questionnaire below will provide a forum for you to explore the most common of these life-style options—marriage.

In Your Marriage, Who Will . . . ?

If you are already married, this exercise may make you more aware of how you and your partner divide various responsibilities. If you are not married, you can use this exercise as a projection, an opportunity to clarify your values and your expectations, and perhaps, someday, as a reference point for discussions with your future spouse.

Directions: For each item listed, check off whose responsibility you think the item is or will become.

Responsibility	Wife's Job	Husband's Job	Do Together	Take Turns
1. Decide where to live	————	————	————	————
2. Earn more money	————	————	————	————
3. Clean the car	————	————	————	————
4. Take the kids to the dentist*	————	————	————	————
5. Cook Thanksgiving dinner	————	————	————	————
6. Change the baby's* diapers	————	————	————	————
7. Talk to the bank manager	————	————	————	————
8. Replace a blown fuse	————	————	————	————
9. Pay the phone bill	————	————	————	————
10. Go to the supermarket	————	————	————	————
11. Send the Christmas cards	————	————	————	————
12. Rake the yard	————	————	————	————
13. Mend clothes	————	————	————	————
14. Choose a new car	————	————	————	————
15. Choose a new refrigerator	————	————	————	————
16. Choose new curtains	————	————	————	————
17. Go to PTA meetings*	————	————	————	————
18. Get up at night when the baby cries*	————	————	————	————
19. Choose where to go for recreation	————	————	————	————
20. Decide when to have sex	————	————	————	————

*We do not intend to imply that all married couples have or should have children. However, even if you intend not to have children, you may find it interesting to fill in these items.

Scoring: The way you filled in the self-assessment today might be different from the way you would fill it in a year from now, or in five or ten years. It is often a mistake to assume that in any one area, one partner must necessarily be less capable than the other. It is nearly always a mistake to assume that people's capabilities and interests do not or will not change.

Reactions: Write in the space below what you have learned about your expectations and thoughts regarding marriage.

From *Well-Being: An Introduction to Health* by John Dorfman, Sheila Kitzinger, and Herbert Schuchman. Copyright © 1980 by Scott, Foresman, and Co. Reprinted by permission of Harper Collins College Publishers.

Spend More Quality Time Together

Quality time (QT) is a precious commodity. It is to relationships what clean air is to the environment—that is, integral.

It is not really true that familiarity breeds contempt; it merely begets forgetfulness of the importance of QT. At some point in your life, you have enjoyed quality time with somebody. There is no need to dwell on what QT is, except to note that it includes a sense of being in the moment, free from the preoccupations of future expectations, plans, and dreams, and past regrets, accomplishments, and delights. We think that QT is evident in relationships marked by:

- shared recreational activities
- holding hands
- writing and receiving a love letter
- giving and receiving a massage
- meditating together before or after making love
- sharing a meal in joy and appreciation
- reading a meaningful statement aloud
- music, art, dance

These are a few thoughts. How might you put some more QT into your relationships? What examples occur to you?

1. _____
2. _____
3. _____
4. _____
5. _____

Source: From D.B. Ardell and M.J. Tagar, *Planning for Wellness,* 1982, Kendall/Hunt Publishing Company, Dubuque, Iowa.

Reviewing Important Concepts

1. It is a difficult task to describe the sexual behavioral profile of a particular society. Describe the limitations of sexuality research and how these limitations can bias our research.
2. Briefly describe the three essential elements of successful love relationships.

3. *In your own words,* briefly summarize each phase of the human sexual response cycle for males and females.

Applying What You've Learned

1. On the basis of your own experiences, circle the ten words or phrases that best define what love means to you now. Put an X by the five words or phrases that you would never associate with love. Complete the questions that follow.

physical attractiveness
self-confidence
compromise
jealousy
loyalty
emotional intimacy
tenderness
sacrifice
marriage
security
kindness
never having to say I'm sorry
honesty
caring about my physical appearance
independence
warm fuzzies
children
compassion
physical intimacy
vulnerability
being there when I need them
responsibility
freedom

a sense of humor
togetherness
trust
respect
open communication
faithfulness
empathy
forgiveness
understanding
possessiveness
sharing
expressing my emotions openly
commitment
putting my partner's needs before my own
dependence
friendship
unconditional acceptance
caring
being able to take out my frustrations
obsessiveness
privacy
self-disclosure

a. Did any of your answers surprise you? Why or why not?

b. Using your ten choices of what love means to you now, draw your version of Sternberg's love triangle. Label each side of your triangle.

c.   Refer to figure 6.6 in your textbook. Which of Sternberg's love triangle combinations comes closest to yours? Draw it next to your triangle (from previous page). Which words from the list would you have to include in order to have your triangle represent complete love? Write these words below. Is it possible for you to include these words/phrases in your definition of love? Why or why not?

2.   Effective communication of thoughts and feelings through words and actions is an essential component of a successful love relationship. One of the surest ways to tear down a person's self-esteem (and eventually a healthy love relationship) is to consistently insult rather than compliment them. The put-down has become as American as apple pie and we have learned to accept it.

Complete the following chart by recording all the insults and compliments you gave or heard others give in one day.

Insults given or heard today

Example: "Do you always have to be such a slob?"

Compliments given or heard today

Example: "Thank you for doing the dishes today."

Source: Data from G. F. Carter and S. B. Wilson, *My Health Status,* 1982, Burgess Publishing Co., Minneapolis, MN.

At the end of the day, compare the two lists. How did the insults and compliments you gave affect your relationship with the people to whom the statements were directed? How did the insults and compliments you heard others give seem to affect the people who received them? How could you communicate differently in the future? Write your answers below.

Stages of Change

Complete Activity for Wellness 6.3 on page 214 of your text to get you thinking about the characteristics you look for in a romantic partner. If you are interested in dating and in improving your date-seeking skills, answer these four questions to determine your stage of change related to dating.

1. I have been happy with my dating situation for more than six months.

2. I have taken action to improve my date-seeking skills within the past six months.

3. I am currently preparing to take action to improve my date-seeking skills in the next month.

4. I would like to take action to improve my dating skills within the next six months.

Scoring

No to all statements   Precontemplation
Yes to statement 4   Contemplation
Yes to statement 3   Preparation
Yes to statement 2   Action
Yes to statement 1   Maintenance

Review table 6.2 on page 225 of *Connections for Health* for tips on moving through the stages of change and developing a more satisfying dating situation.

For Further Study

An enhanced understanding of sexual issues and topics is an important part of being able to appreciate your own sexuality. Satisfaction with your sexual life-style is an important component of high-level wellness. There are many factors which affect sexual life-style. The activities that follow will help you to further explore many of these issues and topics.

Wellness Activities

1. Interview someone who is 65 years or older about the ``rules'' for dating and marriage when he or she was young. What were society's attitudes and expectations for young people?
2. Make an appointment with a campus counselor who counsels married couples. Discuss with the counselor why so many marriages end in divorce. What are the key marital problems the counselor sees in his/her practice?
3. Write a sample marriage contract for yourself containing provisions you feel are important in a marriage. The following are features that could be included: division of assets prior to marriage, budget and income

71

management, the choice to have or not have children, responsibilities of child care, responsibilities of household chores, religion, obligations and rights regarding careers. Be creative; add to this list!

4.   Assemble a panel of people who have different sexual orientations and life-styles: a lesbian, a homosexual, a bisexual, a heterosexual married couple, a divorced person, an older single person. Have the audience write questions for the panel to answer regarding the panel members' sexual orientation and life-styles.

5.   There are people who view being single not as a stepping stone to marriage but as a long-term option or even a permanent life-style. Describe your reaction to this statement. Does this life-style appeal to you? How would your parents, grandparents, friends react if you told them you were choosing to be single as a permanent life-style?

6.   What resources are available on your campus if you wanted information on human sexuality? Describe the different services offered.

7 Parenthood: Pregnancy and Child Care

Parenthood . . . Where Do You Stand?

This chapter will help you enhance your understanding of the reproductive system and your reproductive options. A greater understanding of these topics will affect your level of wellness and serve as a foundation for your future reproductive decisions.

How Well Do You Know the Human Reproductive System?

It is a misconception to think that males and females know all about their respective sexual anatomy just because they are male or female. Put your knowledge to the test by labeling each part of both the male and female reproductive systems illustrated on the next page. When you're through, refer to your textbook (chapter 7) and compare your answers with the diagrams in the chapter. How well did you do?

Personal Life Plan

Parenthood has been called the ultimate responsibility. Before taking the step to parenthood, it is important to seriously consider what it means to be a parent.

The Personal Life Plan will help you explore how pregnancy and parenting might affect your level of wellness. Read each question. Consider the question carefully, then answer it in the space provided.

1. Do I wish to marry? *Yes*

2. If I could choose any age at which to marry, what age would I select? *21-23*

3. How many years of formal education would I like to complete? *2-4*

4. At what point during or after this educational process would I like to marry?

5. Would I like to wait until I'm married to start having intercourse?

6. Would I like to have children one day? *no*

7. How old would I like to be when I have my first child? *I already have 1 → I want more.*

8. How concerned would I be if I (or my partner) were to become pregnant before we were married? *none*

9. If I (or my partner) were to become pregnant when we did not want to be pregnant, what would I do? Raise the child? Adoption? Abortion?

10. How many children would I like to have?

11. Will I be able emotionally and financially to support this family?

12. How would I feel if I were not able to have any children?

13. Would I consider adoption an option were I unable to become pregnant?

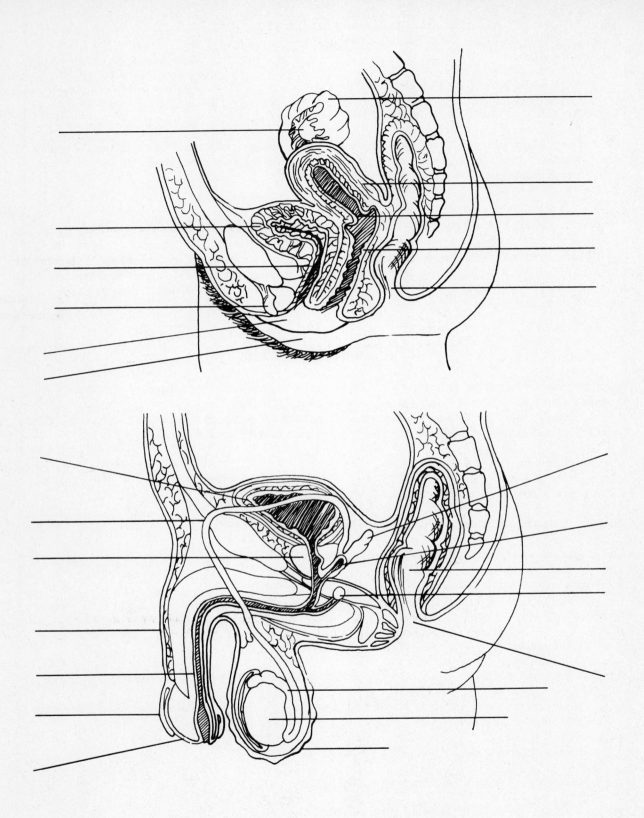

14. What kind of obligation, if any, do I feel toward limiting the size of my family to help limit the pressures of overpopulation?

15. Would I like to work when my children are toddlers? When my children are in their childhood years? When my children are no longer in the home?

16. How do I expect my partner to participate in child rearing?

17. Of all the things I could do in my life, probably the most important thing would be . . . ?

18. This life goal would be affected by marriage in the following ways:

    By child rearing in the following ways:

19. What would it mean to me if my marriage were to end in divorce?

20. Would I like to have sexual intercourse with the person I marry before that marriage occurs?

21. How would I feel if my spouse were to have an intimate sexual relationship outside of our marriage? An intimate emotional relationship?

22. How would I feel if I were to have an intimate sexual relationship outside of my marriage? An intimate emotional relationship?

23. How does my life plan thus far blend with my religious beliefs, with the beliefs of the family and society in which I live, and my personal code of ethics? How does it blend with what I personally feel God would want me to do, with what I personally feel to be right or wrong for me? If these things are in conflict, how can I best reconcile these differences?

In suggesting these as valuable questions, we do not imply that there are any ``correct'' answers. We are simply hoping to stimulate people to consider carefully their own feelings about reproductive issues; the source of these feelings; the way in which these feelings mesh with their values and expectations and the values and expectations of others; and the way they expect these values to guide their lives.

From Robert Hatcher, et al. *Contraceptive Technology 1984–1985,* 12th Revised Edition. Reprinted with permission from Irvington Publishers, Inc., New York, NY.

Reviewing Important Concepts

1. One function of the testes and ovaries is to produce estrogen and testosterone. Delineate the important functions of these hormones.

2. Briefly describe the three stages of labor.

3. At different prenatal periods, the developing infant is called an embryo and a fetus. Explain how these two developmental stages differ.

Applying What You've Learned

1. Based on your study of the male reproductive system, physiologically how would it be possible for a female to become pregnant if a male withdrew his penis from the vagina before he ejaculated?

2. You are at a party with your friend Judy. Judy tells you that she and her husband are planning to have a child as soon as possible. You notice that Judy is drinking some wine and smoking a cigarette. When you ask her about this, she says she'll quit drinking and smoking when she finds out that she is pregnant. Explain to Judy why she should consider quitting before she finds out for sure that she is pregnant.

3. Imagine you or your sexual partner just found out that she is pregnant. Using table 7.2 ``OTCs and the Pregnant Woman,'' identify any medications you have used or are currently using and list them below. List the adverse effects these medications have on the fetus. Which drugs were you aware of that could harm a fetus? Which drugs were you surprised to find on this list? What steps will you have to take in order to insure a safe and healthy fetus? (If you are a male, use the medications you have used or are currently using to answer these questions.)

4. You've been asked to participate in a debate on the topic of prenatal testing. Choose one side, either ``pro'' or ``con,'' and briefly outline the points you'll address in the debate.

Stages of Change

Would you make a good parent? Think about the questions posed in Activity for Wellness 7.1 on page 248 of your text to start thinking about all the challenges involved. If you would like to develop your skills as a caregiver to children, start by answering these four questions to assess your current stage of change.

1. I have been caring for children successfully for more than six months.

2. I have started taking care of children within the past six months.

3. I am currently preparing to start taking care of children in the next month.

4. I would like to take action to learn to care for children within the next six months.

Scoring

No to all statements	Precontemplation
Yes to statement 4	Contemplation
Yes to statement 3	Preparation
Yes to statement 2	Action
Yes to statement 1	Maintenance

Review table 7.7 on page 272 of *Connections for Health* for tips on moving through the stages of change and preparing to become an effective parent or caregiver.

For Further Study

The more you know about the human reproductive system, reproductive options, and parenting, the better position you will be in to make the right decisions for you. The activities and guides below will help you in your decision-making and help you explore your present feelings. It is important to remember that your feelings may change in the future. Use the materials in this section in the future to help you with your wellness decisions.

Wellness Activities

1. For women only: Learn more about your reproductive anatomy. The next time you have a pelvic examination ask your doctor if you can participate by watching the examination using a mirror. Ask your doctor to describe the examination process.
2. Many people feel uncomfortable when using sexual language if they use it at all. To discover your comfort level, try the following exercise. On a piece of paper, write down ten parts of the human reproductive anatomy—both male and female. Say the words out loud. How do you feel? How would you feel if you read this list to a friend, someone of the opposite sex, a group of strangers, your parents?
3. How does it feel to have total responsibility, twenty-four hours a day, for a baby or child? Babysit an infant for an entire day and night. How do you feel about childcare after this experience? Try this activity several times and choose children of different ages. What differences do you notice in caring for babies, toddlers, and young children?
4. Talk with your parents and ask them how they learned to parent. What things would they change, if any, about the way they brought you up?
5. Compare the costs of five over-the-counter pregnancy kits. What process does each brand use to detect pregnancy? How reliable is each brand in detecting pregnancy?
6. Locate at least one article that addresses one of the following ethical issues: artificial insemination, surrogate mothers, re-implantation. What are the arguments raised in the articles? Describe your feelings regarding these arguments.
7. Investigate a prepared childbirth education course offered by your local hospital or public health department. What are the topics covered? When should a woman (or couple) begin attending a prepared childbirth course?
8. Identify the names of several companies that you would like to work for when you graduate. What types of prenatal and paternity leave benefits do they offer to both male and female employees?
9. There are several options regarding childbirth available to expectant parents. Describe the childbirth options you will consider if you decide to become a parent. Explain your reasons for considering these options.

8 Birth Control: Options for Preventing Unintended Pregnancy

Birth Control . . . Where Do You Stand?

The fertility options you use and avoid will have a considerable effect on your level of wellness. Fertility decisions, or indecision, have the potential to give great joy, great sorrow, or both. In order for you to make an informed decision regarding birth control, it is important that you understand the principles of the different birth control methods. The Birth Control Questionnaire will assess your understanding of how various birth control methods work.

One fertility option, abortion, is an important and hotly debated issue. ``What's Your Decision?'' will help you determine your feelings about this issue.

Understanding Birth Control Methods

1. Methods available to the male for controlling conception include
   a. the Norplant.
   b. the cervical cap.
   c. the condom.
   d. the diaphragm.
   e. the IUD.

2. The effectiveness of a method of birth control when used under everyday conditions is called the method's
   a. actual use effectiveness.
   b. theoretical use effectiveness.
   c. absolute use effectiveness.
   d. practical use effectiveness.
   e. reserve use effectiveness.

3. The most serious side effect of the use of birth control pills is
   a. loss of sex drive.
   b. the appearance of liver spots on the skin.
   c. the formation of blood clots.
   d. breakthrough bleeding between menstrual periods.
   e. pregnancy.

4. All of the following are methods used in determining the day of a woman's unsafe period each month EXCEPT the
   a. basal body temperature method.
   b. calendar method.
   c. ovulation method.
   d. symptothermal method.
   e. menstrual method.

5. All of the following are true for the intrauterine device EXCEPT
   a. the insertion of an IUD while a woman is pregnant may cause an abortion.
   b. the IUD is inserted into the vagina.
   c. an occasional pregnancy may occur with the device in place.
   d. most women using it experience no major adverse reactions.
   e. insertion of an IUD may cause cramping.

6. An advantage in using the diaphragm is that
   a. it can be kept in place for several days at a time.
   b. it virtually eliminates the chances of a pregnancy.
   c. its use requires little, if any, motivation.
   d. it has a lower failure rate than the pill.
   e. its use is completely reversible.

7. Spermicides are chemical substances that
   a. kill the egg as soon as fertilization occurs.
   b. aid the movement of sperm through the fallopian tube.
   c. prevent the egg from escaping from the ovary.
   d. after fertilization, kill all other sperm attempting to penetrate the ovum.
   e. kill sperm on contact.

8. One of the disadvantages of using an aerosol foam is that
    a. it must be applied at the same time each day.
    b. its use requires vaginal douching after each intercourse.
    c. it must be applied prior to each intercourse.
    d. the synthetic hormones it contains can upset a woman's own hormonal balance.
    e. it must be used for at least fourteen days before it is safe for the woman to have unprotected intercourse.

9. A tubal ligation is a method of sterilization in which
    a. the uterus is removed.
    b. a ligation of the vas deferens is performed.
    c. the ovaries are removed.
    d. the fallopian tubes are "tied."
    e. the entrance of the cervix is sewed shut.

10. After the male has undergone a vasectomy, he
    a. will produce no more sperm.
    b. can experience orgasm but will not ejaculate.
    c. should refrain from intercourse for the next two weeks.
    d. is free to resume normal sexual activities almost immediately.
    e. will no longer experience orgasm as pleasurable.

11. A birth control method that women can use that also offers protection against sexually transmitted diseases is
    a. the diaphragm.
    b. the birth control pill.
    c. the Norplant.
    d. the female condom.
    e. the cervical cap.

12. One advantage of Depo-Provera is that
    a. it is available over the counter.
    b. it protects against sexually transmitted diseases.
    c. it has no side effects.
    d. it is a good method of birth control for women who are breast-feeding.
    e. it is convenient.

Scoring: The correct answers are listed below.
    1. C   3. C   5. B   7. E   9. D   11. D
    2. A   4. E   6. E   8. C   10. D   12. E

How did you do? Go back to your textbook and review the material you do not fully understand. Knowledge regarding birth control methods is only the first step in making your wellness birth control decision. There are many other personal and social influences that you must also explore.

What's Your Decision?

A woman may decide to have an abortion for many different reasons. Indicate which, if any, of the following reasons you could be the most supportive of by placing the letter in the appropriate place on the continuum. The farther you place your number to the left, the more supportive you are of the decision to have an abortion. Answer the questions that follow.

FOR———————————————————————————————————— AGAINST

a. Incest—Alcoholic and abusive father gets thirteen-year-old daughter pregnant.
b. Mental instability—Woman is grieving over her baby who died of sudden infant death syndrome three weeks ago.

c. Age—Fifty-year-old woman is afraid her baby will have a birth defect.

d. Economics—Unemployed and unskilled woman with three other children becomes pregnant.

e. Rape—Twenty-two-year-old married black female is raped by white male.

f. Health—Woman has had X rays and extensive medication through her second month of pregnancy.

g. Life-style—Married woman wants to complete medical school.

h. Marital difficulty—Woman has filed for legal separation from her husband.

i. You (or your sexual partner)—describe your present life situation: _____

1. Identify which situation you supported the most for having an abortion. Explain your reasoning.

2. Identify the situation you are the most against for having an abortion. Explain your reasoning.

3. If you could not support any of the situations, explain why.

From Deborah A. Miller, *Dimensions of Human Sexuality Student Workbook,* 3rd ed. Copyright © 1991 Wm. C. Brown Communications, Inc. Reprinted by permission of Times Mirror Higher Education Group, Inc., Dubuque, Iowa. All Rights Reserved.

Reviewing Important Concepts

1. Decisions about which birth control method to use, if any, are complicated. Describe the four factors which should be weighed in light of personal and social influences.

2. Why is it important to be aware of the contraindications of birth control methods? How is a contraindication different from a disadvantage of a birth control method?

Applying What You've Learned

1. Suppose you are considering using birth control for the first time. Rank the four factors listed below according to the importance they would play in *your decision*.

    _____ Effectiveness   _____ Safety

    _____ Cost   _____ Reversibility

2. Based on your ranking, which birth control methods might be the most appropriate for you? Why? (Table 8.8 will help you review available methods.)

3. Do you feel the methods you listed above will be compatible with your goals for high-level wellness? Why or why not?

Stages of Change

Are you sexually active? If you are, you and your partner have a responsibility to prevent an unwanted pregnancy. It is important to choose a method of birth control that is effective, and that you are comfortable with. Complete Activity for Wellness 8.1 on page 279 of your text. If you would like to make changes in your method of birth control, answer these four questions to assess your current stage of change.

1. I have been using an effective method of birth control regularly for more than six months.

2. I have taken action to start using a method of birth control within the past six months.

3. I am currently preparing to start using a new method of birth control in the next month.

4. I would like to take action to start using a new method of birth control within the next six months.

Scoring

No to all statements	Precontemplation
Yes to statement 4	Contemplation
Yes to statement 3	Preparation
Yes to statement 2	Action
Yes to statement 1	Maintenance

Review table 8.9 of *Connections for Health* for tips on moving through the stages of change and preventing unwanted pregnancy.

For Further Study

The decision about which birth control method to use, if any, is complicated. The options for birth control are many. Your decision regarding this issue greatly affects your level of wellness. The activities listed below will help you explore your feelings and the options available to you.

Wellness Activities

1. Visit your local health department, Planned Parenthood Clinic, or campus sexuality office to learn about different types of birth control methods and services they have available.
2. Contact a local Roman Catholic Church to see if they offer a natural family planning class. What is the philosophical basis for this type of ``birth control''? How do you feel about this type of family planning? Would you practice this method?
3. Choose a method of birth control and compare the price of using this method among several local pharmacies. Include your campus pharmacy, a hospital pharmacy, and several drug stores.
4. Abortion is one controversial form of birth control. Using the Yellow Pages of your telephone book, locate the listings under ``abortion alternatives'' and ``birth control services.'' Call a few of these agencies and ask the following questions: What is the philosophy of the agency? What types of counseling are available? What services, other than counseling, does the agency offer? What are the costs involved? Write a summary of your findings. What impact has this learning experience had on you? Have your feelings about abortion changed because of information you received as part of this activity?

9 Intentional and Unintentional Injury: Safer Living in a Dangerous World

Injury . . . Where Do You Stand?

Injuries can be intentional or unintentional. Accidents (unintentional injuries) are really the result of a series of events that could be prevented with appropriate attention to certain risk factors. Safety, the minimization of risk, is an important component of wellness: minimizing risk while maximizing your quality of life. ``Cycling in Traffic'' assesses your safety level while engaging in one of the most popular forms of exercise, cycling.

Violence (intentional injury) is a major threat to health and well-being. Take the assessment ``Your Anger Style Inventory'' to help you determine your anger style. Anger can lead to interpersonal violence.

Cycling in Traffic

Are you one of those people who believe that bicycling is a nice idea, but unsafe in traffic? Read the following statements and check your response on the right.

	ALWAYS	SOMETIMES	NEVER
I always ride on the right.	_____	_____	_____
I am predictable; no sudden swerves, no unsignaled turns.	_____	_____	_____
I obey stop signs and lights.	_____	_____	_____
I pay attention and am aware of hazards such as broken glass, potholes.	_____	_____	_____
I watch for inattentive motorists.	_____	_____	_____
I listen to traffic noise and don't use personal stereos while biking.	_____	_____	_____
I wear a safety approved cycling helmet.	_____	_____	_____
I am assertive; I don't let vehicles creep by and force me into parked cars.	_____	_____	_____
I drive defensively, expecting a car to pull out or turn in front of me.	_____	_____	_____
I make myself visible by wearing bright colors and putting reflectors/reflector tape on my bike.	_____	_____	_____

If you checked ALWAYS most of the time, you are following safety rules that will make you a prudent, safe, and secure cyclist. If you checked SOMETIMES, read through the items again and see where you can improve. If you checked NEVER, you are not riding safely. Review all of the items above and change your biking behavior before it's too late.

A sensible, prudent cyclist is quite safe in all but the most extreme traffic situations. You need only two things: (1) complete control of your bicycle and (2) a good understanding of your place in traffic.

Copyright by *Bicycling* Magazine. Reproduced with permission. For subscription information, call 1–800–666–2806.

Your Anger Style Inventory

This quiz will help you determine your anger style, which means the way you usually deal with anger. Consider each statement below and circle the answer that *most closely* represents how you would probably react.

1. You have just found out that a friend of yours is stealing your girlfriend/boyfriend. You would probably:
   a. beat the person up.
   b. decide that the person isn't your friend anymore.
   c. talk with both of them and find out what's going on.
2. You have a friend who has very strong opinions about lots of things. Some of his opinions make you mad. You would probably:
   a. punch him the next time he starts stating his opinions.
   b. ignore it—that's what friendship is about.
   c. argue with him.
3. A guy you know slightly has very strong opinions about lots of things. Some of his opinions make you mad. You would probably:
   a. hit him.
   b. just try to stay away from the guy.
   c. ask him why he feels the way he does.
4. When you are angry, which do you usually do?
   a. think about throwing something or someone against the wall.
   b. go for a walk or run.
   c. talk with a friend who's not involved about how you feel.
5. When you're angry, people who get in your way are likely to:
   a. get pushed aside.
   b. be invited to go with you to a movie or for a walk.
   c. hear all about your problem.
6. It wasn't your fault that you were late getting to school. But because you were late, you missed a test and the teacher won't let you make it up. You would probably:
   a. think about smashing the windshield of the teacher's car.
   b. think, ``Okay, so what if I get a failing grade?''
   c. discuss it with the teacher later when you've calmed down.

7. When you're in a situation that makes you angry, you often think:
   a. No one's going to push **me** around.
   b. All I want to do is get out of here!
   c. I want to clear this up.
8. Lately your boyfriend/girlfriend is nagging you all the time. It's getting on your nerves and making you angry. You would probably decide that:
   a. you've had it—next time you'll hit him or her.
   b. he or she isn't worth it—you'll break up.
   c. this has got to stop—you'll call him or her and talk it out.
9. If you were angry with someone and started thinking of ways to get even with that person, you would probably:
   a. pick the best idea and carry it out.
   b. tell a friend your idea, have a good laugh, but leave it at that.
   c. decide that it's time to let the person know how you feel.
10. You think your friend has let you down in a big way. Next time you see your friend, you would probably:
    a. push him or her out of the way and keep walking.
    b. pretend nothing has happened.
    c. let your friend know you're angry and why.
11. You've heard that a girl you never liked much is going around school telling lies about you. You would probably:
    a. slap her around until she learns some manners.
    b. ignore it—who cares what she says?
    c. tell her to knock it off or else.
12. When you're angry, you often feel like:
    a. hitting someone or something.
    b. taking a nap.
    c. working on the problem so it's no longer a problem.

Scoring: Go through the quiz and count the number of ``a'' answers, ``b'' answers, and ``c'' answers you circled. Enter the amounts for each answer in the blanks below.

A _____   B _____   C _____

Whichever type of answer you circled most often indicates how you usually deal with anger. A description of your anger style follows. While you may have one dominant anger style, you probably use all three at one time or another. No one way of dealing with anger is always right or always wrong, unless it gets you into trouble. The best way to deal with anger depends on the situation.

Violent Anger Expresser (mostly ``a'' answers)—Anger makes you feel violent, either toward people or toward things. Almost everyone feels violent sometimes, but acting violently doesn't solve problems or make bad situations better—and it can easily get you into trouble. Thinking but not acting on violent thoughts probably won't get you into trouble, but it can make you pretty uncomfortable. Consider using your anger in more constructive ways.

Anger Controller (mostly `b'' answers)—You don't try to express your anger—you either ignore it or don't let it bother you. This can be positive in situations that are too minor or too dangerous to do anything about. It can also be positive if you channel the anger into constructive activities, such as exercising. But it can be negative if you do self-destructive things to escape your feelings (such as drinking alcohol or using drugs) or if you don't succeed in ignoring your anger and just carry it around inside you. Before you act, examine the costs and benefits of controlling your anger.

Verbal Anger Expresser (mostly ``c'' answers)—You usually express your anger verbally, either to the person with whom you're angry or to whatever person or thing gets in your way. This can be positive if it is done effectively—it can solve problems or make a bad situation better, which is using anger constructively. Sometimes it helps to get the feelings of anger off your chest. But expressing anger verbally can be negative if it makes a bad situation even worse and leads to more anger or to a fight. Before you express your anger verbally, think about whether this is the time and place to do it.

From Deborah Prothrow-Stith, M.D. *Violence Prevention Curriculum for Adolescents, Teenage Health Teaching Modules,* 1987, Education Development Center. Reprinted by permission of Deborah Prothrow-Stith.

Reviewing Important Concepts

1. Define the term *accident,* and explain why some would argue that there are no accidents.

2. What are the three Es in reducing risks associated with unintentional injury? Choose one type of unintentional injury and use it in your explanation.

3. Why are some individuals willing to take risks that can be a threat to life and health while others don't? Identify and briefly explain two reasons.

Applying What You've Learned

1. Table 9.2 (``Factors Contributing to Unintentional Injury'') in your textbook cites four types of unintentional injuries: traffic, fires, poisoning, and occupational hazards. Choose one of the categories and identify three factors that contribute to its occurrence. Briefly explain how you would control for these risk factors (see suggestions in figure 9.8.).

2. Almost everyone at least fantasizes about suicide at some point in time. However, your friend Roger has been dropping a lot of hints about suicide recently. What positive actions can you take to help him? List at least three.

3. Locate two newspaper articles which reported on a homicide. The homicides could have occurred anywhere. Analyze and describe the relationship between each homicide and the socioeconomic status, race/ethnicity, and gender of the people involved in the space below. Refer to Of Special Interest 9.2: ``Poverty, Race, and Homicide'' to help you.

Stages of Change

If you are age 34 or under, you are more likely to die from an injury than from any other cause. It is important for all of us to do what we can to minimize the chances of injury to ourselves and others. Answer these four questions to assess your current stage of change related to your safety habits.

1. I have been practicing good safety-related habits for more than six months.

2. I have taken action to become safer within the past six months.

3. I am currently preparing to make safety changes in the next month.

4. I would like to improve my safety within the next six months.

Scoring

No to all statements	Precontemplation
Yes to statement 4	Contemplation
Yes to statement 3	Preparation
Yes to statement 2	Action
Yes to statement 1	Maintenance

Review table 9.7 in *Connections for Health* for tips on moving through the stages of change and increasing your daily safety precautions.

For Further Study

While some threats are not within your personal control, there are many options available to you to decrease your risk of injury and death. The activities listed below will help you explore many of the issues regarding intentional and unintentional injuries. Taking responsibility for your safety and the safety of those around you is an important step toward wellness.

Wellness Activities

1. Interview ten people and ask them to name three risky activities. Compare all of the responses. How do you evaluate each of the risks? Do you perceive them as safe or risky? What did you learn by doing this activity? Write a brief paper answering these questions.
2. Air bags are a recent addition to the multitude of options available when you purchase a new automobile. Interview several car salespeople (from different dealers) and ask the following questions. How much do air bags cost? In which models are air bags available? In which models are they standard equipment? Approximately how many air bags do they sell per year?
3. Contact your local chapter of MADD and obtain information about their organization. How did this organization begin? What strategies do they sponsor, locally and nationally, to reduce drunk driving?
4. Take a defensive driving course in your area. Locate one in your area by calling the National Traffic Safety Institute at 800-732-2233 (west of the Mississippi River) or 800-334-1441 (elsewhere). Write a brief paper summarizing what you learned and how you value this learning experience.
5. What mental health resources are available where you live? Consult your campus directory and the yellow pages. Call a few of the resources and ask how they help someone who is talking about suicide. What credentials do the counselors have? Is there a fee involved? What emergency services do they offer?
6. What is it like to live through an atomic bomb attack in your country? How does a devastating act affect the arts (painting, literature, theater) and the philosophy of its people? How do people physically scarred by the fallout fit into society? Robert J. Lifton's *Death in Life: Survivors of Hiroshima,* 2d edition (Chapel Hill, N.C.: University of North Carolina Press, 1991) is a study of how the bombing of Hiroshima and Nagasaki altered a society and culture. Locate a copy of this book and read a few chapters. Write a brief paper describing your reaction (feelings and thoughts) to what you've read.
7. Locate and attend a suicide education class on your campus or in your community. What did you learn about suicide? Did this class clarify any misconceptions you had about suicide? Do you feel suicide education classes reduce or increase suicide rates? Explain your rationale. How did attending this class affect you?
8. The Prevention WorkGroup on Assault and Homicide of the Surgeon-General's Workshop on Violence and Public Health recommends that the public be made aware that alcohol consumption may be hazardous to health because of its association with violence. Make a short video or newspaper ad that will educate fellow students and increase their awareness about this issue.
9. Do you think there should be a ban on handguns? What is currently being done at the national and state levels to legislate a ban? Contact at least two organizations to get differing opinions on handgun bans (e.g., National Rifle Association, National Safety Council). Briefly outline each organization's position; then choose and defend your position.

10. How safe is flying on an airplane? Take the ``Airline Passenger's Safety Quiz'' in *The University of California, Berkeley Wellness Letter,* February 1990, pp. 4-5. Hand in your quiz and include a brief summary of your results and an explanation of what you learned to help you travel more safely.

10 Disorders of the Cardiovascular System: Influencing Your Odds

Cardio-respiratory Diseases . . . Where Do You Stand?

Check Your Healthy Heart "I.Q."

Answer "true" or "false" to the following questions to test your knowledge of heart disease and its risk factors. Be sure to check the answers and explanations that follow to see how well you do.

1. **T** F The risk factors for heart disease that you *can do something about* are: high blood pressure, high blood cholesterol, smoking, obesity, and physical inactivity.
2. T F A stroke is often the first symptom of high blood pressure, and a heart attack is often the first symptom of high blood cholesterol.
3. T F A blood pressure greater than or equal to 140/90 mm Hg is generally considered to be high.
4. T F High blood pressure affects the same number of blacks as it does whites.
5. T F The best ways to treat and control high blood pressure are to control your weight, exercise, eat less salt (sodium), restrict your intake of alcohol, and take your high blood pressure medicine, if prescribed by your doctor.
6. T F A blood cholesterol level of 240 mg/dL is desirable for adults.
7. T F The most effective dietary way to lower the level of your blood cholesterol is to eat foods low in cholesterol.
8. T F Lowering blood cholesterol levels can help people who have already had a heart attack.
9. T F Only children from families at high risk of heart disease need to have their blood cholesterol levels checked.
10. T F Smoking is a major risk factor for four of the five leading causes of death including heart attack, stroke, cancer, and lung diseases such as emphysema and bronchitis.
11. T F If you have had a heart attack, quitting smoking can help reduce your chances of having a second attack.
12. **T** F Someone who has smoked for 30 to 40 years probably will not be able to quit smoking.
13. **T** F The best way to lose weight is to increase physical activity and eat fewer calories.
14. **T** F Heart disease is the leading killer of men **and** women in the United States.

1. **TRUE** High blood pressure, smoking, and high blood cholesterol are the three most important risk factors for heart disease. On the average, each one doubles your chance of developing heart disease. So, a person who has all three of these risk factors is 8 times more likely to develop heart disease than someone who has none. Obesity increases the likelihood of developing high blood cholesterol and high blood pressure, which increase your risk for heart disease. Physical inactivity increases your risk of heart attack. Regular exercise and good nutrition are essential to reducing high blood pressure, high blood cholesterol, and overweight. People who exercise are also more likely to cut down or stop smoking.

2. **TRUE** A person with high blood pressure or high blood cholesterol may feel fine and look great; there are often no signs that anything is wrong until a stroke or heart attack occurs. To find out if you have high blood pressure or high blood cholesterol, you should be tested by a doctor, nurse, or other health professional.

3. **TRUE** A blood pressure of 140/90 mm Hg or greater is generally classified as high blood pressure. However, blood pressures that fall below 140/90 mm Hg can sometimes be a problem. If the diastolic pressure, the second or lower number, is between 85–89, a person is at increased risk for heart disease or stroke and should have his/her blood pressure checked at least once a year by a health professional. The higher your blood pressure, the greater your risk of developing heart disease or stroke. Controlling high blood pressure reduces your risk.

4. FALSE   High blood pressure is more common in blacks than in whites. If affects 29 out of every 100 black adults compared to 26 out of every 100 white adults. Also, with aging, high blood pressure is generally more severe among blacks than among whites, and therefore causes more strokes, heart disease, and kidney failure.

5. TRUE   Recent studies show that life-style changes can help keep blood pressure levels normal even into advanced age and are important in treating and preventing high blood pressure. Limit high-salt foods which include many snack foods, such as potato chips, and salted pretzels, and salted crackers; processed foods, such as canned soups; and condiments, such as ketchup and soy sauce. Also, it is **extremely important** to take blood pressure medication, if prescribed by your doctor, to make sure your blood pressure stays under control.

6. FALSE   A total blood cholesterol level of under 200 mg/dL is **desirable** and usually puts you at a lower risk for heart disease. A blood cholesterol level of 240 mg/dL or above is **high** and increases your risk of heart disease. If your cholesterol level is high, your doctor will want to check your levels of LDL-cholesterol ("bad" cholesterol) and HDL-cholesterol ("good" cholesterol). A HIGH level of LDL-cholesterol increases your risk of heart disease, as does a LOW level of HDL-cholesterol. A cholesterol level of 200–239 mg/dL is considered **borderline-high** and usually increases your risk for heart disease. If your cholesterol is borderline-high, you should speak to your doctor to see if additional cholesterol tests are needed. All adults 20 years of age or older should have their blood cholesterol level checked at least once every 5 years.

7. FALSE   Reducing the amount of cholesterol in your diet is important; however, eating foods **low in saturated fat** is the most effective dietary way to lower blood cholesterol levels, along with eating less total fat and cholesterol. Choose low-saturated fat foods, such as grains, fruits, and vegetables; low-fat or skim milk and milk products; lean cuts of meat; fish; and chicken. Trim fat from meat before cooking; bake or broil meat rather than fry; use less fat and oil; and take the skin off chicken and turkey. Reducing overweight will also help lower your level of LDL-cholesterol as well as increase your level of HDL-cholesterol.

8. TRUE   People who have had one heart attack are at much higher risk for a second attack. Reducing blood cholesterol levels can greatly slow down (and, in some people, even reverse) the buildup of cholesterol and fat in the walls of the coronary arteries and significantly reduce the chances of a second heart attack.

9. TRUE   Children from "high risk" families, in which a parent has high blood cholesterol (240 mg/dL or above) or in which a parent or grandparent has had heart disease at an early age (at 55 years of age or younger), should have their cholesterol levels tested. If a child from such a family has a cholesterol level that is high, it should be lowered under medical supervision, primarily with diet, to reduce the risk of developing heart disease as an adult. For most children, who are not from high-risk families, the best way to reduce the risk of adult heart disease is to follow a low-saturated fat, low cholesterol eating pattern. All children over the age of 2 years and all adults should adopt a heart-healthy eating pattern as a principal way of reducing coronary heart disease.

10. TRUE   Heavy smokers are 2 to 4 times more likely to have a heart attack than nonsmokers, and the heart attack death rate among all smokers is 70 percent greater than that of nonsmokers. Older male smokers are also nearly twice as likely to die from stroke than older men who do not smoke, and these odds are nearly as high for older female smokers. Further, the risk of dying of lung cancer is 22 times higher for male smokers than male nonsmokers and 12 times higher for female smokers than female nonsmokers. Finally, 80 percent of all deaths from emphysema and bronchitis are directly due to smoking.

11. TRUE   One year after quitting, ex-smokers cut their extra risk for heart attack by about half or more, and eventually the risk will return to normal in healthy ex-smokers. Even if you have already had a heart attack, you can reduce your chances of having a second attack if you quit smoking. Ex-smokers can also reduce their risk of stroke and cancer, improve blood flow and lung function, and help stop diseases like emphysema and bronchitis from getting worse.

12. FALSE   Weight control is a question of balance. You get calories from the food you eat. You burn off calories by exercising. Cutting down on calories, especially calories from fat, is key to losing weight. Combining this with a regular physical activity, like walking, cycling, jogging, or swimming, not only can help in losing weight but also in maintaining weight loss. A steady weight loss of ½ to 1 pounds a week is safe for most adults, and the weight is more likely to stay off over the long run. Losing weight, if you are overweight, may also help reduce your blood pressure, lower your LDL-

cholesterol, and raise your HDL-cholesterol. Being physically active and eating fewer calories will also help you control your weight if you quit smoking.

14. TRUE   Coronary heart disease is the #1 killer in the United States. Approximately 489,000 Americans died of coronary heart disease in 1990, and approximately half of these deaths were women.

Source: Data prepared by the National Heart, Lung, and Blood Institute, National Institutes of Health Publication No. 92-2724, Revised, October 1992. U.S. Department of Health and Human Services, Bethesda, MO.

Your Stroke Odds

You can assess your risk of a stroke in the next 10 years and compare the odds with those of other people your age. The new self-test is based on data collected over 36 years on 5,734 patients in Framingham, Mass.

IDENTIFY THE RISK FACTORS:

Age

Your age	Points	Your age	Points
Under 57	0	72–74	6
57–59	1	75–77	7
60–62	2	78–80	8
63–65	3	81–83	9
66–68	4	84–86	10
69–71	5		

Blood pressure[1]

Men		Women			
Add 2 points if under treatment for hypertension		Not being treated for hypertension		Being treated for hypertension	
Pressure	Points	Pressure	Points	Pressure	Points
95–105	0	95–104	0	95–104	6
106–116	1	105–114	1	105–114	6
117–126	2	115–124	2	115–124	7
127–137	3	125–134	3	125–134	7
138–148	4	135–144	4	135–144	7
149–159	5	145–154	5	145–154	8
160–170	6	155–164	6	155–164	8
171–181	7	165–174	7	165–174	8
182–191	8	175–184	8	175–184	9
192–202	9	185–194	9	185–194	9
203–213	10	195–204	10	195–204	10

History of diabetes?
No: 0 points   Yes: 2 points (men) 3 points (women)

Are you a smoker?
No: 0 points   Yes: 3 points

---

[1]Use systolic blood pressure, the higher of the two numbers in a blood-pressure reading (140 is the systolic pressure in a reading of 140 over 100, for example).
From *U.S. News & World Report,* April 13, 1992. Reprinted by permission.

History of heart attack or heart disease?[2]
No: 0 points   Yes: 3 points (men) 2 points (women)

Do you have an irregular heartbeat?[3]
No: 0 points   Yes: 4 points (men) 6 points (women)

Do you have an enlarged heart?[4]
No: 0 points   Yes: 6 points (men) 4 points (women)

ADD UP YOUR POINTS:

Age_____   Heart disease _____
Blood pressure_____   Irregular heartbeat _____
Diabetes _____   Enlarged heart _____
Smoker _____   TOTAL POINTS _____

FIND YOUR STROKE RISK OVER THE NEXT 10 YEARS:

Men		Women	
Points	**Risk**	**Points**	**Risk**
1	2.6%	1	1.1%
2	3.0%	2	1.3%
3	3.5%	3	1.6%
4	4.0%	4	2.0%
5	4.7%	5	2.4%
6	5.4%	6	2.9%
7	6.3%	7	3.5%
8	7.3%	8	4.3%
9	8.4%	9	5.2%
10	9.7%	10	6.3%
11	11.2%	11	7.6%
12	12.9%	12	9.2%
13	14.8%	13	11.1%
14	17.0%	14	13.3%
15	19.5%	15	16.0%
16	22.4%	16	19.1%
17	25.5%	17	22.8%
18	29.0%	18	27.0%
19	32.9%	19	31.9%
20	37.1%	20	37.3%
21	41.7%	21	43.4%
22	46.6%	22	50.0%
23	51.8%	23	57.0%
24	57.3%	24	64.2%
25	62.8%	25	71.4%
26	68.4%	26	78.2%
27	73.8%	27	84.4%
28	79.0%		
29	83.7%		
30	87.9%		

COMPARE WITH THE RISK FOR THE AVERAGE PERSON YOUR AGE:

Men		Women	
Age	**Risk**	**Age**	**Risk**
55–59	5.9%	55–59	3.0%
60–64	7.8%	60–64	4.7%
65–69	11.0%	65–69	7.2%
70–74	13.7%	70–74	10.9%

[2]Includes angina (chest pain), coronary insufficiency (narrowing of the coronary blood vessels), intermittent claudication (narrowing of arteries in the legs) and heart failure.
[3]Atrial fibrillation, a type of rapid, irregular heartbeat.
[4]Left ventricular hypertrophy, or enlargement of the heart's left ventricle. Reduces the heart's pumping ability, increases the risk of blood clots.
USN&WR—Basic data: American Heart Association, the Framingham Heart Study.

| 75–79 | 18.0% | 75–79 | 15.5% |
| 80–84 | 22.3% | 80–84 | 23.9% |

HOW TO CUT THE RISK

High blood pressure
Multiplies stroke risk: 300 percent
Preventive steps: Older persons with systolic blood pressure of 160 or higher should bring it down as low as 140. Diastolic blood pressure of 90 or greater should be reduced to the 70-to-80 range. Blood pressure-lowering strategies include antihypertensive drugs, weight loss and, for some people, low-sodium and high-potassium diets.

Heart disease
Multiplies stroke risk: 500 percent
Preventive steps: Use diet, medication or both to keep total blood cholesterol below 200 milligrams per deciliter. Low-density lipoprotein, the "bad" cholesterol, should be kept below 130. Vigorous exercise three times a week cuts the risk by 60 percent. For people with atrial fibrillation, the blood thinner warfarin may cut the added risk to about 70 percent; aspirin may also work well.

Smoking
Multiplies risk: For most strokes, 100 to 300 percent. For strokes caused by bleeding, up to 1,000 percent.
Preventive steps: Quitting before age 50 cuts risk nearly to a nonsmoker's in two to five years.

Prior stroke
Multiplies stroke risk: 900 percent
Preventive steps: Aspirin and Ticlid, a prescription anticlotting drug, prevent 22 to 25 percent of repeat strokes. Endarterectomy, in which surgeons ream out clogged neck arteries, cuts the risk by 60 percent.

Gender
Multiplies stroke risk: For men, at least 19 percent
Preventive steps: Aspirin seems to protect men more than women in people who have had a mild "warning stroke," or transient ischemic attack.

Race
Multiplies stroke risk: 60 percent for blacks among men over age 40, 100 percent for blacks among women over age 40
Preventive steps: Stop smoking, treat high blood pressure. Screen children with sickle cell anemia with an ultrasound test that reveals narrowed arteries to the brain. Such children may benefit from periodic blood transfusions.

Diabetes mellitus
Multiplies stroke risk: 500 percent
Preventive steps: None. Diabetics should focus on other risk factors.

Heredity
Multiplies stroke risk: 400 percent
Preventive steps: Since you can't change your parents, anyone with a family history of stroke should look for other risk factors that can be reduced.

USN&WR—Basic data: National Stroke Association, American Heart Association, U.S. Department of Health and Human Services.

Your Risk of Cerebrovascular and Cardiovascular Disease

As mentioned in chapter 4, your waist-to-hip ratio (WHR) is an important measure of risk due to obesity. Refer to Activity for Wellness 4.1. Write your WHR in one of the blanks below depending on whether it is below or above 1.0.

MY WHR IS LESS THAN 1.0	MY WHR IS MORE THAN 1.0
_____	_____

The risk of cerebrovascular and cardiovascular disease increases dramatically when the circumference of the waist starts to exceed that of the hips (1.0).

Based on your WHR, is your risk increased due to obesity?   YES   NO

Reviewing Important Concepts

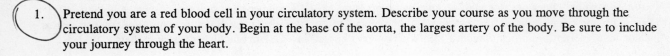

1. Pretend you are a red blood cell in your circulatory system. Describe your course as you move through the circulatory system of your body. Begin at the base of the aorta, the largest artery of the body. Be sure to include your journey through the heart.

2. Risk factors increase one's chances of developing a disease. Describe the major risk factors for heart disease. Identify which of the risk factors can be modified so that risk may be reduced.

Applying What You've Learned

1. Certain dietary factors have been statistically associated with heart disease and some cancers. Dietary fat, including cholesterol, and vitamins A and C are discussed in your textbook. Review the preventive strategies for each nutrient/vitamin and alcohol. Refer back to the dietary worksheets in chapter 3 of this workbook and analyze your diet with regard to these nutrients and vitamins. Enter your nutritional values, where applicable, in the blanks below. Complete the remaining question.

Total fat _____   Saturated fat _____   Cholesterol _____
Sodium _____   Vitamin A _____   Vitamin C _____

DO YOU EAT HIGH-FIBER FOODS?____ Identify the HIGH-FIBER foods currently in your diet:

_____

IS YOUR ALCOHOL CONSUMPTION MINIMAL _____ MODERATE _____ HEAVY _____?
(This is a subjective assessment of your consumption.)

What are the strengths and weaknesses of your diet with regard to the preventive dietary strategies for cancer and heart disease?

2. List five foods you could eliminate, reduce, or increase in your diet that might help you to limit your risk of cardiovascular heart disease (CHD). How easy would it be for you to make these changes?

Food	Very Easy	Will Take Time to Get Used to	Difficult
1. _____	_____	_____	_____
2. _____	_____	_____	_____
3. _____	_____	_____	_____
4. _____	_____	_____	_____
5. _____	_____	_____	_____

Stages of Change

During your college years you are forming habits that will affect your health for years to come. Cardiovascular disease is the #1 killer in America, but there are many things you can do to minimize your risk of contracting it. Complete Activity for Wellness 10.1 in your text to determine your risk of cardiovascular disease. If a high-fat diet is one of your risk factors, answer these questions to begin reducing the amount of fat in your diet.

1. I have been eating a low-fat (less than 30% of calories from fat) diet for more than six months.

2. I have started to limit my fat intake within the past six months.

3. I am currently preparing to limit my fat intake within the next month.

4. I would like to take action to limit my fat intake within the next six months.

Scoring

No to all statements	Precontemplation
Yes to statement 4	Contemplation
Yes to statement 3	Preparation
Yes to statement 2	Action
Yes to statement 1	Maintenance

Review table 10.2 in *Connections for Health* for tips on moving through the stages of change and reducing dietary fat and cardiovascular disease risk.

For Further Study

Heart disease and diabetes are only a few of the noncommunicable diseases that may be roadblocks to high-level wellness. Your goal is to minimize your risk in order to maximize your opportunity for high-level wellness. Explore the activities listed that follow; they can help you achieve your goal.

Wellness Activities

1. Go to the student health center and have your blood pressure checked. What is a ``normal'' blood pressure reading? What do the two numbers mean? How often should you have your blood pressure checked? Ask the person taking your blood pressure to describe how a blood pressure reading is taken.
2. Learn CPR (cardiopulmonary resuscitation). Contact your local American Heart Association, American Red Cross, or your school to find out when a class is being offered.
3. Contact the cardiac rehabilitation department of your local hospital. Ask them if you can visit the center while it is being used. What types of people do they see coming to their program? Based on their observations, are the employees of the hospital seeing many patients who had risk factors that could have been modified before their heart problems presented? Which ones? What changes does the cardiac program suggest their patients make?
4. Virtually all the studies on preventing heart disease have been done on men. How do women differ from men when it comes to heart disease? One article, ``A Woman's Heart'' by Patricia Long (*In Health,* March/April 1991, pp. 53–58), describes how women's risks differ. Use this article and others to describe the gender differences for heart disease risk factors. What is being done to include women in clinical trials and federally funded studies?

11 Cancer and Other Noncommunicable Disease Threats to Wellness: The Body Under Siege

Cancer and Other Noncommunicable Diseases . . . Where Do You Stand?

Self-responsibility and personal involvement are essential components in the prevention of noncommunicable diseases such as heart disease, cancer, and diabetes. These diseases threaten a person's quest for high-level wellness. You can begin to take responsibility and involve yourself by completing the activities that follow in this chapter.

What Is Known . . . What Is Suspected . . . What Is Myth about Cancer Risk Factors

You may have been led to believe that almost everything causes cancer, but that isn't so. Cancer risk factors vary in their effect on individuals. Your hereditary makeup and exposure to certain substances could increase your chances of getting cancer.

Below is a list of factors that may or may not cause cancer. Determine if each factor is a myth about cancer, a suspected factor that can increase your risk, or a known factor that can increase your risk. Write your answer in the blanks next to each factor.

Factor	*Myth, Suspected, or Known Risk Factor*
Age	_____
Fluoride	_____
Alcohol	_____
Bumps, Bruises	_____
Diet	_____
D.E.S. (Diethylstilbestrol)	_____
Asbestos	_____
Family History of Breast and Colon Cancer	_____
Cigars, Pipes, and Chewing Tobacco	_____
Radiation	_____
Sun	_____
Cigarettes	_____
Pesticides, Fungicides	_____
Cancer is Contagious	_____
Occupation	_____
Estrogen for Menopause	_____

From the American Cancer Society, "What Is Known . . . What Is Suspected . . . What Is Myth . . . "Revised 1988. Reprinted by permission.

Answers: Factors Known to Increase Cancer Risk

Age	Risk increases with age.
Alcohol	Increased risk with excessive use, especially if you smoke.
Asbestos	Five-fold increased risk of lung cancer if occupational exposed. If you smoke, the risk is much higher.
Cigarettes	Ten-fold increased risk of lung cancer.
Cigar, Pipes, and Chewing Tobacco	Increased risk of mouth, larynx, and esophageal cancer.
D.E.S.	Increased risk of vaginal cancer for daughters of women who took DES during pregnancy.
Estrogen for Menopause	Increased risk of endometrial cancer with long-term use.
Family History of Breast and Colon Cancer	Increased risk for these cancers.
Occupation	Exposure to industrial agents (nickel, chromate, asbestos, vinyl chloride, etc.) increases risk.
Radiation	Increased risk with excessive exposure to X rays. If you've had radiation therapy early in life, there may be increased risk, which your doctor will evaluate.
Sun	Increased risk of skin cancer with overexposure and no sunscreen protection.

Factors Suspected to Increase Cancer Risk

Diet	High fat, low fiber may be related to cancer of several sites. Various elements of diet are being studied.
Occupation	In addition to the known industrial agents, certain other chemicals and dusts are being studied.
Pesticides, Fungicides	Potential risk if protective equipment is not used.

Myths about Cancer

Bumps, Bruises	Bruises, bumps do not cause cancer.
Cancer is Contagious	Cancer is not contagious.
Fluoride	Fluoridated water does not cause cancer.

Adapted from: American Cancer Society. ``What Is Known . . . What Is Suspected . . . What Is Myth . . .'' Revised 1988.

Check Your Asthma "I.Q."

The following true-or-false statements test what you know about asthma. Be sure to read the correct answers and explanations that follow.

1. T F Asthma is a common disease among children and adults in the United States.
2. T F Asthma is an emotional or psychological illness.
3. T F The way that parents raise their children can cause asthma.
4. T F Asthma episodes may cause breathing problems, but these episodes are not really harmful or dangerous.
5. T F Asthma episodes usually occur suddenly without warning.
6. T F Many different things can bring on an asthma episode.
7. T F Asthma cannot be cured, but it can be controlled.
8. T F There are different types of medicine to control asthma.
9. T F People with asthma have no way to monitor how well their lungs are functioning.
10. T F Both children and adults can have asthma.
11. T F Tobacco smoke can make an asthma episode worse.
12. T F People with asthma should not exercise.

Answers to the Asthma "I.Q." Quiz

1. TRUE Asthma is a common disease among children and adults in the United States, and it is increasing. About 10 million people have asthma, of whom 3 million are under 18 years of age.

2. FALSE Asthma is not an emotional or psycological disease, although strong emotions can sometimes make asthma worse. People with asthma have sensitive lungs that react to certain things, causing the airways to tighten, swell, and fill with mucus. The person then has trouble breathing and may cough and wheeze.

3. FALSE The way parents raise their children does not cause asthma. It is not caused by a poor parent-child relationship or by being overprotective.

4. FALSE Asthma episodes can be very harmful. People can get very sick and need hospitalization. Some people have died from asthma episodes. Frequent asthma episodes, even if they are mild, may cause people to stop being active and living normal lives.

5. FALSE Sometimes an asthma episode may come on quite quickly. However, before a person has any wheezing or shortness of breath there are usually symptoms such as a cough, a scratchy throat, or tightness in the chest. Most patients learn to recognize these early symptoms and can take medicine to prevent a serious episode.

6. TRUE For most people with asthma, an episode can start from many different "triggers." Some of these things are pollen from trees or grasses; molds or house dust; weather changes; strong odors; cigarette smoke; and certain foods. Other triggers include being upset; laughing or crying hard; having a cold or the flu; or being near furry or feathered animals. Each person with asthma has an individual set of asthma "triggers."

7. TRUE There is no cure yet for asthma. However, asthma patients can control it to a large degree by:
   - Getting advice from a doctor who treats asthma patients
   - Learning to notice early signs of an asthma episode and to start treatment
   - Avoiding things that cause asthma episodes
   - Taking medicine just as the doctor says
   - Knowing when to get medical help with a severe episode.

8. TRUE Several types of medicines are available to control asthma. Some people with mild asthma need to take medication only when they have symptoms. But most people need to take medicine every day to prevent symptoms and also to take medicine when symptoms do occur. A doctor needs to decide the best type of medicine for each patient and how often it should be taken. Asthma patients and their doctors need to work together to manage the disease.

9. FALSE People with asthma can monitor how well their lungs are functioning with a peak flow meter. This small device can be used at home, work, or school. The peak flow meter may show that the asthma is getting worse before the usual symptoms appear.

99

10. TRUE   Both children and adults can have asthma. Sometimes, but not always, symptoms will go away as children get older. However, many children continue to have asthma symptoms throughout adulthood. In some cases, symptoms of asthma are not recognized until a person is an adult.

11. TRUE   Smoke from cigarettes, cigars and pipes can bring on an asthma attack. Indoor smoky air from fireplaces and outdoor smog can make asthma worse. Some can also "set off" other triggers. Smokers should be asked not to smoke near someone with asthma. Moving to another room may help, but smoke travels from room to room. No smoking is best for everyone!

12. FALSE   Exercise is good for most people—with or without asthma. When asthma is under good control, people with asthma are able to play most sports. For people whose asthma is brought on by exercise, medicines can be taken before exercising to help avoid an episode. A number of Olympic medalists have asthma.

Source: Data Prepared by the National Heart, Lung, and Blood Institute, National Asthma Education Program, National Institutes of Health Publication No. 90-1128, January 1990. U.S. Department of Health and Human Services, Bethesda, MD.

Reviewing Important Concepts

1.   List four categories of carcinogenic exposure and describe two examples for each category.

2.   Describe eight behaviors associated with cancer risk.

Applying What You've Learned

1.   Can people who have a noncommunicable disease such as cancer or diabetes achieve high-level wellness? If so, what are some things they could do to progress toward their optimal level?

2. It is very likely that many times during your day you are exposed to a variety of cancer risks. Use the chart below to record all of the possible cancer risks you are exposed to in any one twenty-four hour period.

   Describe where you are, what you are doing, the cancer risk, the type of cancer risk (0 = occupational; M = medical; S-C = socio-cultural), and what you could do to reduce or eliminate your risk. Refer to your textbook for examples of cancer risks. An example is provided to get you started.

My Possible Cancer Risks				
Where	Activity	Cancer Risk	Type	Changes I Could Make
yard	sunbathing	sun rays	S-C	use sunscreen (contains SPF)

3. List five foods you could eliminate, reduce, or increase in your diet that might help you to limit your risk of cancer. How easy would it be for you to make these changes?

Food	Very Easy	Will Take Time to Get Used to	Difficult
1. _____	_____	_____	_____
2. _____	_____	_____	_____
3. _____	_____	_____	_____
4. _____	_____	_____	_____
5. _____	_____	_____	_____

4. Beth is a sun lover and enjoys sporting a deep tan during the summer. Explain the potential problems of sunbathing to her. What skin care products could she use to protect herself from the sun's harmful rays? Describe three guidelines Beth should follow to minimize her risk if she insists on pursuing her golden tan.

Stages of Change

Do you perform cancer self-examinations every month? Complete Activity for Wellness 11.1, 11.2, and 11.3 in your text to learn techniques for some important self-exams. Then answer these four questions to assess your current stage of change.

1. I have been performing monthly self-exams for more than six months.

2. I have started performing monthly self-exams within the past six months.

3. I am currently preparing to start performing regular self-exams in the next month.

4. I would like to start performing self-exams within the next six months.

Scoring

No to all statements	Precontemplation
Yes to statement 4	Contemplation
Yes to statement 3	Preparation
Yes to statement 2	Action
Yes to statement 1	Maintenance

Review table 11.8 of *Connections for Health* for tips on moving through the stages of change to increase your chances of detecting cancer early.

For Further Study

Cancer is a noncommunicable disease that may be a roadblock to high-level wellness. Your goal is to minimize your risk in order to maximize your opportunity for high-level wellness. Explore the activities and guides listed that follow; they can help you achieve your goal.

Wellness Activities

1. Visit your student health center and ask a health professional to teach you how to do a breast self-examination or a testes self-examination. Demonstrate the technique to the health professional to make sure you're doing it correctly.
2. Get a diabetes test or a Pap test through your local health department or student health center. Ask how the test works. How many people are detected through the test? How do you interpret the results?
3. New cures for cancer make the headlines every day. Review the newspapers and news magazines and locate two new claims for cancer cures. What claims are being made? Are there scientific data to substantiate these claims?
4. Interview several people about their sunbathing habits. Do they pursue the golden tan? Do they use sunscreen with SPF? If not, why? Do they follow any of the recommendations listed in chapter 11 of your textbook?

12 Communicable Diseases: Threats to Wellness Old and New

Communicable Diseases . . . Where Do You Stand?

Infectious diseases are threats to high-level wellness. The prevention and control of infectious diseases has become more important than ever with the advent of AIDS and the increasing incidence of communicable diseases.

Immunization of Adults: A Call to Action

Are your immunizations current? Review your medical records to make sure you've received all the necessary immunizations. Where can you go in your area for immunizations? Is there a cost?

Personal Immunization Record

Name: _____ Sex: _____ Birthdate: _____

Address: _____

Vaccine	Date Given Month/Day/Year	Doctor or Clinic Phone Number	Date Next Dose Due
Tetanus and Diphtheria toxoids (Td) for Adult Use			
Pneumococcal			
Measles*			
Mumps*			
Rubella*			
Polio (specify OPV or eIPV)			
Hepatitis B			

Influenza   _____   _____   _____
             _____   _____   _____
             _____   _____   _____
             _____   _____   _____
             _____   _____   _____
             _____   _____   _____

Other   _____   _____   _____
             _____   _____   _____
             _____   _____   _____

Source: From "Immunization of Adults: A Call to Action" September 1986, Revised September 1991, Revised May 1994.
U.S. Department of Health and Human Services, National Immunization Program, Atlanta, Georgia.
*These vaccines are frequently combined as measles-mumps-rubella (MMR) or measles-rubella (MR).

How Much Do You Know about Sexually Transmitted Diseases?

Sexually transmitted diseases are roadblocks to high-level wellness. You can minimize your risk of infection by becoming knowledgeable about the various STDs, their symptoms, and the preventive measures you can take. Read each question below and circle the correct answer.

1. STDs are most effectively transmitted by
   a. airborne droplets.
   b. direct contact.
   c. contaminated objects.
   d. contaminated swimming pools.
   e. contaminated food.

2. Gonorrhea has the potential to cause all of the following EXCEPT
   a. sterility in a male.
   b. cancer.
   c. sterility in a female.
   d. blindness in infants.
   e. a form of arthritis.

3. All of the following are true about HIV/AIDS EXCEPT
   a. heterosexual sex can transmit the virus.
   b. the virus can be spread by mosquitoes.
   c. having sex with multiple partners increases risk of exposure.
   d. using condoms during sex helps prevent the spread of HIV.
   e. sharing needles is one way to spread the virus.

4. Primary syphilis is characterized by
   a. small water-filled blisters.
   b. one or more large sores.
   c. urethral discharge.
   d. a rash on the palms of the hands.
   e. all of the above.

5. Between attacks, herpes virus apparently stays in the
   a. nerves.
   b. blood.
   c. liver.
   d. heart.
   e. penis.

6. Of the following, the most common STD is
   a. AIDS.
   b. herpes.
   c. Chlamydia.
   d. gonorrhea.
   e. syphilis.

7. All of the following are ways to lower your risk of contracting HIV EXCEPT
   a. avoiding shaking hands with people in high risk groups.
   b. using latex condoms every time you have sex.
   c. not sharing needles.
   d. practicing abstinence or mutual monogamy.
   e. using and storing condoms properly.

8. The ultimate responsibility for prevention of STDs lies with
   a. the public health department.
   b. the churches.
   c. the physician.
   d. the schools.
   e. the individual.

9. Symptoms of herpes typically include

a. small, fluid-filled blisters on the genitals.
b. one large chancre on the penis.
c. a rash all over the body.
d. patches of falling hair.
e. all of the above are true.

10. All of the following are true of genital herpes except
    a. it is caused by viruses.
    b. it is often a lifelong infection.
    c. there is currently no real cure.
    d. it commonly causes male and female sterility.
    e. it can be painful in both sexes.

11. Venereal warts are caused by
    a. a spirochete.
    b. a virus.
    c. untreated gonorrhea.
    d. untreated syphilis.
    e. herpes.

12. Late or tertiary syphilis is capable of damaging
    a. the brain.
    b. the spinal cord.
    c. the aorta.
    d. the optic nerves.
    e. all of the above are true.

Scoring: Check your answers with the key below. How did you do? Refer back to your textbook to review the concepts you do not fully understand.

1. b 2. b 3. b 4. b   5. a   6. c
7. a 8. e 9. a 10. d   11. b   12. e

From Curtis O. Byer and Louis W. Shainberg, *Dimensions of Human Sexuality, Instructor's Manual,* 2d edition. Copyright © 1988 Wm. C. Brown Communications, Inc. Reprinted by permission of Times Mirror Higher Education Group, Inc., Dubuque, Iowa. All Rights Reserved.

Could You Negotiate Safer Sex?

"Agree" (A) or "Disagree" (D) with the statements presented below. Indicate the items for which you are "Unsure" (U) of your response. Compare your responses to those of a friend. Discuss each item for which you said you were unsure of your response. Are there items for which you and a friend disagree? What changes or adaptations would you or your friend have to make in order to take on a "safer" orientation toward sex with a partner?

I believe that:

I could use a condom effectively. _____
I could buy condoms without embarrassment. _____
If my partner did not want to use a condom during sexual intercourse, I could convince him/her to use one.
_____

Consumption of alcohol or use of other recreational drugs would in no way affect my affirmation to use a condom or to convince my partner to respect my wishes. _____
Having to remember to buy, carry, and use condoms would interfere with sexual spontaneity. _____
If I suggested using a condom, my partner would think that I must have had many previous sexual partners.
_____

I would feel comfortable insisting on using a condom with a new sexual partner. _____
I would not feel self-conscious putting a condom on myself (or on my partner). _____
I would be able to discuss use of condoms with a partner even before we had any physical intimacy such as touching, caressing, or kissing. _____
If I suggested using a condom, my partner would think I lacked trust in him/her. _____
Using a condom during sexual intercourse would interfere with sexual pleasure or sexual functioning. _____
Using condoms is an activity primarily for people who have many sexual partners. _____
Having to use a condom might subsequently prove to be embarrassing to me or my partner if the mechanics of using one resulted in loss of erection. _____
I could tactfully remove and dispose of a condom after sexual intercourse. _____
I could convince my partner that use of a condom can be a stimulating part of sexual foreplay. _____

Reviewing Important Concepts

1. All infectious diseases have a cycle of progression that may aid in transmission and spread of the disease. Choose an STD and trace it through the infectious disease cycle. Give examples to illustrate how the STD is carried through each part of the cycle.

2. AIDS has had a disproportionate impact on people of color, women, and other minority groups. Describe how AIDS has affected these groups differently. What is being predicted for women during the late 1990s?

3. As a result of widespread immunization practices, many diseases have been reduced significantly in occurrence. Why is it important that these immunization practices *not* be discontinued?

4. Part of the reason STDs pose a problem of such great magnitude stems from the fact that treatment of the infected individual solves only half the STD problem. Describe the other problems involved in controlling STDs.

From L. D. McAllister, *STD, Including AIDS, Teacher's Guide,* New York City Department of Health, Bureau of STD Control, Education Unit, New York, NY.

Applying What You've Learned

1. Some people may not know what to say when telling a sex partner that he or she could have an STD. The exercise below will allow you to examine possible ways.

   Situation: Frank just learned that he has an STD. He wants to tell his partner, Ruth, that she might be infected, too, and that she should get medical care. In the spaces below, write one or two examples of what Frank might say to Ruth in his talk with her.
   a. What things could Frank say to get the conversation started? That is, how could he begin?

   b. How could he tell Ruth that he has an STD?

   c. What could Frank say in telling Ruth that she also might have the STD?

106

d.   How could he encourage her to get help?

e.   Describe the best settings (for example, time and place) for a person telling a sex partner about an STD infection.

f.   How might Ruth react to Frank?

g.   What are some possible results of this talk for Frank?

h.   What are some possible results of this talk for Ruth?

i.   Combining some of these ideas, write a short script of Frank's talk with Ruth.

Source: McAllister, D. L. *STD, Including AIDS, Teacher's Guide*. New York City Department of Health, Bureau of STD Control, Education Unit, 158 E. 115th St., Room 413, New York, N.Y. 10029.

2.   List five ways YOU can reduce your chances of becoming infected with the HIV virus.

3.   You have been asked to develop a presentation for incoming freshmen about postponing sexual involvement and condom use for those not choosing abstinence. Your goal is to inform and motivate students. Outline your talk below using factors found to influence condom use among college students.

4.   Your textbook lists several personal prevention methods that provide protection against most STDs. List the methods you feel you could easily and comfortably use to provide adequate protection against STDs. Which methods would you not feel comfortable using?

Stages of Change

If you are sexually active, you are at risk for contracting a host of sexually transmitted diseases, including HIV. In this day and age, practicing safer sex is essential. Answer these four questions to assess your current stage of change related to safer sex practices.

1.   I have been practicing safer sex every time I have sex for more than six months.

2.   I have started practicing safer sex within the past six months.

3.   I am currently preparing to start practicing safer sex within the next month.

4.   I would like to start practicing safer sex within the next six months.

Scoring

No to all statements	Precontemplation
Yes to statement 4	Contemplation
Yes to statement 3	Preparation
Yes to statement 2	Action
Yes to statement 1	Maintenance

Review table 12.8 of *Connections for Health* for tips on moving through the stages of change and becoming more responsible about practicing safer sex every time you have sex.

For Further Study

Despite public and private health efforts, infectious diseases still pose a threat to wellness. The best protection, however, is prevention. Increase your level of wellness by using the activities below to help you minimize your personal risk.

Wellness Activities

1. Interview someone at the student health center on your campus. What are the STDs he or she sees most frequently? What action is being taken to reduce the spread of STDs on campus?
2. Talk with someone from your local public health department in charge of contact investigation. Ask him or her to describe how they contact sexual partners of someone who has an STD. What problems does he or she encounter with contact investigation?
3. What STDs are required by law to be reported in your state? Who is supposed to report the STD?
4. Conduct a media update on Acquired Immune Deficiency Syndrome (AIDS). Review newspapers and magazines for new developments regarding diagnosis and cures. What actions are being taken to give the public reliable information about AIDS?
5. Investigate what your college or university is doing to encourage condom use as a preventive measure against the spread of AIDS and other STDs.

13 Coming to Terms with Death and Loss: A Wellness Perspective

Coming to Terms with Death . . . Where Do You Stand?

Understanding death and dying is an important step in appreciating the richness of life. It can also help us to relate in a positive, caring way to other people who have suffered the loss of a loved one. Take time to do the exercises below; explore your feelings and attitudes. It can help you achieve a higher level of wellness.

Assess Your Attitudes toward Your Death

Complete the following sentences. You may want to question people of other age groups to determine differences in attitudes.

1. Before I could die happily, I feel I would have to . . .
2. My greatest fear about my own death is . . .
3. If I were to die today, my biggest regret would be . . .
4. I would like the following things around me when I die . . .
5. When I think of my own death, the saddest thing is . . .
6. Before I die, I would like to . . .
7. After I die, I would like to . . .
8. When I die, I hope that . . .
9. I would like to have at my bedside when I die . . .
10. When I die, I will be glad to get away from . . .
11. When I die, I would like my funeral to be . . .
12. I want to die at age _____ because . . .
13. If I were to die tomorrow, my biggest accomplishment would be . . .
14. I would like to die at home if . . .
15. I want the cause of my death to be . . .
16. I would consider suicide when . . .
17. I want to be permitted to die when . . .

Reviewing Important Concepts

1. Death is the cessation of physical life processes. The process of dying involves three stages. Describe each of these stages, and explain how they differ from each other. At what point is a reversal of the symptoms of death possible?

2. Briefly outline Kübler-Ross's five psychological stages of death and dying. Do these stages apply to everyone? Explain.

Applying What You've Learned

1. Robert D. Russell discusses five philosophies or perspectives on life and death that have emerged in modern America. Which philosophy comes closest to what you believe about life and death? Why? Briefly describe the people, institutions (church, school, etc.), and/or events that have shaped your philosophy.

2. You and a friend have just heard that Kim, a friend close to both of you, is dying. Using Kübler-Ross's five stages of death and dying, describe how you and your friend can help Kim as she goes through each stage of this process. (In the case where conversation is helpful, write what you would actually say to Kim.)

3. We seldom think seriously about our own funeral. By planning ahead, one can avoid burdening those left behind with decisions, when they may already be deeply burdened with feelings of loss, sorrow, and grief. To help you consider some possible arrangements, complete the checklist that follows.

My Funeral

Preparation of My Body

_____ I do not want to be embalmed so that mourning can be extended for a long period of time.

_____ I do not want an open casket.

_____ I am willing to have an autopsy made.

_____ I wish to leave the following organs if they can be used to help other people: _____

_____ I am willing to leave my whole body to medical science so that it may be used for scientific study.

_____ Though my body cannot be present, I wish to have a funeral.

Type of Funeral

I want to be waked for _____ days at _____ (insert name of funeral home).

I want a church service held at _____ (name of church).

I want the following musical pieces to be played at my wake and funeral: _____
_____
_____

I want the following passages read at my wake and funeral: _____

I would like _____ to read the above passages.

_____ I want flowers at my funeral.

In lieu of flowers, I would prefer donations to the following charities, churches, or associations made in my name:
_____

If flowers are sent to my funeral, I would like them to be delivered to _____ (nursing homes, hospitals, schools, churches) for the enjoyment of others.

I would like the following friends to be pallbearers:
_____
_____
_____

Special requests: _____
_____
_____

Disposition of My Body

I want to be _____ buried _____ cremated.

I want to be buried at _____ (location).

_____ I want an elaborate casket.

_____ I want a simple, plain, and inexpensive casket.

_____ I want to be buried at sea, the source from which all life springs. Therefore, I do not need a casket.

_____ I would like my ashes scattered _____ (location).

_____ I would like my ashes to be buried _____ (location).

_____ I would like my ashes kept in a cremation container and kept by _____ (person's name).

_____ I would like a simple gravestone.

_____ I would like a memorial with my name to be placed _____ (location).

_____ I do not want any tombstone or marker at my grave.

Other desires: _____
_____
_____
_____

Other Considerations Not Covered:
_____
_____
_____

Stages of Change

If you were to die suddenly, would you want to be an organ donor? While many people have thought about this, fewer have taken steps to complete a uniform donor card. Answer these four questions to assess your current stage of change related to organ donation.

1. I have had a uniform donor card for more than six months.

2. I have taken action to obtain a uniform donor card within the past six months.

3. I am currently preparing to obtain a donor card within the next month.

4. I would like to get a donor card within the next six months.

Scoring

No to all statements	Precontemplation
Yes to statement 4	Contemplation
Yes to statement 3	Preparation
Yes to statement 2	Action
Yes to statement 1	Maintenance

Review table 13.4 of *Connections for Health* for tips on moving through the stages of change toward getting a uniform donor card and possibly saving lives.

For Further Study

A careful examination of ``death education'' may, in fact, be a course in ``life education.'' Use the following activities to help you come to terms with this aspect of life. It will enable you to progress in a positive direction on the wellness continuum.

Wellness Activities

1. Decisions about dying have traditionally been deliberations between a doctor and the patient. Since the early 1970s patients' rights have become a legal issue as well. Some court action has given new power to patients and their families while other court action has taken away power. What decisions should be made by a patient? When should the legal system become involved? What is the difference between natural death and wrongful death? The article in the May/June 1988 issue of *Hippocrates,* ``The Judge'' (pp. 54–62) offers some observations. Use this and other articles to answer the questions poised on page 113.

2. What services are available in your community to help bereaved persons (hospitals, churches, etc.)? How do you find out about these services? Is there a cost involved?

3. Visit a hospital or nursing home, and question the staff about their policies about dying. Are patients who are terminally ill told? Are there specially trained personnel to help terminal patients? What is their policy concerning living wills? How do other patients react when someone has died?

4. Do your parents and friends have wills? When were they written? Ask them if they are willing to discuss the contents of the wills with you. Are older people more likely to have wills made than younger people? Why?

5. Contact several funeral homes in your community. Ask the directors to describe the range of services and costs. What preparations can be made in advance? Does this funeral home cater to a specific religion or ethnic population? If so, are there any special customs that are followed?

6. Interview someone from another culture. Ask him or her to explain how death is viewed in his or her culture. What words or phrases are used to say that someone has died? What funeral customs are practiced?

7. The medical directive, a durable power of attorney, allows you to appoint someone to make medical decisions for you if you should become unable to make them yourself. Using the source below, make a copy of the form and complete it. It asks you to consider four different situations that involve mental incompetence. For each situation you will be asked to indicate your wishes concerning possible medical interventions. What impact has doing this exercise had on you? Attach your medical directive with your explanation. (Emanuel, Linda L. and Emanuel, Ezekiel J. ``The Medical Directive: A New Comprehensive Advance Care Document,'' *Journal of the American Medical Association* 261:3288–93, June 9, 1989.)

Drug Use and Drug Abuse . . . Where Do You Stand?

Drugs are everywhere in our environment and are a part of everyone's life-style. Responsible drug use, including recreational and self-medication, is an important key to high-level wellness.

Don't Swallow 'til You've Asked These Questions

Are you getting all the facts you need when you take medication? The next time you take medicine, ask yourself the questions listed below. Place a check mark in the box if you can answer the question. You're a wise consumer if you can answer every question. Call your doctor or pharmacist for information regarding the questions you are unable to answer.

- ☐ 1. Do I really need this medication?
- ☐ 2. What is the medication for? How will it help me?
- ☐ 3. What are the unwanted side effects of this medicine? If they occur, what should I do? Which should be reported?
- ☐ 4. Are there any other medicines (prescription or nonprescription) that should not be taken while this medicine is being taken?
- ☐ 5. How should I take this medicine (before meals, with meals, after meals)? Does ``every six hours'' mean every six hours while awake? etc.
- ☐ 6. Can I stop taking the medication early if the symptoms disappear?
- ☐ 7. How soon should I expect results?
- ☐ 8. Can I drink alcohol while taking this medication?
- ☐ 9. Are there any dietary changes I should make while taking this medication? (Example: people on oral contraceptives often are advised to take vitamin B_6 supplements, people taking diuretics often are advised to increase the potassium in their diets, etc.)
- ☐ 10. Can you prescribe a generic drug rather than a brand name drug so I can save money?
- ☐ 11. What should I do if I accidentally miss a dose? (Should I skip it or take a double dose next time?)
- ☐ 12. Are there any foods I should avoid while taking this medicine? (Some antibiotics are not as effective if you take them too close to the time you eat/drink dairy products, etc.)
- ☐ 13. Is it safe to operate machinery or drive while taking this medicine (i.e., will the drug make me sleepy)?
- ☐ 14. Does the medication come in another form (if you have trouble swallowing tablets, downing syrups, etc.)?
- ☐ 15. Should the prescription be refilled; if so, under what circumstances?

From The Hope Health Letter published by The Hope Heart Institute, Kalamazoo, MI. Reprinted by permission

Marijuana Assessment Questionnaire

Denial of marijuana dependence and addiction stems from misconceptions of the harmlessness of this drug. Current research clearly documents the physical, psychological, and emotional harm of marijuana in the 1990s.

This questionnaire is a tool to help those who might have a problem, or those individuals and family members concerned with others who might have a problem with marijuana. Check the box before any question to which you would answer yes.

☐   1. Are you smoking marijuana
        ☐   in the morning
        ☐   on a daily basis
        ☐   during work/school time
        (one or more checks is a yes answer)

☐   2. While under the influence of marijuana, do you experience any of the following symptoms:
        ☐   irritability   ☐   restlessness
        ☐   anxiety   ☐   sweating
        ☐   tremors   ☐   feeling loss of control
        ☐   insomnia   ☐   nausea, vomiting

☐   3. As a result of marijuana use, do you experience a loss of initiative and ambition and/or a withdrawal from customary interests and interpersonal relationships?

☐   4. After using marijuana, have you experienced:
        ☐   a clouding of mental processes
        ☐   impaired thinking and confusion
        ☐   flashbacks
        ☐   fear of brain damage
        ☐   delusions

☐   5. Have others commented on your poor driving skills while under the influence of marijuana, and/or have you noticed impairment in perceptual motor skills, driving decision making, and/or tracking and reaction time?

☐   6. As a result of using marijuana, have you experienced any adverse negative consequences (e.g., problems at work/school, accidents, difficulty in relationships, or mood swings)?

☐   7. Do you think about using marijuana often? (i.e., Do events, time of day, or particular daily situations trigger the desire to use marijuana?)

☐   8. Have you been unable to stop using marijuana for 3 months or longer without substituting other drugs, alcohol, or medication?

☐   9. Do you use marijuana with cocaine, alcohol, and/or other drugs?

☐   10. Do other members of your family have problems with marijuana, alcohol, and/or other drugs?

☐   11. Do you use marijuana to alleviate stress, loneliness, depression, boredom, and/or problems in relationships?

☐   12. Did you start using marijuana at a young age, and/or have you been using marijuana regularly for several years?

If you checked three or more of these questions, consult a specialist in drug and alcohol assessment and treatment for further evaluation.

Cocaine Assessment Questionnaire

Check the box before any question to which you would answer yes.

☐   1.   Are you using more cocaine than you plan to use, and do you find that you are enjoying it less? That is, your tolerance is developing and despite not feeling very well, you continue to use.

☐   2.   Are you experiencing three or more of the following physical signs?
- ☐ Excessive periods of fatigue
- ☐ Itching, scratching, and/or skin lesions
- ☐ Sinus problems and nose bleeds
- ☐ Trouble breathing and/or catching your breath
- ☐ Chest pains and palpitations
- ☐ Tremors and poor coordination
- ☐ Decreased appetite or weight loss
- ☐ Light spots on the periphery of your vision
- ☐ Headaches
- ☐ Sleep disturbances, sleepiness, or excessive sleeping
- ☐ Hoarseness

☐   3.   Do you feel apathetic, disinterested, and/or depressed? Have you lost the ability to concentrate?

☐   4.   Do you experience mood swings, irritability, short temper, emotional outbursts, rage or excessive sadness, paranoid and/or frantic bizarre behavior?

☐   5.   As a result of cocaine use, have you been absent, late, or exhibited inappropriate behavior at work?

☐   6.   Are family members and friends suggesting that you have a problem with cocaine and/or are you lying about your frequency of cocaine use?

☐   7.   Are you reducing outside interests, withdrawing from, or in conflict with friends and family members?

☐   8.   Are you experiencing financial and/or legal problems as a direct or indirect result of cocaine use?

☐   9.   Are you injecting or freebasing cocaine?

☐   10.   The morning after cocaine use, are you feeling depressed, remorseful, guilty, and/or shameful about your behavior the night before?

    If you checked the boxes before two or more of these questions, you may have a potentially serious cocaine problem. Pursue further evaluation with a chemical dependency professional.

Copyright © Richard Fields, Ph.D., FACES, Bellevue, WA.

Reviewing Important Concepts

1.   Drugs may have a synergistic effect on one another. Explain this concept, and describe why it is important to be aware of this potential problem when taking drugs. Use examples to illustrate your explanation.

(2) The American Psychological Association considers substance abuse and substance dependence to be different. Describe the essential features of each category and how these categories differ.

3. Describe how psychoactive drugs differ from other drugs.

4. Athletes use drugs recreationally and as ergogenic aids. Which drugs does your textbook cite as being frequently used by athletes? What are the ethical and safety issues involved with drugs and sports?

Applying What You've Learned

1. You are asked to speak to a group of students about the responsibilities of drug use. Select one of the three areas of responsibility and outline your talk below. Describe ways in which the students can model these responsible behaviors.

2. Your roommate, Paul, claims he is drug-free. He will take medication if ill, but he will not take any other type of drug. You point out to Paul that he is a very heavy coffee drinker. Explain to Paul why the caffeine in his coffee is considered a psychoactive drug.

3. Following is a list of reasons people use psychoactive drugs. Read each motive, then write several possible alternatives to drug use. Answer the questions that follow the chart on the next page.

Motive for drug use	Possible alternatives
Need for relaxation/ Need to unwind	Playing music, walking, meditation
To escape boredom/ To get out of a bad mood	
Peer pressure/ To gain acceptance	
To feel "high"/ Desire to stimulate senses (sight, sound, taste, touch)	
To relieve depression	
To feel less inhibited	
Kicks/Risks/Adventure/ Trying something new	
To discover meaningful value/ The meaning of life/ Nature of the universe	
Need for more energy	

a. Can you think of additional reasons for using drugs? What are they?

b. Which reasons might influence you personally? What alternatives, corresponding to these reasons, exist for you?

c. If you were trying to convince yourself not to use drugs, what arguments would be most persuasive?

d. If you were to develop a plan of regular activities for yourself in order to reduce your susceptibility to drug use, what would you include? Consider realistically the time, energy, and money that these activities require. Make sure the activities you choose are practical ones for you.

Stages of Change

How many times in the last week have you taken drugs? Don't forget to include caffeine, aspirin, over-the-counter and prescription medicines, tobacco, and alcohol in your count. Why did you take each of these drugs? Are you using drugs responsibly? Answer these four questions to assess your current stage of change related to your drug usage.

1.   I have maintained changes in my drug-taking behavior for more than six months.

2.   I have taken action to use drugs more responsibly within the past six months.

3.   I am currently preparing to change my drug-taking behavior within the next month.

4.   I would like to take action to use drugs more responsibly within the next six months.

Scoring

No to all statements	Precontemplation
Yes to statement 4	Contemplation
Yes to statement 3	Preparation
Yes to statement 2	Action
Yes to statement 1	Maintenance

Review table 14.7 of *Connections for Health* for tips on moving through the stages of change and thinking critically about all the drugs you take.

For Further Study

The decision for responsible use of drugs is yours. Use the activities below to help you get in touch with many of the issues regarding drugs and drug use—they will help you on your road to high-level wellness. Learning more about psychoactive drugs, drug-taking behavior, and alternatives to drug-taking will help you in your decisions regarding your life-style. There are many ways of experiencing ``natural highs'' without chemical assistance. In order to achieve high-level wellness, you can begin exploring activities and interests that will help you find fulfillment. The list below will provide a starting place for you.

Wellness Activities

1.   Interview a pharmacist about overuse and misuse of over-the-counter drugs. What are the most frequently misused over-the-counter drugs seen in the pharmacy? What role does the pharmacist play in helping to reduce overuse and misuse by customers?
2.   One federal agency that is primarily concerned with drugs and drug use is the Food and Drug Administration. Write to the FDA for information on their roles and responsibilities in serving the public.
3.   Conduct a ``spring house cleaning'' in your medicine cabinet. Do you know what each medication was prescribed for? How old are the medications? (Throw out old medications by flushing them down the toilet.)
4.   Are you in touch with the drug-taking environment on your campus? Interview ten to fifteen students on your campus. Ask them about their attitudes toward drug-taking, how their family and peers influence their decisions about drug-taking and the availability of drugs. Ask these questions with regard to illicit, prescription, and over-the-counter drugs.
5.   Interview an addictions counselor (on your campus or locate one in the yellow pages) about the clients he/she helps. How has drugs/alcohol changed the clients' lives? Ask the counselor to describe the childhood of a typical client. What do the clients need to do in order to get their lives back together?
6.   Attend a Narcotics Anonymous or Cocaine Anonymous meeting. What role did drugs play in these people's lives? How have they changed their lives in order to remain drug-free?
7.   Does your campus have a drug problem? If so, what measures are the university administrators taking to reduce drug abuse? How effective do you believe these measures are?

8. Take a course on body massage or sensory awareness training to increase the level of awareness of your senses.

9. There are many activities that you can participate in that can result in ``natural highs.'' The following is a list of suggestions. Be creative and add to this list.

scuba diving	skydiving
biofeedback training	guided fantasy and daydreams
sensory deprivation tanks	self-hypnosis
relaxation	rappeling
wilderness backpacking	snow or water skiing

10. It has been said that the most widely used drug in our society is caffeine. Often caffeine is ``hidden'' in foods and medications. In order to find out if caffeine is in a product, you must read the product label. Examine the foods and the over-the-counter medications in your home for caffeine. Any surprises?

11. During the 1970s, there was a much different attitude toward psychoactive drugs than there is today. One book written during this time was *The Natural Mind: A New Way of Looking at Drugs and the Higher Consciousness* by Andrew Weil (Boston, Mass. Houghton Mifflin, 1973). Locate this book at the library and browse through it. Describe Weil's philosophy and attitude toward drugs. How does Weil's philosophy compare to the 1990s attitude and philosophy toward drugs? Compare your philosophy and attitude to Weil's.

12. Interview an athletic coach about drug use among athletes on campus. Is use prevalent? How does the university enforce the NCAA-instituted drug education and drug-testing program? What other things do the coaches do to discourage the use of drugs? If an athlete is caught using drugs, what are the repercussions of his/her actions? (You could also ask the same questions found on page 119, emphasizing steroid use.)

15   Tobacco: Smoking and Smokeless Threats to Well-Being

Tobacco . . . Where Do You Stand?

There has been much written and said about the dangers of tobacco—yet people continue to use tobacco in many forms (cigarettes, pipe, snuff, chew). By becoming aware of smoking behavior, we take the first step to increasing our level of wellness.

If you are a smoker, you may wish to stop smoking or reduce the amount you smoke. If you are a nonsmoker, there are many ways in which you can support smokers in their attempt to quit. The following assessments will help both the smoker and the nonsmoker become more aware of smoking behavior.

Check Your Smoking I.Q.

An Important Quiz for Older Smokers

If you or someone you know is an older smoker, you may think that there is no point in quitting now. Think again. By quitting smoking now, you will feel more in control and have fewer coughs and colds. On the other hand, with every cigarette you smoke, you increase your chances of having a heart attack, a stroke, or cancer. Need to think about this more? Take this older smokers' I.Q. quiz. Just answer ``true'' or ``false'' to each statement below. The correct answers follow.

1. T F If you have smoked for most of your life, it's not worth stopping now.
2. T F Older smokers who try to quit are more likely to stay off cigarettes.
3. T F Smokers get tired and short of breath more easily than nonsmokers the same age.
4. T F Smoking is a major risk factor for heart attack and stroke among adults 60 years of age and older.
5. T F Quitting smoking can help those who have already had a heart attack.
6. T F Most older smokers don't want to stop smoking.
7. T F An older smoker is more likely to smoke **more** cigarettes than a younger smoker.
8. T F Someone who has smoked for 30 to 40 years probably won't be able to quit smoking.
9. T F Very few older adults smoke cigarettes.
10. T F Lifelong smokers are more likely to die of diseases like emphysema and bronchitis than nonsmokers.

Answers to the Check Your Smoking I.Q. Quiz

1. FALSE   Nonsense! You have every reason to quit now and quit for good—even if you've been smoking for years. Stopping smoking will help you live longer and feel better. You will reduce your risk of heart attack, stroke, and cancer; improve blood flow and lung function; and help stop diseases like emphysema and bronchitis from getting worse.

2. TRUE   Once they quit, older smokers are far more likely than younger smokers to stay away from cigarettes. Older smokers know more about both the short- and long-term health benefits of quitting.

3. TRUE   Smokers, especially those over 50 years old, are much more likely to get tired, feel short of breath, and cough more often. These symptoms can signal the start of bronchitis or emphysema, both of which are suffered more often by older smokers. Stopping smoking will help reduce these symptoms.

4. TRUE   Smoking is a major risk factor for four of the five leading causes of death including heart disease, stroke, cancer, and lung diseases like emphysema and bronchitis. For adults 60 and over, smoking is a major risk factor for six of the top 14 causes of death. Older male smokers are nearly twice as likely to die from stroke as older men who do not smoke. The odds are nearly as high for older female smokers. Cigarette smokers of any age have a 70 percent greater heart disease death rate than do nonsmokers.

5. TRUE   The good news is that stopping smoking does help people who have suffered a heart attack. In fact, their chances of having another attack are smaller. In some cases, ex-smokers can cut their risk of another heart attack by half or more.

6. FALSE   Most smokers would prefer to quit. In fact, in a recent study, 65 percent of older smokers said that they would like to stop. What keeps them from quitting? They are afraid of being irritable, nervous, and tense. Others are concerned about cravings for cigarettes. Most don't want to gain weight. Many think it's too late to quit—that quitting after so many years of smoking will not help. But this is **not** true.

7. TRUE   Older smokers usually smoke cigarettes than younger people. Plus, older smokers are more likely to smoke high nicotine brands.

8. FALSE   You may be surprised to learn that older smokers are actually **more** likely to succeed at quitting smoking. This is more true if they're already experiencing long-term smoking-related symptoms like shortness of breath, coughing, or chest pain. Older smokers who stop want to avoid further health problems, take control of their life, get rid of the smell of cigarettes, and save money.

9. FALSE   One out of five adults age 50 or older smokes cigarettes. This is more than 11 million smokers, a fourth of the country's 43 million smokers! About 25 percent of the general U.S. population still smokes.

10. TRUE   Smoking greatly increases the risk of dying from diseases like emphysema and bronchitis. In fact, over 80 percent of all deaths from these two diseases are directly due to smoking. The risk of dying from lung cancer is also a lot higher for smokers than nonsmokers: 22 times higher for males, 12 times higher for females.

How did you do?

10 correct
Congratulations! You could have written this quiz! Since you already know so much about the effects of smoking on older adults, share this information with your family and friends. If you smoke, you also know enough to quit—today!

8–9 correct
Excellent. If you got at least eight right, then you have at least eight good reasons to stop smoking—or never start. Ask your doctor or nurse for more information.

Fewer than 8 correct
Take a little more time to review the facts in this quiz. Then, talk to your doctor or nurse soon about the benefits of stopping smoking.

For more information, write:
NHLBI Smoking Education Program, 4733 Bethesda Avenue, Suite 530, Bethesda, MD 20814-4820

Source: Prepared by the National Heart, Lung, and Blood Institute Smoking Education Program. National Institutes of Health Publication No. 91-3031, October 1991. U.S. Department of Health and Human Services, Bethesda, MD.

The Fagerstrom Nicotine Tolerance Scale

The Fagerstrom Nicotine Tolerance Scale was designed to help smokers determine their levels of physical dependence on nicotine, the addictive substance in tobacco. Answer each question. Then figure your score using the scoring key on the following page.

		A	B	C
1.	How soon after you wake up do you smoke your first cigarette?	After 30 min.	Within 30 min.	—
2.	Do you find it difficult to refrain from smoking in places where it is forbidden, such as the library, theater, doctor's office?	No	Yes	—
3.	Which of all the cigarettes you smoke in a day is the most satisfying one?	Any other than the first one in the morning	The first one in the morning	—
4.	How many cigarettes a day do you smoke?	1–15	16–25	More than 26
5.	Do you smoke more during the morning than during the rest of the day?	No	Yes	—
6.	Do you smoke when you are so ill that you are in bed most of the day?	No	Yes	—
7.	Does the brand you smoke have low, medium, or high nicotine content?	Low	Medium	High
8.	How often do you inhale the smoke from your cigarette?	Never	Sometimes	Always

Scoring:

1. Assign no points for each answer in column A
2. Assign 1 point for each answer in column B
3. Assign 2 points for each answer in column C (note that not all questions have an answer in column C).
4. Total the number of points

The questionnaire has a range of 0–11 points, with 0 indicating minimum physical dependence and 11 points maximum physical dependence.

Reprinted from K-O Fagerstrom, *Addictive Behaviors, Vol. 3,* Copyright 1969, Pages No. 235-241., with kind permission from Elsevier Science Ltd., The Boulevard, Langford Lane, Kidlington OX5 1GB, UK.

Monitoring Your Smoking Behavior

Learn about your smoking habit by using a simple tool called a ``packwrap.'' A packwrap is designed to make it easy for you to measure how much and when you smoke. Photocopy the sample packwrap on the next page, and wrap it around your cigarette pack.

Each time you smoke, make a mark in the appropriate box. Write down the time of day in the appropriate column. Make a note of where you are when you smoke. For example, if you're at your desk at 9:00 A.M. and smoke a cigarette, you would make the following notation: 9 A.M.-D (for desk). Find a short pencil that will fit into your cigarette pack so you'll always be prepared.

Monitor your smoking behavior for one week and then answer the following questions:

a. How much are you really smoking? Any surprises?
b. What time of the day are you most likely to smoke?
c. Where (location/activity) are you smoking?

Time	Sun.	Mon.	Tues.	Wed.	Thur.	Fri.	Sat.	
Total								

Reviewing Important Concepts

1. Describe the differences between mainstream and sidestream smoke.

2. What is involuntary smoking? List three possible health risks associated with involuntary smoking.

3. Describe the numerous undesirable health effects that are associated with smokeless tobacco use.

Applying What You've Learned

1. Robert started smoking at age sixteen, almost ten years ago. He's decided he wants to quit. He comes to you for advice. Explain the different ways Robert might choose to stop smoking. List some of the community resources Robert could call for further information. How can you help Robert quit smoking and remain a nonsmoker? Describe three things you can do.

2. Betty asked Judy if she wanted a ride home for Christmas break. The trip was six hours and Betty would enjoy the company in addition to sharing expenses. One concern Judy has is that Betty is a cigarette smoker. The thought of a six-hour trip in a smoke-filled car is not appealing to Judy. What options does Judy have?

3. A call from home has brought interesting news. Your dad has decided, after all these years, to quit smoking. Both you and your mom are happy, but your mom is apprehensive. She is concerned about the withdrawal symptoms associated with quitting. She asks you for help. What are three common withdrawal symptoms your dad may experience? What things can your dad do to minimize their effects? Give her two tips on what to do to help your dad stay off cigarettes for good.

Stages of Change

If you are a smoker, you probably know that there are many compelling reasons to quit. You may have even tried unsuccessfully to quit in the past. But the best step for you to take toward becoming a nonsmoker depends on your current stage of change. Answer these four questions honestly.

1. I quit smoking more than six months ago.

2. I quit smoking within the past six months.

3. I am currently preparing to quit smoking in the next month.

4. I would like to quit smoking within the next six months.

Scoring

No to all statements	Precontemplation
Yes to statement 4	Contemplation
Yes to statement 3	Preparation
Yes to statement 2	Action
Yes to statement 1	Maintenance

Review table 15.8 of *Connections for Health* for tips on moving through the stages of change toward becoming a nonsmoker.

For Further Study

Quit smoking. Reduce the amount you smoke. Help someone quit. Help someone stay stopped. You can increase your level of wellness by choosing one of these options and acting on your choice. The following activities are designed to help you on your road to success.

Wellness Activities

1. Call your local American Lung Association or American Cancer Society and request a packet of materials to help people quit smoking. Review the materials. Describe the techniques they suggest for smokers.
2. Imagine you are a visitor from a foreign country where no one smokes. Visit a shopping mall and observe the people smoking. What do you see? (Remember: you've never seen anybody smoke before!)
3. Interview several ex-smokers. What were their quitting experiences like? How long have they been nonsmokers? How do they feel being nonsmokers? Compare the different experiences and answers. Are there any common themes? Ask each person how having others supporting their decision helped them in their efforts to quit.
4. Does cigarette advertising induce people to smoke? Research this question and write a brief paper summarizing each issue. Include your opinion about this issue.

16   Alcohol: Risks and Responsibilities

Alcohol . . . Where Do You Stand?

Alcohol is a drug that, when abused or misused, can cause great problems for individuals and society. Alcohol and wellness can, however, co-exist. The assessments below will help you identify how your cultural norms influence your drinking behavior and how much you know about the effects of alcohol. Take the first step to responsible alcohol use by finding out where you stand.

Understanding Your Culture

It's important to analyze your own culture to determine all the influences it has on you and your drinking behavior. Check over the following list to see what culture traps might be keeping you, or someone you know, from making an independent decision about drinking.

It is the norm in one or more groups that I belong:

☐   for people to drink more alcohol than is good for them.

☐   for the host or hostess at a party to check repeatedly to make sure everyone's glass is full and drinks are being continually pushed.

☐   to persuade guests to stay for one or more rounds or have one more for the road.

☐   to mention with pride one's ability to consume large amounts of alcohol.

☐   to have a drink when one doesn't really want to, just because the others are.

☐   for people who feel overburdened to seek relief through alcohol.

☐   for drinking contests to be considered an amusing entertainment.

☐   to consider drinking a sign of maturity and worldliness.

☐   for people to be offended by someone who refuses a drink.

☐   for people to drink more alcohol than is good for them every day or almost every day.

☐   to see alcohol as a necessary part of every social occasion.

☐   for people to think it's funny to see their friends intoxicated.

☐   for parents to consider drinking alcohol as proof of adult status.

Now that you think it through, how much do you think culture influences your drinking? Test it over the next two weeks. See how many examples you can identify in your group situations. Watch for these examples of cultural attitudes and norms at lunch, after work, at parties. Before you have that drink, pause for that millisecond—click—and make sure it's your own decision.

From Robert Allen, *Lifeagain,* 1981. Copyright © 1981. Human Resources Institute, Morristown, NJ. Reprinted by permission.

To Your Health:
The Effects of Alcohol on Body Functions

This quiz will help you to assess how well you understand the effects of alcohol on your body. After you answer all of the questions, check your responses with the correct responses which are found at the end of the questions section. Then place a check in the blank to the right of the question for every correct answer. Score one point for every correct answer. Add the total number of correct answers to find your score.

1.   Ethanol and ether have similar effects. Are they classified as depressants or stimulants?   ____

2.   True or false: Alcohol is not digested like other foods.   ____

3. About 20 percent of the alcohol you consume is absorbed through your stomach. From where is the other 80 percent absorbed? _____
4. Alcohol affects behavior through which part of the body? _____
5. How does alcohol get to the brain? _____
6. Ninety percent of the ethanol in one's body is oxidized. This means the body produced heat and energy by combining alcohol with oxygen and ultimately converts the mixture to water and carbon dioxide. Will taking a cold shower or drinking hot coffee speed up oxidation? _____
7. Name three factors that affect the absorption rate of alcohol in the body. _____
8. How do the nonalcoholic substances (such as water, sugar, salts, and other carbohydrates found in beer) affect the rate of alcohol absorption in the body? _____
9. Are champagne and other sparkling wines absorbed faster or slower than noncarbonated wines?
10. True or false: There is approximately the same amount of ethanol in a 1-ounce shot of 100-proof distilled spirits, a 4-ounce glass of table wine, and a 12-ounce can of beer. _____
11. Generally speaking, a larger person must drink more alcohol than a smaller person to become intoxicated. What factor influences intoxication once the alcohol has been absorbed in the bloodstream? _____
12. An average person needs an hour to oxidize ½ ounce of ethanol. The average drink usually contains ½ ounce of ethanol. If you wish to drink, but avoid intoxication, how far apart should you space your drinks? _____
13. Which of the following are impaired by intoxication: judgment, memory, coordination, auditory and visual perception? _____
14. True or false: Two people of the same weight and physical condition will have the same physical and psychological reactions to an equal amount of alcohol. _____
15. True or false: One person will have the same physical and psychological reactions to alcohol every time he or she drinks the same amount. _____
16. Ethanol provides heat and energy through oxidation. Because of this chemical property, ethanol may be classified as both a drug and a_____. _____
17. What is the condition in which a person requires increasing amounts of alcohol in order to achieve the same effect as formerly was achieved by much smaller quantities of alcohol? _____

Answers:

1. Depressants
2. True
3. From the small intestine
4. The brain
5. It is carried to the brain through the bloodstream
6. No
7. Concentration of alcohol in beverage consumed; amount of alcohol consumed; rate of consumption; amount of food in stomach; nonalcoholic substance in beverage; emotions (i.e., stress, fear, anger); carbonation in beverage.

8. Slow, decrease
9. Faster
10. True
11. Body weight
12. About 1 hour
13. Any of the above
14. False
15. False
16. Food
17. Tolerance

Your total number correct _____

If you didn't answer all of the questions correctly, go back to your textbook and review the information in chapter 5.

From *An Ounce of Prevention,* DHEW Publication No. (ADM) 77-454A, 1977. National Institute on Alcohol Abuse and Alcoholism.

Social Self-Assessment

The National Institute on Alcohol Abuse and Alcoholism summarized the existing literature and found that the following factors were indicative of the fewest problems with alcohol as an adult. How do you stack up with these factors? Remember, these are associated with the lowest rates of problems associated with drinking.

You are least likely to have problems with alcohol if:

[ ]   1.   you were exposed to alcohol in relatively small quantities early in life by your family or within the context of a religious or cultural group.

[ ]   2.   your family members viewed alcohol as a food and consumed small quantities primarily at mealtime.

[ ]   3.   your parents set a good example by practicing responsible drinking behaviors.

]]   4.   your family did not view drinking alcoholic beverages as a means of demonstrating maturity, adulthood, or masculinity/feminity.

[ ]   5.   abstinence was accepted as a legitimate choice with respect to the consumption of alcoholic beverages.

[ ]   6.   drunkenness was not an acceptable form of behavior.

[ ]   7.   alcohol was viewed as a beverage and not as the central focus of a group activity.

[ ]   8.   rules and rituals associated with drinking were known and understood by all group members; they were both reasonable and agreeable to those members.

Source: National Institute on Alcohol Abuse and Alcoholism.

Reviewing Important Concepts

1.   People often mistakenly believe that alcohol absorption and metabolism are the same. How do these two processes differ?

2.   Describe the seven factors that influence the rate of alcohol absorption in the body.

3.   There are consequences to irresponsible use of alcohol. Give several examples of these consequences.

4.   Describe responsible alcohol use.

5. In 1981 the U.S. Surgeon General issued an advisory that pregnant women should not drink alcohol due to its teratogenic effects on the developing fetus. Describe Fetal Alcohol Syndrome (FAS) and how it affects children born with this syndrome.

Applying What You've Learned

You are going to a Christmas party. There will be lots of eggnog being served made from a ``secret'' family recipe. You discover while talking with your host that the ``secret'' in the eggnog is grain alcohol. To find out what your blood alcohol concentration is after one hour of drinking at the Christmas party, complete the following steps.

1. During the first hour, I drank _____ glasses of eggnog, 1.5 ounces each.

2. How many ounces of absolute alcohol are in the drinks you've had so far? Remember, there are 13.6 grams of absolute alcohol in every 1.5 ounce serving of spirits.

   _____ × 13.6 gms. absolute alcohol = _____
   Number of glasses eggnog   Total gms. absolute alcohol [A]

3. _____ [A] grams of absolute alcohol enters your blood stream as it is being consumed. You need to determine the volume of water in which this alcohol dissolves. Alcohol is water soluble, not fat soluble. Individuals vary in their water content based on body type. Using the chart below, circle the water content of your body based on your body type.

Body Type	Water Content
lean, muscular male	70% or .70
muscular, female	60% or .60
average male or female	60% or .60
obese male or female	50% or .50

4. My weight is _____ pounds. The space that alcohol enters is equal to:

   _____ × _____ = _____
   Body water content   Weight   Pounds of water [B]

   Each pound of water represents approximately .4545 liters of water, therefore:

   .4545 liters × _____ = _____
                              [B]   Liters of water [C]

5. The legal blood alcohol concentration (BAC) in most states is .10 percent. This means there is 1 part alcohol per 1000 parts blood. BAC levels are measured in milligrams percent. Therefore, you need to convert from grams to milligrams (1 gram = 1000 milligrams). To make the conversion to milligrams/liter divide the number of grams of absolute alcohol [A] by the distribution volume:

$$\underline{\hspace{4cm}} \times 1,000 = \underline{\hspace{6cm}}$$
$$\text{[A]} \qquad\qquad\qquad\qquad \text{Number of milligrams of absolute alcohol [D]}$$

$$\underline{\hspace{3cm}} \div \underline{\hspace{3cm}} = \text{milligram/liter [E]}$$
$$\text{[D]} \qquad\qquad \text{[C]}$$

Divide by 10 to get the amount per 100 milliliters (mL):

$$\underline{\hspace{3cm}} \div 10 = \underline{\hspace{6cm}}$$
$$\text{[E]} \qquad\qquad\qquad \text{Amount of absolute alcohol per 100 milliliters body water [F]}$$

6. Blood absorbs 80 percent of the alcohol in body tissue water. Complete the following to obtain the amount of alcohol in your blood:

$$\underline{\hspace{3cm}} \times .80 = \underline{\hspace{3cm}} \text{mg/100 mL blood}$$
$$\text{[F]} \qquad\qquad\qquad \text{[G]}$$

7. Your blood alcohol concentration, after consuming _____ glasses of eggnog is _____ mg/100mL blood. [G]

8. To convert the amount of alcohol in your blood to milligrams percent, divide by 1000.

$$\underline{\hspace{3cm}} \text{mg/100 mL blood} \div 1000 = \underline{\hspace{3cm}} \text{percent BAC}$$
$$\text{[G]} \qquad\qquad\qquad\qquad \text{[H]}$$

9. In healthy individuals, the liver reduces BAC at an average of 0.015 percent per hour. Therefore, after one hour your BAC is:

$$\underline{\hspace{3cm}} \text{percent} - .015 \text{ percent} = \underline{\hspace{3cm}} \text{percent}$$
$$\text{[H]} \qquad\qquad\qquad\qquad\qquad \text{[I]}$$

Summary

1. You are a _____ (insert body type and sex), weighing _____ pounds. You consumed _____ glasses of eggnog in the first hour of the Christmas party. The amount of eggnog you drank will give you a blood alcohol concentration of _____ [I] after one hour.

(Note: Eating food prior to drinking alcohol delays and reduces peak blood alcohol level. In this example, we have assumed a fasted state. In addition, we have assumed that the eggnog was consumed rapidly. Remember that responsible drinking behavior includes pacing your drinks and establishing reasonable limits on the number of drinks you consume.)

2. A friend wants to go home and asks you for a ride. Should you drive? Refer to table 16.3 ``Psychological and Physical Effects of Various Blood-Alcohol Concentration Levels'' and table 16.4 ``Blood-Alcohol Concentration and Driver Impairment'' in your textbook. Based on what you know from reading these charts, do you think it would be safe to drive? How long should you wait before driving?

3.   It is important to make plans for alternative transportation in case you have too much to drink. In this case, you have decided that it is not safe for you to drive. What other alternatives can you choose from so that you and your friend can get home safely? List at least four alternatives.

4.   When we consider the effects of alcohol on the body, there are two other factors that play an important role other than amount of absolute alcohol in the body. Describe these factors.

Stages of Change

Alcohol is a major factor in the social life on many college campuses. Have you ever thought about what parties and gatherings would be like at your school if alcohol were not served? Answer these four questions to assess your current stage of change related to your attitudes toward alcohol use on your campus.

1.   I have been hosting and attending alcohol-free events for more than six months.

2.   I have started hosting alcohol-free events within the past six months.

3.   I am planning an alcohol-free event within the next month.

4.   I would like to host an alcohol-free event in the next six months.

Scoring

No to all statements   Precontemplation
Yes to statement 4   Contemplation
Yes to statement 3   Preparation
Yes to statement 2   Action
Yes to statement 1   Maintenance

Review table 16.8 of *Connections for Health* for tips on how to challenge an alcohol-based campus culture by supporting alcohol-free events.

For Further Study

Acting responsibly when you use alcohol, if you use it at all, and encouraging similar behavior in your friends and family will increase your chances of attaining high-level wellness. The activities listed below will help you discover more about responsible alcohol use.

Wellness Activities

1. Attend a local Alcoholics Anonymous meeting in your area. Check your telephone directory for an A.A. chapter near you. How are the meetings conducted? Describe membership requirements and fees. Pay special attention to the types of people attending the meetings.
2. Examine several alcohol advertisements. What messages, images, and life-styles are being promoted?
3. What laws in your state are aimed at curbing irresponsible alcohol use? What were the major arguments for enacting these laws? Are the laws enforceable? Do you believe that it's the role of the legislature to regulate alcohol use?
4. Mothers Against Drunk Drivers (M.A.D.D.) is an organization that is responding to the increase in traffic deaths due to drunk drivers. Contact your local chapter of M.A.D.D., and find out what they are doing to curb drunk driving.

17 Better Consumerism: Rx for Wellness

Consumerism . . . Where Do You Stand?

The health care system, with its practitioners, resources, services, and products can be an intimidating system. By becoming an active, responsible consumer, you can approach the health care system with self-confidence and a feeling of being in control.

You can become an active, responsible consumer by asking questions, performing background research, and identifying people and agencies who can help you and to whom you can take complaints. Find out where you stand and how you can achieve a higher level of wellness by completing the activities in this chapter.

Measure Your Assertiveness

Learning how to be assertive takes practice. Measure your assertiveness by completing the questionnaire below.

Directions: Indicate how characteristic or descriptive of you each of the following statements is by using the code given below.

+3 very characteristic of me, extremely descriptive
+2 rather characteristic of me, quite descriptive
+1 somewhat characteristic of me, slightly descriptive
−1 somewhat uncharacteristic of me, slightly nondescriptive
−2 rather uncharacteristic of me, quite nondescriptive
−3 very uncharacteristic of me, extremely nondescriptive

_____ 1. Most people seem to be more aggressive and assertive than I am.
_____ 2. I have hesitated to make or accept dates because of ``shyness.''
_____ 3. When the food served at a restaurant is not done to my satisfaction, I complain about it to the waiter or waitress.
_____ 4. I am careful to avoid hurting other people's feelings, even when I feel that I have been injured.
_____ 5. If a salesman had gone to considerable trouble to show me merchandise that is not quite suitable, I have a difficult time saying ``no.''
_____ 6. When I am asked to do something, I insist upon knowing why.
_____ 7. There are times when I look for a good, vigorous argument.
_____ 8. I strive to get ahead as well as most people in my position.
_____ 9. To be honest, people often take advantage of me.
_____ 10. I enjoy starting conversations with new acquaintances and strangers.
_____ 11. I often don't know what to say to attractive persons of the opposite sex.
_____ 12. I will hesitate to make phone calls to business establishments and institutions.
_____ 13. I would rather apply for a job or for admission to a college by writing letters than by going through with personal interviews.
_____ 14. I find it embarrassing to return merchandise.
_____ 15. If a close and respected relative were annoying me, I would smother my feelings rather than express my annoyance.
_____ 16. I have avoided asking questions for fear of sounding stupid.
_____ 17. During an argument I am sometimes afraid that I will get so upset that I will shake all over.
_____ 18. If a famed and respected lecturer makes a statement which I think is incorrect, I will have the audience hear my point of view as well.
_____ 19. I avoid arguing over prices with clerks and salespeople.
_____ 20. When I have done something important or worthwhile, I manage to let others know about it.
_____ 21. I am open and frank about my feelings.

_____22. If someone has been spreading false and bad stories about me, I see him/her as soon as possible to ``have a talk'' about it.
_____23. I often have a hard time saying ``no.''
_____24. I tend to bottle up my emotions rather than make a scene.
_____25. I complain about poor service in a restaurant and elsewhere.
_____26. When I am given a compliment, I sometimes just don't know what to say.
_____27. If a couple near me in a theater or at a lecture were conversing rather loudly, I would ask them to be quiet or to take their conversation elsewhere.
_____28. Anyone attempting to push ahead of me in a line is in for a good battle.
_____29. I am quick to express an opinion.
_____30. There are times when I just can't say anything.

Scoring

1. Change the signs (+ or -) for items 1, 2, 4, 5, 9, 11, 12, 13, 14, 15, 16, 17, 19, 23, 24, 26, and 30.
2. Total the plus (+) items.
3. Total the minus (–) items.
4. Subtract the minus total from the plus total to obtain your score.

Your score can range from – 0 through zero to +90. The higher the score (closer to +90), the more assertively you usually behave. The lower the score (close to – 0), the more nonassertive is your typical behavior. This particular scale does not measure aggressiveness.

From: S.A. Rathus. ``A 30-Item Schedule for Assessing Assertive Behavior'' in *Behavior Therapy,* 4:398-406, 1973. Academic Press, Orlando, FL. Reprinted by permission.

Family Medical Record

The National Foundation-March of Dimes, as part of its comprehensive efforts toward prevention of birth defects, urges everyone to keep a family health record. Scientists are learning more of how inherited traits and environmental factors influence the unborn and the newborn. This makes an accurate family health history valuable in routine medical consultations and as a diagnostic tool for physicians. Your medical record also will be useful in filling out insurance forms, school and travel records.

Important Telephone Numbers

Physicians:
Dr. _____ _____
Dr. _____ _____
Dr. _____ _____
Dr. _____ _____
Dentists:
Dr. _____ _____
Dr. _____ _____
Pharmacist_____ _____

Police Emergency _____
Fire Emergency _____
Ambulance Service _____
Poison Control Center _____
Health Insurance Agt. _____
Medicare Information _____
Medicare Information _____
Local Medical Society _____

Designed by The National Foundation-March of Dimes in collaboration with the American Medical Association and Woman's Day. Reprinted by permission of March of Dimes Birth Defects Foundation.

Family Health History

Information about the health of your immediate family can prove helpful in early diagnosis and treatment of diseases that are known either to be genetic or to occur more commonly in some families. Make a note of *any* serious or chronic diseases in your family, with special attention to those listed at the right. It also helps to note the age when the disease first occurred.

Be sure to include:

Allergies	Diabetes	Heart defects	Mental retardation	Visual defects
Arthritis	Epilepsy	Hypertension	Obesity	Other recurring
Cancer	Hearing defects	Mental illness	Tuberculosis	family diseases

Name	Birth Date	Blood Type & Rh	Occupation	Diseases, Etc. and Cause	If Deceased, Age
HUSBAND					
his father					
his mother					
WIFE					
her father					
her mother					

Children's Birth Record

Be sure to note such details as duration of pregnancy, length of labor, cesarean delivery, use of forceps, newborn respiratory distress, jaundice or birth defects. If you are Rh negative and the child was Rh positive, were you given the Rh vaccine?

Name	Date	Sex	Wt.	Blood Type & Rh	APGAR Score	Hospital, City	Physician	Details

Incomplete Pregnancies

A complete history includes details of spontaneous or induced abortions, miscarriages and stillbirths. If you are Rh negative and the fetus was Rh positive, it is important to know if you were given the Rh vaccine.

Termination	Duration	Circumstances	Termination	Duration	Circumstances

Immunization Schedule and Record

The American Academy of Pediatrics recommends that children be immunized and given tuberculin testing according to the immunization schedule below. Vaccine combinations and schedules are improved frequently, however, so that a physician can recommend what is best for you. As each immunization is completed, it should be recorded on page 139.

Immunization Schedule

2 months	Diphtheria/Tetanus/Pertussis (whooping cough) vaccine, first shot; polio vaccine, first dose	15–18 months	Rubeola (measles) and rubella (German measles) vaccines; polio booster; DTP booster
4 months	Polio vaccine, second dose; DTP	4–6 years	Polio booster; DTP booster
6 months	Polio vaccine, completed; DTP	14–16 years	Tetanus/diphtheria toxoid (adult form)
12 months	Tuberculin test	Thereafter	Tetanus/diphtheria toxoid every 10 years

Immunization Record

Enter month and year of completed series, boosters, single immunizations

Immunizations	Child	Child	Child	Child	Child	Mother	Father
DTP completed							
boosters							
polio completed							
boosters							
tuberculin test							
rubeola (measles)							
rubella (German measles)							
mumps							
tetanus/diphtheria toxoid							
other							

Periodic Physical Examinations

Name	Date	Physician/Clinic	Ht.	Wt.	Blood Pressure	Findings, Advice or Instructions

Individual Problems, Medications, Allergies

Note any medications that are taken regularly; any substances that must be avoided for medical reasons; and any allergies.

Name	Conditions	Special Instructions or Medications

Record of Family Illnesses

List accidents, surgery and illnesses, including chicken pox, mononucleosis, hepatitis, measles, rubella, mumps, strep throat and whooping cough. If there was surgery, specify what was done, and note any history of X-rays, medications and special diet. A record of blood transfusions is vital for a woman who is Rh negative.

Name	Date	Nature of Illness, Injury of Surgery	Physician	Office, Clinic, Hospital	Treatment

Health and Accident Insurance Information

Name	Policy Number	Date Issued	Company	Type of Coverage	Premium	Payments Rec'd	Payments Rec'd

Reviewing Important Concepts

1. Describe the deceptive/fraudulent sales techniques that can mislead unsuspecting and poorly informed consumers.

2. What consumer skills can be learned and practiced to minimize the probability of being ``ripped off''?

3. Your textbook describes many of the problems related to the delivery of health care in the U.S. Briefly describe at least five of these barriers which prevent effective and efficient delivery of health care services to all Americans.

4. There are many mechanisms for paying for health care received in the U.S. Briefly describe both the public and private mechanisms available.

Applying What You've Learned

1. Your friend Paul has just been ``suckered'' into purchasing a set of contact lenses and two pairs of sunglasses. The contacts were advertised for $49.95. Paul walked out of the store with a bill for $250.00. To top it all, the sunglasses are in colors he doesn't like. As you listen to Paul's experience, you realize he is in dire need of some consumer skills to defend himself in the marketplace.
   Describe how Paul could have used the following skills when he went shopping for his contacts: assertiveness, bargaining and bidding, budgeting, comparison shopping, data collection.

2. Dissatisfied with a health product or service? Write a letter using the space below. Be brief, to the point, and include the pertinent facts. State your proposal for a fair and just settlement.

3. Locate a recent newspaper or magazine article that discusses a new ``scientific'' finding regarding a health topic (for example: diet, diseases and cures, exercise). List the questions a responsible, well-informed consumer would ask himself or herself after reading the article. Answer the questions with regard to your article. How do you now interpret the new scientific findings?

Stages of Change

As a student, health care may not seem like something you need to be concerned about. But it is likely that you or someone close to you will need to become involved in the health care system within the next few years. When that time comes you will be at a great advantage if you are well informed. Answer these four questions to assess your current stage of change related to knowledge about health care.

1. I have been involved with action to promote health care for more than six months.

2. I have started to become active in health care issues in the past six months.

3. I am preparing to become involved in health care issues within the next month.

4. I would like to gain knowledge about health care issues and become involved in the next six months.

Scoring

No to all statements	Precontemplation
Yes to statement 4	Contemplation
Yes to statement 3	Preparation
Yes to statement 2	Action
Yes to statement 1	Maintenance

Review table 17.4 of *Connections for Health* for tips on becoming knowledgeable about the health care system and working toward access to health care for all.

For Further Study

As a consumer, you have many resources available to assist you—but you need to know where to find them. In addition, there are many consumer skills that can be learned and practiced to minimize being ``ripped off.'' The activities that follow will help you achieve ``self-advocacy,'' an important attitude for consumers to possess that can lead to high-level wellness.

Wellness Activities

1. Take an assertiveness course offered by your university or continuing adult education program. Practice your assertiveness skills by role playing with a friend. Be creative and think of different situations, real or imagined.
2. Compare five advertisements for various health products. What types of marketing techniques are used to sell these products?
3. Are you ``blindly'' loyal to certain brand name healthcare products? Make a list of the over-the-counter drugs (analgesics, cough syrups, etc.), skin care products and hair care products you use. Why did you buy each particular brand? List your reasons, then decide if you have ``blind loyalty'' to each product. What other products, if any, could you buy instead that would work just as well?
4. Take a first-aid class offered by your school or the American Red Cross to develop your self-care skills.
5. Donate blood at your local blood bank, hospital, or American Red Cross. What's done with the blood after you donate it? What tests are conducted to screen for infectious diseases such as AIDS or hepatitis?
6. Many hospitals have physician referral systems to help you select a doctor. Choose a hospital in your area that offers this service. (The service is free.) Phone the receptionist and ask how the system is set up. What kinds of information do they keep on each doctor? What are the most common questions asked? How many calls do they get each week? Would this be the single best way to select a physician? Why?
7. In order to get a ``handle'' on hospital costs in your area, survey several hospitals. Ask the price of regular rooms, intensive care rooms, routine blood tests, etc. Write a brief report describing your findings.
8. Learn how to take your own blood pressure. Contact your campus wellness center or the American Heart Association. How has this learning experience changed your perception of self-care? Describe what impact this learning experience has had on your life.

Aging . . . Where Do You Stand?

The challenge of high-level wellness doesn't end when you turn 30, 50, or 65—it continues through all stages of your life. This challenge will require you to cope with changes in your physical, social, and economic status, in addition to environmental changes in the world. Where do you stand now with regard to aging well? This chapter will help you answer this question.

Aging Well

Look at the line below. At the far left, place today's date and your current age. On the extreme right end of the line, record what you think is a ``ripe old age,'' an age that you feel you can achieve—with a little luck and a lot of good living. On the line between the two extremes, you will notice five goals. In the space provided below, write down five things you would like to accomplish before you leave this good life.

Your Age and Today's Date 5-6-99 19 yrs. old.   Five Goals 1 2 3 4 5   90 yrs.   Ripe Old Age

Goals:

1. Get married
2. Have 2-3 more children
3. Have a home built in the country.
4. Live economically well.
5. Stay married to Mike until death.

   What did you write for a ripe old age? Sixty-five? Ninety? From the physiological point of view, most authorities agree that the human body is capable of achieving the ripe old age of 120 years. After that, there are no guarantees. Naturally, most of us will be struck down before that age due to disease, injury, accidents, or a score of other perils of this life. But 120 years is your ultimate potential, and many people may realistically expect to achieve the age of 100. So, as you go about achieving the five goals you identified on the continuum above, add a sixth goal: to live long and well.

Source: From C.T. Kuntzelman, *Living Well Workbook,* 1981. Reprinted by permission of Livingwell, Inc., Houston, TX.

Age, Prejudice, and Discrimination

In each of the following situations, two people are listed as having asked you for your advice and opinion. In the space provided, write how you would respond to each person.

What would you do if:

1. She came to you and said she was contemplating marriage?

    Your 21-year-old niece: _go for it_

    Your 71-year-old grandmother: _____

2. He told you he wanted to become a nurse?

    Your 21-year-old nephew: _____

    Your 60-year-old uncle: _____

3. He said he wanted to learn how to bowl?

    Your 18-year-old cousin: _____

    Your 80-year-old father: _____

4. He said he was joining an art class?

    Your 16-year-old brother: _____

    Your 73-year-old grandfather: _____

5. She was planning to campaign actively for a presidential candidate?

    Your 22-year-old niece: _____

    Your 75-year-old friend: _____

6. She was going to start college after being out of school for years?

    Your 36-year-old aunt: _____

    Your 60-year-old aunt: _____

7. She wanted to learn a trade?

    Your 20-year-old sister: _____

    Your 65-year-old mother: _____

8. She started coming home at 2:00 or 3:00 in the morning?

    Your 21-year-old sister: _____

    Your 70-year-old grandmother: _____

9. He became an old-movie buff and started to travel around to see old movies wherever they were shown?

    Your 16-year-old brother: _____

    Your 60-year-old grandfather: _____

10. All he ever did for recreation was play cards?

Your 25-year-old cousin: _____

Your 70-year-old uncle: _____

In which of the situations did your answers vary the most? Why do you believe the variance occurred?

Did your answer vary by whether the person was related to you or not?

What criteria (besides age) did you use in responding to the individuals' requests?

If you were the older person in each situation, what response would you prefer?

Reviewing Important Concepts

1. Primary aging is the unavoidable result of chronology that affects all species. Briefly describe the biological changes that occur in humans as they age.

2. Although everyone experiences some degree of change as a result of aging, these changes do not necessarily have to impact negatively on mental and physical wellness. Describe the adaptations one can make to reduce the negative effects of aging.

3. Good health accompanied by a comfortable life-style is a fundamental goal for most people regardless of age. However, this basic need is not always easily fulfilled for some older adults. Describe the personal and social barriers to wellness that many older adults experience.

Applying What You've Learned

1. Imagine for a moment that you are capable of seeing into the future.
    A. Picture in your mind a typical afternoon during your seventy-fifth year. In the space below draw a picture of yourself. Include your surroundings, your activities, any people or companions who are with you, and your physical appearance. Be as detailed as possible.

    B. Now evaluate your drawing, and consider the following facts:
        1. Of men over 65, 85 percent have living spouses. Of women over 65, only 40 percent have living spouses. Did you include a spouse in the picture?
        2. Contrary to popular opinion, only a small proportion of elderly (about 5 percent) live in institutions. Where were you living?
        3. Of all people, 65 and older, only about 14 percent are active in the work force. Did you picture yourself as working?
        4. Although most persons past 65 retain hearing sufficient for normal activities, the aged are three times more likely than younger persons to have a significant hearing loss. Did you depict yourself with a hearing aid?

The quality of your later life is largely dependent on how you take care of yourself today. How are you going to prepare yourself for high-level wellness in later life?

Source: From R. Reed-Flora and T.A. Long, *Health Behaviors,* 1982, West Publishing Company.

2. Appropriate adaptations in your home environment can reduce the negative effects of aging and improve safety. Place yourself 40 years into the future. Look around your home and list the changes that you would make so that your adaptation to the aging process was positive and enhanced your wellness. Be sure to check your entrance ways!

3. Research has delineated at least four predominant patterns of successful aging high in life satisfaction. Using these theories, describe what steps you can take now so that you can have a high level of life satisfaction as you grow older.

4. You have been asked to give a brief presentation to a group of middle-aged adults. The goal of this presentation is to teach the participants how to avoid disability in the later years. Identify the thirteen risk factors discussed in your textbook. Briefly explain what each person can do to minimize their risk so they can achieve a high level of wellness in later years.

Stages of Change

Have you ever helped an elderly relative or friend? Younger people can do a great deal to help older adults with daily tasks or by just being a friend. But sometimes the generation gap can seem wide. Answer these four questions to assess your current stage of change related to becoming a supporter of the elderly.

1. I have been helping an older person regularly for more than six months.

2. I have started helping an older person within the past six months.

3. I am preparing to start supporting an older person in the next month.

4. I would like to start helping an older person within the next six months.

Scoring

No to all statements	Precontemplation
Yes to statement 4	Contemplation
Yes to statement 3	Preparation
Yes to statement 2	Action
Yes to statement 1	Maintenance

Review table 18.5 of *Connections for Health* for tips on becoming a supportive caregiver to the elderly.

For Further Study

Living longer enhances the probability of having to cope with change and make adaptations to maximize the quality of life. The activities below will help you prepare for these changes and adaptations so you can achieve high-level wellness in later life.

Wellness Activities

1. Norma Farber, a grandmother, wrote a children's book, *How Does It Feel to Be Old?* (E. P. Dutton, 1979) which explains how it feels to be old. Read this book and describe how it has changed your ideas of old age (if at all).

2. Does old age mean you're useless, boring, and retired? Here's a list of a few people who were achievers in advanced age:

   At 100, Grandma Moses was painting.
   At 91, Adolph Zukor was chairman of Paramount Pictures.
   At 85, Coco Chanel was the head of a fashion design firm.
   At 81, Benjamin Franklin effected the compromise that led to the adoption of the U.S. Constitution.

   Go to the library and see if you can find five more people who were achievers in advanced age.

3. Visit a retirement community near your home. What types of people are living there? Strike up a conversation with some of the residents. How do they spend their time? Why did they decide to move there? What are the advantages and disadvantages of living in this retirement community?

4. Describe the services available to assist older adults in your community. How are these services funded and staffed? Who is eligible to receive these services?

5. Talk with a retirement planner about planning for your retirement. What advice does the retirement planner give you? When are you going to begin to implement your plan?

6. Conduct a life review with an older person. Begin the interview with childhood memories and talk about each life stage. Would this person live his/her life any differently? What advice can they give you about enjoying life to the fullest? Record your conversation, then write a summary including your impressions on the aging process. Remember to give a copy to your interviewee.

7. Aging brings about significant biological changes. Try one of the exercises below to gain insight into how an older person has to adapt their life-style to accommodate these changes. (The change the activity simulates is in parentheses.)

   a. Turn your thermostat down to 63 degrees. (Decreased basal metabolic rate)
   b. Wear gloves for an entire day. Try opening a ``childproof'' container. (Decreased feeling in fingers)
   c. Put small balls of tin foil in your shoes. (Arthritis)
   d. Cook a meal without using any additional seasonings. Make sure there is no salt added to canned items. (Decreased taste)
   e. Borrow a pair of eyeglasses that distort your depth perception. Try climbing stairs or crossing a street while your vision is affected. Be careful—take someone with you when you try this! (Depth perception)

8. High health care costs are a barrier to high-level wellness for an older adult. Survey local nursing homes and home health agencies in your community. How much do these services cost? What services do they provide? Do they take patients with Alzheimer's disease?

19   Ecology: Establishing a Healthy Environment

Ecology . . . Where Do You Stand?

Environmental sensitivity is an important dimension of high-level wellness. People erroneously believe that there is nothing they can do about the environmental crisis. However, you can play an important and significant role in improving the health of the environment, thereby improving your level of wellness.

Everywhere you turn, someone is talking about an environmental problem they say is the most critical. Which environmental problems do we concern ourselves with? Experts say we may be angry and frightened about the wrong environmental risks. They say that the risks that are killing us are ones which the public (for the most part) is not that concerned about. Complete the activity below and find out how you and experts rate the health risks associated with environmental problems.

Rating Risks

How do you rate health risks associated with environmental problems? The following is a list of health risks associated with environmental problems. Rate each risk using the following categories: high, medium, medium-to-low, low. Write your rating in the blank to the right.

Environmental Problem	Your Rating	EPA Rating
1. Hazardous waste sites		
2. Exposure to work-site chemicals		
3. Industrial pollution of waterways		
4. Nuclear accident radiation		
5. Radioactive waste		
6. Chemical leaks from underground storage tanks		
7. Pesticides		
8. Pollution from industrial accidents		
9. Water pollution from farm run-off		
10. Tap-water contamination		
11. Industrial air pollution		
12. Ozone-layer destruction		
13. Coastal-water contamination		
14. Sewage-plant contamination		
15. Vehicle exhaust		
16. Oil spills		
17. Acid rain		
18. Water pollution from urban run-off		
19. Damaged wetlands		
20. Genetic alteration		

Environmental Problem	Your Rating	EPA Rating
21. Nonhazardous waste sites	_____	_____
22. Greenhouse effect	_____	_____
23. Indoor air pollution	_____	_____
24. X-ray radiation	_____	_____
25. Indoor radon	_____	_____
26. Microwave oven radiation	_____	_____

The list you just reviewed is from a recent national opinion poll by the Roper Organization. The items are listed according to **how the American public rated** twenty-six health risks associated with environmental problems. In 1987, a task force of U.S. Environmental Protection Agency officials rated health risks associated with environmental problems. (Four of the risks were not rated.) Below you'll find how the EPA officials rated the risks.

EPA Rating	*Question Numbers*
High	2, 7, 10, 11, 12, 15, 17, 23, 25
Medium	9, 18
Medium-to-low	1, 6, 8, 14, 16, 21
Low	3, 13, 19, 20, 22
Not ranked	4, 5, 24, 26

Transfer the EPA ratings to the column labeled ``EPA rating'' in the list above. Place an asterisk (*) next to the items which you and the EPA agree on. Review how you rated the risks and how the EPA rated the risks. Answer the questions that follow.

1. Briefly explain how your ratings differ from the EPA's. Why do you believe your ratings differed?

2. Of the risks ranked ``high'' by the EPA, which are risks that affect your personal environment (i.e., where you live or go to school)?

3. Of the risks ranked ``high'' by you, which are risks that affect your personal environment (i.e., where you live or go to school)?

4. Which of the environmental problems identified in questions 2 and 3 would you be willing to spend your time and energy on in order to help the environment?

5.   Identify three actions which you could take to lessen the impact of this environmental problem.

From *American Healthy,* © 1990 by Christine Russell. Reprinted by permission.

Reviewing Important Concepts

1.   Explain the inherent dangers at each extreme of the adaptation continuum. What skills have we lost or never learned as a result of our technology and dependency on institutions?

2.   What are Barry Commoner's Four Laws of Ecology? Give examples of each law as it relates to your environment.

Applying What You've Learned

1.   Rifkin challenges us to ``take an entire day to observe everything you come in contact with: things you see, hear, touch, smell, feel, or consume; things that you change; and things you exchange. Then try to trace each experience or item in both directions, back to its original source and forward to its final destination.''
       List two items or experiences that occur in your day. Trace each back to its original source and forward to its final destination. What Law of Ecology has each item/experience affected?

2. In order to maintain a sustainable earth society, we need to be located approximately between 2.0 and 3.5 on the Adaptation Continuum. What changes, if any, would *you* have to make in order to locate yourself on the continuum between these two points?

3. Save all of your trash and recyclables for one week. Answer the questions that follow.
    a. PACKAGING—Examine the packaging you threw away. Identify at least three products that contain excess packaging. Are there similar products you could purchase that use less? List your options for each product.

    b. RECYCLABLES—Identify and list the items that you could recycle.

    plastic
    glass
    paper
    metal
    cardboard

    c. PLASTICS—Even though plastics are recyclable, their production generates hazardous waste. Are there any products you could stop buying in order to reduce plastic production?

    d. AEROSOL SPRAY PRODUCTS—Which of these products are available in pump bottles rather than in aerosol cans? Which of these products could you do without?

e. JUNK MAIL—How much junk mail are you receiving? Weigh it to find out.

f. FOOD WASTES—What kinds of food and how much of it are you throwing away? How can you reduce or eliminate this type of waste?

Stages of Change

Do you care about our environment? Many college students are very concerned about the future of the earth and the kind of world we will leave our children. Just think about the impact students could have if they all became advocates for the environment. Answer these four questions to assess your current stage of change related to becoming an environmental advocate.

1. I have been actively advocating for the environment for more than six months.

2. I have started to become an environmental advocate within the past six months.

3. I am preparing to become an advocate within the next month.

4. I would like to start advocating for the environment within the next six months.

Scoring

No to all statements	Precontemplation
Yes to statement 4	Contemplation
Yes to statement 3	Preparation
Yes to statement 2	Action
Yes to statement 1	Maintenance

Review table 19.9 of *Connections for Health* for tips on moving through the stages of change and becoming involved with environmental policy issues.

For Further Study

The quality of our environment rests heavily on what we, as individuals, are willing to do. Where do you begin? What changes can you make that will help move us toward a sustainable earth society? The activities listed below can help you on your way toward high-level wellness.

Wellness Activities

1. Make a list of the environmental changes you want on your campus. How do you propose to change the attitudes of unconcerned students so that they will feel more responsible for how the campus appears?

   What do you believe the college administrators can do to improve the campus environment? What do you believe the faculty should do to improve the campus environment? How can the student government become actively involved on a day-to-day basis with enforcing environmental rules and regulations on the campus?

   Does your campus have an environmental policy that is written and included in the student and faculty handbook? If not, investigate why not. If so, is it up to date?

   Source: Carter, G. F., and Wilson, S. B. *My Health Status*. Minneapolis, Minn.: Burgess Publishing Co., 1982.

2. Industrial consumption patterns are often wasteful and do not follow nature's patterns, thus having a great negative impact on the environment. There are many political action groups whose purpose is to reverse the negative effect of industry and work for a sustainable earth society.

   Listed below are six environmental action groups. Write to one of these organizations and find out what it is doing to ``clean up'' our environment.

   Environmental Defense Fund
   1616 P St., N.W., Suite 150
   Washington, D.C. 20036

   Worldwatch Institute
   1776 Massachusetts Ave.
   Washington, D.C. 20036

   Environmental Action
   Foundation (EAF)
   1525 New Hampshire Ave., N.W.
   Washington, D.C. 20036

   National Coalition Against
   the Misuse of Pesticides
   530 7th St., S.E.
   Washington, D.C. 20003

   Citizen's Clearinghouse
   for Hazardous Waste
   P.O. Box 926
   Arlington, Va. 22216

   Greenhouse Crisis Foundation
   1130 17th St., N.W., Suite 630
   Washington, D.C. 20036

3. Collect aluminum cans from along a road and bring them to a recycling machine or recycling center. How much money were the cans worth? What types of cans did you find? What other types of litter did you notice on the roadside?

4. Today, it is very easy to forget what ``energy-saving'' devices and items we could actually do without. Look through your kitchen and bathroom cabinets, and identify those items that represent created needs. How easy would it be for you to give up using these items? What would you use instead?

5. It has been said that radon is our worst radiation hazard. Radon is colorless, odorless and tasteless. The only way to tell if your house has a dangerously high level of radon gas is to test it. Write for the publication ``A Citizen's Guide to Radon: What It Is and What to Do About It'' (OPA-86-004) from the Superintendent of Documents, U.S. Government Printing Office, Washington, D.C. 20402. Read the booklet and then test your home. What are the results? What action, if any, do you need to take?

6. What recycling efforts are being implemented in your community? Do you have a recycling center or curb-side recycling? What items do they recycle? Find out what impact recycling has on the landfills in your areas.

7. STOP JUNK MAIL! According to the authors of *50 Simple Things You Can Do To Save the Earth* (Earthworks Press, 1989), if you save up all the junk mail you receive in one year it would be the equivalent of one and a half trees. Write to Mail Preference Service, Direct Marketing Assn., 11 West 42nd St., P.O. Box 3861, New York, N.Y. 10163-3861, and request that your name not be added to any new mailing lists. You'll have to write to individual companies that are currently sending you mail to have your name removed from their lists.

8. Many consumers are looking for products marked ``recyclable'' or ``biodegradable.'' Two nonprofit groups that are working toward eco-labeling are Green Seal (Palo Alto, Calif.) and Green Cross Certification Co. (Oakland, Calif.). Write to one or both of these groups, and answer the following questions. What is the group

trying to accomplish? What kind of label is the group designing? How does a product qualify for one of these labels? How is the accuracy of an eco-label certified? How soon will consumers see these labels on products? What makes this label and the group behind it trustworthy?

Appendix A: Wellness Project

The Wellness Project will help you develop and implement a plan that will enable you to improve the behavior you identified in chapter 1. You will be asked to implement the plan for two weeks during the semester. We hope that you will continue to improve the behavior for a longer period of time and make it part of your life-style. In addition, we encourage you to use this process with other life-style behaviors and continue your quest for high-level wellness.

It is important for you to familiarize yourself with the entire project before beginning. Take a moment right now to read the descriptions of each phase and review the wellness contract that follows. A sample wellness contract is provided at the end of this appendix (A). If you have any questions, ask your instructor.

Area for Improvement

By completing the exercises in chapter 1, you identified a behavior for improvement. Enter the behavior you wish to improve in the blank provided on the wellness contract.

Goal

In broad, general terms, describe your goal in the blanks provided on the wellness contract.

Current Status

Refer to your textbook and workbook. Use the information in the personal assessments to describe your current status in the blanks provided on the wellness contract.

Research

Read text chapter that pertains to my goal & summarize. (ch. 2)

Before you can develop your plan of action, you will have to identify resources and review the literature related to your area of improvement. By reviewing the appropriate literature, you will increase your knowledge about the behavior you have chosen to improve.

1. Locate at least four articles from professional journals and books that relate to your goal. You may find that you will have to use more than four articles in order to get the information you need. You can use your textbook as one of the resources. (See the recommended readings in your textbook and this workbook.) Enter the references under the heading titled ``Resources.''
2. Review each article using ``Applying Critical Thinking Approaches to Reports of Health News'' in chapter 1 of this workbook as a guide.
3. Write a short summary of each article. Briefly discuss the credibility of the source, factors in the study design and interpretation of results (if applicable), and how the article applies to your goal.
4. After reviewing and synthesizing all the information, write a brief paper that answers the following questions:
   a. What strategies do the experts suggest you can use to improve this area of wellness?
   b. Does the literature suggest that there may be risks associated with this behavior? If so, explain the risks.
   c. Does the literature suggest benefits associated with this behavior? If so, explain the benefits.
5. Attach your findings to the wellness project so that your instructor can review them.

Turn in one page of notes from chapter. front & back.

Objectives

After reviewing the literature, you are ready to plan your two-week behavior change project. Begin by stating your objectives and outlining the specific steps you will take to accomplish your goal. These steps, which you will record in a journal (described below), will be used as standards for judging the success of your project. The objectives should be measurable.

Make sure your plan is realistic and based on sound information. Write your objectives in the space provided on the wellness contract.

Scheduling

A change in behavior requires a change in your schedule. Scheduling describes how you plan to rearrange your commitments and time so that you can achieve your objectives. For each objective you stated, you should list a day, time, and place when you will accomplish it. Enter your schedule in the blanks provided on the wellness contract.

Reinforcing and Enabling Factors

Reinforcing and enabling factors are those factors you identified in chapter 1 (Supports and Barriers-to-Action) that will support you and help you achieve your goal. List these factors in the space provided on the wellness contract.

Barriers

Barriers are the factors you identified in chapter 1 (Supports and Barriers-to-Action) that may be roadblocks to your wellness goal. List these factors in the space provided on the wellness contract.

Your Commitment

Before you begin your project, you need to identify a time period during which you will carry out your objectives. The minimum time commitment should be two weeks. However, we encourage you to carry out your project for as long as possible.

In addition to specifying a time period, you need to identify a supporter: someone you choose to help you meet your goal. Explain to your supporter what you are trying to accomplish and identify ways your supporter can help you be successful in your efforts.

Both you and your supporter need to sign the wellness project. Submit the contract to your instructor for comment and approval.

Wellness Journal

DO NOT DO Journal!!

YOU ARE READY TO BEGIN! In order to document your progress and experiences, you will need to keep a wellness journal. The wellness journal is a day-by-day account of your implementation of the contract. Use a daily diary to record your feelings as you go through the behavior change process. You will also want to keep a chart, where appropriate, to monitor your progress.

Summary of Wellness Journal

DO not DO

Write a summary of your experience. Identify the reasons for your successes and failures. Discuss the possibility of continuing this project and having it become part of your life-style. What factors will influence you to continue this project? What factors may prove to be roadblocks?

Personal Wellness Contract

Area for Improvement: _____

Goal: _____

Current Status:

_____

_____

_____

Resources:

_____

_____

_____

_____

_____

_____

_____

_____

Objectives:

_____

_____

_____

_____

_____

_____

Scheduling:

_____

_____

_____

_____

_____

Reinforcing and Enabling Factors:

_____

_____

_____

Barriers:

_____

_____

_____

I will complete this action between _____ and _____.

_____   _____
           My signature   My supporter's signature

Personal Wellness Contract

Area for improvement: _stress/environment_

Goal: to reduce my stress level

Current Status:

My dorm room is a mess. I feel uncomfortable (stressed) whenever I'm there. I suffer from several of the signs of stress listed in the Stress Symptom Inventory in the work book. It's hard for me to study because the room is disorganized and cluttered. After reading Chapter 19 of the textbook, I realize my room is an example of the second law of thermodynamics — entropy.

Resources:

1. Lakein, A. How to Get Control of Your Time and Your Life. New York: Signet Books, 1975.

2. Tubesing, D. and Tubesing, N. Healthy Balance: A Do It Yourself Guide to Whole Person Wellbeing. Minneapolis, Minn.: Augsburg Publishing House, 1991.

3. Winston, S. Getting Organized. The Easy Way to Put Your Life in Order. New York: Warner Books, 1979.

4. Mullen, D., Gold, R., Belcastro, P., and McDermott, R. Connections for Health, 3rd ed. Dubuque, Iowa: Wm. C. Brown Publishers, 1992.

Objectives:

1. I will completely clean my room (spring cleaning).

2. I will hang/put away my clothes whenever I change them.

3. I will make my bed each morning.

4. Instead of stacking papers and things, I will put them in the appropriate place the first time.

Scheduling:

1. Spring cleaning—next Saturday from 8:30 — 10:30 a.m.
2. Take an extra 5 minutes at night before I get into bed to put clothes in closet or hamper.
3. Make bed before I shower in the morning.
4. Set my alarm 10 minutes earlier.

Reinforcing and Enabling Factors:

1. I used to be more organized, I know I can be again.
2. I don't have a roommate to contribute to my messiness.
3. I don't like this feel of being stressed out when I'm in my room.
4. My friend Lindsey will check on my room once a day and motivate me to meet my objectives.

Barriers:

1. I don't have a roommate to nag me into organization.
2. I'm lazy and tired at night.
3. I usually run late in the mornings.

I will complete this action between ___ May 1 ___ and ___ May 14 ___

___ Gina Lazzara ___
My signature

___ Lindsey Annerino ___
My supporter's signature

B Nutritive Values of Food

Table 2. Nutritive Value of the Edible Part of Food
(Tr indicates nutrient present in trace amount.)

Item No.	Foods, approximate measures, units, and weight (weight of edible portion only)			Water	Food energy	Pro-tein	Fat	Fatty acids		
								Satu-rated	Mono-unsatu-rated	Poly-unsatu-rated
	Beverages		Grams	Per-cent	Cal-ories	Grams	Grams	Grams	Grams	Grams
	Alcoholic:									
	Beer:									
1	Regular----------------------	12 fl oz---------	360	92	150	1	0	0.0	0.0	0.0
2	Light------------------------	12 fl oz---------	355	95	95	1	0	0.0	0.0	0.0
	Gin, rum, vodka, whiskey:									
3	80-proof---------------------	1-1/2 fl oz-----	42	67	95	0	0	0.0	0.0	0.0
4	86-proof---------------------	1-1/2 fl oz-----	42	64	105	0	0	0.0	0.0	0.0
5	90-proof---------------------	1-1/2 fl oz-----	42	62	110	0	0	0.0	0.0	0.0
	Wines:									
6	Dessert----------------------	3-1/2 fl oz-----	103	77	140	Tr	0	0.0	0.0	0.0
	Table:									
7	Red-------------------------	3-1/2 fl oz-----	102	88	75	Tr	0	0.0	0.0	0.0
8	White-----------------------	3-1/2 fl oz-----	102	87	80	Tr	0	0.0	0.0	0.0
	Carbonated:[2]									
9	Club soda--------------------	12 fl oz---------	355	100	0	0	0	0.0	0.0	0.0
	Cola type:									
10	Regular----------------------	12 fl oz---------	369	89	160	0	0	0.0	0.0	0.0
11	Diet, artificially sweetened	12 fl oz---------	355	100	Tr	0	0	0.0	0.0	0.0
12	Ginger ale--------------------	12 fl oz---------	366	91	125	0	0	0.0	0.0	0.0
13	Grape------------------------	12 fl oz---------	372	88	180	0	0	0.0	0.0	0.0
14	Lemon-lime--------------------	12 fl oz---------	372	89	155	0	0	0.0	0.0	0.0
15	Orange-----------------------	12 fl oz---------	372	88	180	0	0	0.0	0.0	0.0
16	Pepper type------------------	12 fl oz---------	369	89	160	0	0	0.0	0.0	0.0
17	Root beer--------------------	12 fl oz---------	370	89	165	0	0	0.0	0.0	0.0
	Cocoa and chocolate-flavored beverages. See Dairy Products (items 95-98).									
	Coffee:									
18	Brewed-----------------------	6 fl oz---------	180	100	Tr	Tr	Tr	Tr	Tr	Tr
19	Instant, prepared (2 tsp powder plus 6 fl oz water)----------	6 fl oz---------	182	99	Tr	Tr	Tr	Tr	Tr	Tr
	Fruit drinks, noncarbonated:									
	Canned:									
20	Fruit punch drink------------	6 fl oz---------	190	88	85	Tr	0	0.0	0.0	0.0
21	Grape drink------------------	6 fl oz---------	187	86	100	Tr	0	0.0	0.0	0.0
22	Pineapple-grapefruit juice drink---------------------	6 fl oz---------	187	87	90	Tr	Tr	Tr	Tr	Tr
	Frozen:									
	Lemonade concentrate:									
23	Undiluted------------------	6-fl-oz can-----	219	49	425	Tr	Tr	Tr	Tr	Tr
24	Diluted with 4-1/3 parts water by volume----------	6 fl oz---------	185	89	80	Tr	Tr	Tr	Tr	Tr
	Limeade concentrate:									
25	Undiluted------------------	6-fl-oz can-----	218	50	410	Tr	Tr	Tr	Tr	Tr
26	Diluted with 4-1/3 parts water by volume----------	6 fl oz---------	185	89	75	Tr	Tr	Tr	Tr	Tr
	Fruit juices. See type under Fruits and Fruit Juices.									
	Milk beverages. See Dairy Products (items 92-105).									
	Tea:									
27	Brewed-----------------------	8 fl oz---------	240	100	Tr	Tr	Tr	Tr	Tr	Tr
	Instant, powder, prepared:									
28	Unsweetened (1 tsp powder plus 8 fl oz water)--------	8 fl oz---------	241	100	Tr	Tr	Tr	Tr	Tr	Tr
29	Sweetened (3 tsp powder plus 8 fl oz water)-------------	8 fl oz---------	262	91	85	Tr	Tr	Tr	Tr	Tr

[1]Value not determined.
[2]Mineral content varies depending on water source.

166

Nutrients in Indicated Quantity

Cholesterol	Carbohydrate	Calcium	Phosphorus	Iron	Potassium	Sodium	Vitamin A value		Thiamin	Riboflavin	Niacin	Ascorbic acid	Item No.
							(IU)	(RE)					
Milligrams	Grams	Milligrams	Milligrams	Milligrams	Milligrams	Milligrams	International units	Retinol equivalents	Milligrams	Milligrams	Milligrams	Milligrams	
0	13	14	50	0.1	115	18	0	0	0.02	0.09	1.8	0	1
0	5	14	43	0.1	64	11	0	0	0.03	0.11	1.4	0	2
0	Tr	Tr	Tr	Tr	1	Tr	0	0	Tr	Tr	Tr	0	3
0	Tr	Tr	Tr	Tr	1	Tr	0	0	Tr	Tr	Tr	0	4
0	Tr	Tr	Tr	Tr	1	Tr	0	0	Tr	Tr	Tr	0	5
0	8	8	9	0.2	95	9	(1)	(1)	0.01	0.02	0.2	0	6
0	3	8	18	0.4	113	5	(1)	(1)	0.00	0.03	0.1	0	7
0	3	9	14	0.3	83	5	(1)	(1)	0.00	0.01	0.1	0	8
0	0	18	0	Tr	0	78	0	0	0.00	0.00	0.0	0	9
0	41	11	52	0.2	7	18	0	0	0.00	0.00	0.0	0	10
0	Tr	14	39	0.2	7	3 32	0	0	0.00	0.00	0.0	0	11
0	32	11	0	0.1	4	29	0	0	0.00	0.00	0.0	0	12
0	46	15	0	0.4	4	48	0	0	0.00	0.00	0.0	0	13
0	39	7	0	0.4	4	33	0	0	0.00	0.00	0.0	0	14
0	46	15	4	0.3	7	52	0	0	0.00	0.00	0.0	0	15
0	41	11	41	0.1	4	37	0	0	0.00	0.00	0.0	0	16
0	42	15	0	0.2	4	48	0	0	0.00	0.00	0.0	0	17
0	Tr	4	2	Tr	124	2	0	0	0.00	0.02	0.4	0	18
0	1	2	6	0.1	71	Tr	0	0	0.00	0.03	0.6	0	19
0	22	15	2	0.4	48	15	20	2	0.03	0.04	Tr	4 61	20
0	26	2	2	0.3	9	11	Tr	Tr	0.01	0.01	Tr	4 64	21
0	23	13	7	0.9	97	24	60	6	0.06	0.04	0.5	4 110	22
0	112	9	13	0.4	153	4	40	4	0.04	0.07	0.7	66	23
0	21	2	2	0.1	30	1	10	1	0.01	0.02	0.2	13	24
0	108	11	13	0.2	129	Tr	Tr	Tr	0.02	0.02	0.2	26	25
0	20	2	2	Tr	24	Tr	Tr	Tr	Tr	Tr	Tr	4	26
0	Tr	0	2	Tr	36	1	0	0	0.00	0.03	Tr	0	27
0	1	1	4	Tr	61	1	0	0	0.00	0.02	0.1	0	28
0	22	1	3	Tr	49	Tr	0	0	0.00	0.04	0.1	0	29

[3] Blend of aspartame and saccharin; if only sodium saccharin is used, sodium is 75 mg; if only aspartame is used, sodium is 23 mg.

[4] With added ascorbic acid.

Item No.	Foods, approximate measures, units, and weight (weight of edible portion only)			Water	Food energy	Pro-tein	Fat	Fatty acids		
								Satu-rated	Mono-unsatu-rated	Poly-unsatu-rated
			Grams	Per-cent	Cal-ories	Grams	Grams	Grams	Grams	Grams
	Dairy Products									
	Butter. See Fats and Oils (items 128-130).									
	Cheese:									
	Natural:									
30	Blue-----------------------	1 oz------------	28	42	100	6	8	5.3	2.2	0.2
31	Camembert (3 wedges per 4-oz container)-----------------	1 wedge-------	38	52	115	8	9	5.8	2.7	0.3
	Cheddar:									
32	Cut pieces------------------	1 oz------------	28	37	115	7	9	6.0	2.7	0.3
33		1 in³----------	17	37	70	4	6	3.6	1.6	0.2
34	Shredded--------------------	1 cup-----------	113	37	455	28	37	23.8	10.6	1.1
	Cottage (curd not pressed down):									
	Creamed (cottage cheese, 4% fat):									
35	Large curd---------------	1 cup-----------	225	79	235	28	10	6.4	2.9	0.3
36	Small curd---------------	1 cup-----------	210	79	215	26	9	6.0	2.7	0.3
37	With fruit---------------	1 cup-----------	226	72	280	22	8	4.9	2.2	0.2
38	Lowfat (2%)---------------	1 cup-----------	226	79	205	31	4	2.8	1.2	0.1
39	Uncreamed (cottage cheese dry curd, less than 1/2% fat)--------------------	1 cup-----------	145	80	125	25	1	0.4	0.2	Tr
40	Cream-----------------------	1 oz------------	28	54	100	2	10	6.2	2.8	0.4
41	Feta------------------------	1 oz------------	28	55	75	4	6	4.2	1.3	0.2
	Mozzarella, made with:									
42	Whole milk---------------	1 oz------------	28	54	80	6	6	3.7	1.9	0.2
43	Part skim milk (low moisture)---------------	1 oz------------	28	49	80	8	5	3.1	1.4	0.1
44	Muenster-------------------	1 oz------------	28	42	105	7	9	5.4	2.5	0.2
	Parmesan, grated:									
45	Cup, not pressed down------	1 cup-----------	100	18	455	42	30	19.1	8.7	0.7
46	Tablespoon----------------	1 tbsp----------	5	18	25	2	2	1.0	0.4	Tr
47	Ounce--------------------	1 oz------------	28	18	130	12	9	5.4	2.5	0.2
48	Provolone-------------------	1 oz------------	28	41	100	7	8	4.8	2.1	0.2
	Ricotta, made with:									
49	Whole milk---------------	1 cup-----------	246	72	430	28	32	20.4	8.9	0.9
50	Part skim milk------------	1 cup-----------	246	74	340	28	19	12.1	5.7	0.6
51	Swiss----------------------	1 oz------------	28	37	105	8	8	5.0	2.1	0.3
	Pasteurized process cheese:									
52	American-------------------	1 oz------------	28	39	105	6	9	5.6	2.5	0.3
53	Swiss----------------------	1 oz------------	28	42	95	7	7	4.5	2.0	0.2
54	Pasteurized process cheese food, American --------------	1 oz------------	28	43	95	6	7	4.4	2.0	0.2
55	Pasteurized process cheese spread, American------------	1 oz------------	28	48	80	5	6	3.8	1.8	0.2
	Cream, sweet:									
56	Half-and-half (cream and milk)	1 cup-----------	242	81	315	7	28	17.3	8.0	1.0
57		1 tbsp----------	15	81	20	Tr	2	1.1	0.5	0.1
58	Light, coffee, or table--------	1 cup-----------	240	74	470	6	46	28.8	13.4	1.7
59		1 tbsp----------	15	74	30	Tr	3	1.8	0.8	0.1
	Whipping, unwhipped (volume about double when whipped):									
60	Light-----------------------	1 cup-----------	239	64	700	5	74	46.2	21.7	2.1
61		1 tbsp----------	15	64	45	Tr	5	2.9	1.4	0.1
62	Heavy-----------------------	1 cup-----------	238	58	820	5	88	54.8	25.4	3.3
63		1 tbsp----------	15	58	50	Tr	6	3.5	1.6	0.2
64	Whipped topping, (pressurized)	1 cup-----------	60	61	155	2	13	8.3	3.9	0.5
65		1 tbsp----------	3	61	10	Tr	1	0.4	0.2	Tr
66	Cream, sour-----------------------	1 cup-----------	230	71	495	7	48	30.0	13.9	1.8
67		1 tbsp----------	12	71	25	Tr	3	1.6	0.7	0.1

168

Cholesterol	Carbohydrate	Calcium	Phosphorus	Iron	Potassium	Sodium	Vitamin A value		Thiamin	Riboflavin	Niacin	Ascorbic acid	Item No.
							(IU)	(RE)					
Milligrams	Grams	Milligrams	Milligrams	Milligrams	Milligrams	Milligrams	International units	Retinol equivalents	Milligrams	Milligrams	Milligrams	Milligrams	
21	1	150	110	0.1	73	396	200	65	0.01	0.11	0.3	0	30
27	Tr	147	132	0.1	71	320	350	96	0.01	0.19	0.2	0	31
30	Tr	204	145	0.2	28	176	300	86	0.01	0.11	Tr	0	32
18	Tr	123	87	0.1	17	105	180	52	Tr	0.06	Tr	0	33
119	1	815	579	0.8	111	701	1,200	342	0.03	0.42	0.1	0	34
34	6	135	297	0.3	190	911	370	108	0.05	0.37	0.3	Tr	35
31	6	126	277	0.3	177	850	340	101	0.04	0.34	0.3	Tr	36
25	30	108	236	0.2	151	915	280	81	0.04	0.29	0.2	Tr	37
19	8	155	340	0.4	217	918	160	45	0.05	0.42	0.3	Tr	38
10	3	46	151	0.3	47	19	40	12	0.04	0.21	0.2	0	39
31	1	23	30	0.3	34	84	400	124	Tr	0.06	Tr	0	40
25	1	140	96	0.2	18	316	130	36	0.04	0.24	0.3	0	41
22	1	147	105	0.1	19	106	220	68	Tr	0.07	Tr	0	42
15	1	207	149	0.1	27	150	180	54	0.01	0.10	Tr	0	43
27	Tr	203	133	0.1	38	178	320	90	Tr	0.09	Tr	0	44
79	4	1,376	807	1.0	107	1,861	700	173	0.05	0.39	0.3	0	45
4	Tr	69	40	Tr	5	93	40	9	Tr	0.02	Tr	0	46
22	1	390	229	0.3	30	528	200	49	0.01	0.11	0.1	0	47
20	1	214	141	0.1	39	248	230	75	0.01	0.09	Tr	0	48
124	7	509	389	0.9	257	207	1,210	330	0.03	0.48	0.3	0	49
76	13	669	449	1.1	307	307	1,060	278	0.05	0.46	0.2	0	50
26	1	272	171	Tr	31	74	240	72	0.01	0.10	Tr	0	51
27	Tr	174	211	0.1	46	406	340	82	0.01	0.10	Tr	0	52
24	1	219	216	0.2	61	388	230	65	Tr	0.08	Tr	0	53
18	2	163	130	0.2	79	337	260	62	0.01	0.13	Tr	0	54
16	2	159	202	0.1	69	381	220	54	0.01	0.12	Tr	0	55
89	10	254	230	0.2	314	98	1,050	259	0.08	0.36	0.2	2	56
6	1	16	14	Tr	19	6	70	16	0.01	0.02	Tr	Tr	57
159	9	231	192	0.1	292	95	1,730	437	0.08	0.36	0.1	2	58
10	1	14	12	Tr	18	6	110	27	Tr	0.02	Tr	Tr	59
265	7	166	146	0.1	231	82	2,690	705	0.06	0.30	0.1	1	60
17	Tr	10	9	Tr	15	5	170	44	Tr	0.02	Tr	Tr	61
326	7	154	149	0.1	179	89	3,500	1,002	0.05	0.26	0.1	1	62
21	Tr	10	9	Tr	11	6	220	63	Tr	0.02	Tr	Tr	63
46	7	61	54	Tr	88	78	550	124	0.02	0.04	Tr	0	64
2	Tr	3	3	Tr	4	4	30	6	Tr	Tr	Tr	0	65
102	10	268	195	0.1	331	123	1,820	448	0.08	0.34	0.2	2	66
5	1	14	10	Tr	17	6	90	23	Tr	0.02	Tr	Tr	67

Table 2. Nutritive Value of the Edible Part of Food (Continued)

(Tr indicates nutrient present in trace amount.)

Item No.	Foods, approximate measures, units, and weight (weight of edible portion only)			Water	Food energy	Protein	Fat	Fatty acids		
								Saturated	Monounsaturated	Polyunsaturated
			Grams	Percent	Calories	Grams	Grams	Grams	Grams	Grams
	Dairy Products—Con.									
	Cream products, imitation (made with vegetable fat):									
	Sweet:									
	Creamers:									
68	Liquid (frozen)------------	1 tbsp----------	15	77	20	Tr	1	1.4	Tr	Tr
69	Powdered------------------	1 tsp-----------	2	2	10	Tr	1	0.7	Tr	Tr
	Whipped topping:									
70	Frozen--------------------	1 cup-----------	75	50	240	1	19	16.3	1.2	0.4
71		1 tbsp----------	4	50	15	Tr	1	0.9	0.1	Tr
72	Powdered, made with whole milk--------------------	1 cup-----------	80	67	150	3	10	8.5	0.7	0.2
73		1 tbsp----------	4	67	10	Tr	Tr	0.4	Tr	Tr
74	Pressurized--------------	1 cup-----------	70	60	185	1	16	13.2	1.3	0.2
75		1 tbsp---------	4	60	10	Tr	1	0.8	0.1	Tr
76	Sour dressing (filled cream type product, nonbutterfat)--	1 cup-----------	235	75	415	8	39	31.2	4.6	1.1
77		1 tbsp----------	12	75	20	Tr	2	1.6	0.2	0.1
	Ice cream. See Milk desserts, frozen (items 106-111).									
	Ice milk. See Milk desserts, frozen (items 112-114).									
	Milk:									
	Fluid:									
78	Whole (3.3% fat)-------------	1 cup-----------	244	88	150	8	8	5.1	2.4	0.3
	Lowfat (2%):									
79	No milk solids added-------	1 cup-----------	244	89	120	8	5	2.9	1.4	0.2
80	Milk solids added, label claim less than 10 g of protein per cup----------	1 cup-----------	245	89	125	9	5	2.9	1.4	0.2
	Lowfat (1%):									
81	No milk solids added-------	1 cup-----------	244	90	100	8	3	1.6	0.7	0.1
82	Milk solids added, label claim less than 10 g of protein per cup----------	1 cup-----------	245	90	105	9	2	1.5	0.7	0.1
	Nonfat (skim):									
83	No milk solids added-------	1 cup-----------	245	91	85	8	Tr	0.3	0.1	Tr
84	Milk solids added, label claim less than 10 g of protein per cup----------	1 cup-----------	245	90	90	9	1	0.4	0.2	Tr
85	Buttermilk-------------------	1 cup-----------	245	90	100	8	2	1.3	0.6	0.1
	Canned:									
86	Condensed, sweetened---------	1 cup-----------	306	27	980	24	27	16.8	7.4	1.0
	Evaporated:									
87	Whole milk----------------	1 cup-----------	252	74	340	17	19	11.6	5.9	0.6
88	Skim milk-----------------	1 cup-----------	255	79	200	19	1	0.3	0.2	Tr
	Dried:									
89	Buttermilk-------------------	1 cup-----------	120	3	465	41	7	4.3	2.0	0.3
	Nonfat, instantized:									
90	Envelope, 3.2 oz, net wt.[6]	1 envelope------	91	4	325	32	1	0.4	0.2	Tr
91	Cup-----------------------	1 cup-----------	68	4	245	24	Tr	0.3	0.1	Tr
	Milk beverages:									
	Chocolate milk (commercial):									
92	Regular---------------------	1 cup-----------	250	82	210	8	8	5.3	2.5	0.3
93	Lowfat (2%)------------------	1 cup-----------	250	84	180	8	5	3.1	1.5	0.2
94	Lowfat (1%)------------------	1 cup-----------	250	85	160	8	3	1.5	0.8	0.1

[5]Vitamin A value is largely from beta-carotene used for coloring.
[6]Yields 1 qt of fluid milk when reconstituted according to package directions.

170

Cholesterol	Carbohydrate	Calcium	Phosphorus	Iron	Potassium	Sodium	Vitamin A value		Thiamin	Riboflavin	Niacin	Ascorbic acid	Item No.
							(IU)	(RE)					
Milligrams	Grams	Milligrams	Milligrams	Milligrams	Milligrams	Milligrams	International units	Retinol equivalents	Milligrams	Milligrams	Milligrams	Milligrams	
0	2	1	10	Tr	29	12	[5]10	[5]1	0.00	0.00	0.0	0	68
0	1	Tr	8	Tr	16	4	Tr	Tr	0.00	Tr	0.0	0	69
0	17	5	6	0.1	14	19	[5]650	[5]65	0.00	0.00	0.0	0	70
0	1	Tr	Tr	Tr	1	1	[5]30	[5]3	0.00	0.00	0.0	0	71
8	13	72	69	Tr	121	53	[5]290	[5]39	0.02	0.09	Tr	1	72
Tr	1	4	3	Tr	6	3	[5]10	[5]2	Tr	Tr	Tr	Tr	73
0	11	4	13	Tr	13	43	[5]330	[5]33	0.00	0.00	0.0	0	74
0	1	Tr	1	Tr	1	2	[5]20	[5]2	0.00	0.00	0.0	0	75
13	11	266	205	0.1	380	113	20	5	0.09	0.38	0.2	2	76
1	1	14	10	Tr	19	6	Tr	Tr	Tr	0.02	Tr	Tr	77
33	11	291	228	0.1	370	120	310	76	0.09	0.40	0.2	2	78
18	12	297	232	0.1	377	122	500	139	0.10	0.40	0.2	2	79
18	12	313	245	0.1	397	128	500	140	0.10	0.42	0.2	2	80
10	12	300	235	0.1	381	123	500	144	0.10	0.41	0.2	2	81
10	12	313	245	0.1	397	128	500	145	0.10	0.42	0.2	2	82
4	12	302	247	0.1	406	126	500	149	0.09	0.34	0.2	2	83
5	12	316	255	0.1	418	130	500	149	0.10	0.43	0.2	2	84
9	12	285	219	0.1	371	257	80	20	0.08	0.38	0.1	2	85
104	166	868	775	0.6	1,136	389	1,000	248	0.28	1.27	0.6	8	86
74	25	657	510	0.5	764	267	610	136	0.12	0.80	0.5	5	87
9	29	738	497	0.7	845	293	1,000	298	0.11	0.79	0.4	3	88
83	59	1,421	1,119	0.4	1,910	621	260	65	0.47	1.89	1.1	7	89
17	47	1,120	896	0.3	1,552	499	[7]2,160	[7]646	0.38	1.59	0.8	5	90
12	35	837	670	0.2	1,160	373	[7]1,610	[7]483	0.28	1.19	0.6	4	91
31	26	280	251	0.6	417	149	300	73	0.09	0.41	0.3	2	92
17	26	284	254	0.6	422	151	500	143	0.09	0.41	0.3	2	93
7	26	287	256	0.6	425	152	500	148	0.10	0.42	0.3	2	94

[7]With added vitamin A.

Table 2. Nutritive Value of the Edible Part of Food (Continued)

(Tr indicates nutrient present in trace amount.)

Item No.	Foods, approximate measures, units, and weight (weight of edible portion only)			Water	Food energy	Pro-tein	Fat	Fatty acids		
								Satu-rated	Mono-unsatu-rated	Poly-unsatu-rated
			Grams	Per-cent	Cal-ories	Grams	Grams	Grams	Grams	Grams
	Dairy Products—Con.									
	Milk beverages:									
	Cocoa and chocolate-flavored beverages:									
95	Powder containing nonfat dry milk	1 oz	28	1	100	3	1	0.6	0.3	Tr
96	Prepared (6 oz water plus 1 oz powder)	1 serving	206	86	100	3	1	0.6	0.3	Tr
97	Powder without nonfat dry milk	3/4 oz	21	1	75	1	1	0.3	0.2	Tr
98	Prepared (8 oz whole milk plus 3/4 oz powder)	1 serving	265	81	225	9	9	5.4	2.5	0.3
99	Eggnog (commercial)	1 cup	254	74	340	10	19	11.3	5.7	0.9
	Malted milk:									
	Chocolate:									
100	Powder	3/4 oz	21	2	85	1	1	0.5	0.3	0.1
101	Prepared (8 oz whole milk plus 3/4 oz powder)	1 serving	265	81	235	9	9	5.5	2.7	0.4
	Natural:									
102	Powder	3/4 oz	21	3	85	3	2	0.9	0.5	0.3
103	Prepared (8 oz whole milk plus 3/4 oz powder)	1 serving	265	81	235	11	10	6.0	2.9	0.6
	Shakes, thick:									
104	Chocolate	10-oz container	283	72	335	9	8	4.8	2.2	0.3
105	Vanilla	10-oz container	283	74	315	11	9	5.3	2.5	0.3
	Milk desserts, frozen:									
	Ice cream, vanilla:									
	Regular (about 11% fat):									
106	Hardened	1/2 gal	1,064	61	2,155	38	115	71.3	33.1	4.3
107		1 cup	133	61	270	5	14	8.9	4.1	0.5
108		3 fl oz	50	61	100	2	5	3.4	1.6	0.2
109	Soft serve (frozen custard)	1 cup	173	60	375	7	23	13.5	6.7	1.0
110	Rich (about 16% fat), hardened	1/2 gal	1,188	59	2,805	33	190	118.3	54.9	7.1
111		1 cup	148	59	350	4	24	14.7	6.8	0.9
	Ice milk, vanilla:									
112	Hardened (about 4% fat)	1/2 gal	1,048	69	1,470	41	45	28.1	13.0	1.7
113		1 cup	131	69	185	5	6	3.5	1.6	0.2
114	Soft serve (about 3% fat)	1 cup	175	70	225	8	5	2.9	1.3	0.2
115	Sherbet (about 2% fat)	1/2 gal	1,542	66	2,160	17	31	19.0	8.8	1.1
116		1 cup	193	66	270	2	4	2.4	1.1	0.1
	Yogurt:									
	With added milk solids:									
	Made with lowfat milk:									
117	Fruit-flavored[8]	8-oz container	227	74	230	10	2	1.6	0.7	0.1
118	Plain	8-oz container	227	85	145	12	4	2.3	1.0	0.1
119	Made with nonfat milk	8-oz container	227	85	125	13	Tr	0.3	0.1	Tr
	Without added milk solids:									
120	Made with whole milk	8-oz container	227	88	140	8	7	4.8	2.0	0.2
	Eggs									
	Eggs, large (24 oz per dozen):									
	Raw:									
121	Whole, without shell	1 egg	50	75	75	6	5	1.6	1.9	0.7
122	White	1 white	33	88	15	4	0	0.0	0.0	0.0
123	Yolk	1 yolk	17	49	60	3	5	1.6	1.9	0.7
	Cooked:									
124	Fried in margarine	1 egg	46	69	90	6	7	1.9	2.7	1.3
125	Hard-cooked, shell removed	1 egg	50	75	75	6	5	1.6	2.0	0.7
126	Poached	1 egg	50	75	75	6	5	1.5	1.9	0.7
127	Scrambled (milk added) in margarine	1 egg	61	73	100	7	7	2.2	2.9	1.3

[8]Carbohydrate content varies widely because of amount of sugar added and amount and solids content of added flavoring. Consult the label if more precise values for carbohydrate and calories are needed.

Nutrients in Indicated Quantity

Cholesterol	Carbohydrate	Calcium	Phosphorus	Iron	Potassium	Sodium	Vitamin A value		Thiamin	Riboflavin	Niacin	Ascorbic acid	Item No.
							(IU)	(RE)					
Milligrams	Grams	Milligrams	Milligrams	Milligrams	Milligrams	Milligrams	International units	Retinol equivalents	Milligrams	Milligrams	Milligrams	Milligrams	
1	22	90	88	0.3	223	139	Tr	Tr	0.03	0.17	0.2	Tr	95
1	22	90	88	0.3	223	139	Tr	Tr	0.03	0.17	0.2	Tr	96
0	19	7	26	0.7	136	56	Tr	Tr	Tr	0.03	0.1	Tr	97
33	30	298	254	0.9	508	176	310	76	0.10	0.43	0.3	3	98
149	34	330	278	0.5	420	138	890	203	0.09	0.48	0.3	4	99
1	18	13	37	0.4	130	49	20	5	0.04	0.04	0.4	0	100
34	29	304	265	0.5	500	168	330	80	0.14	0.43	0.7	2	101
4	15	56	79	0.2	159	96	70	17	0.11	0.14	1.1	0	102
37	27	347	307	0.3	529	215	380	93	0.20	0.54	1.3	2	103
30	60	374	357	0.9	634	314	240	59	0.13	0.63	0.4	0	104
33	50	413	326	0.3	517	270	320	79	0.08	0.55	0.4	0	105
476	254	1,406	1,075	1.0	2,052	929	4,340	1,064	0.42	2.63	1.1	6	106
59	32	176	134	0.1	257	116	540	133	0.05	0.33	0.1	1	107
22	12	66	51	Tr	96	44	200	50	0.02	0.12	0.1	Tr	108
153	38	236	199	0.4	338	153	790	199	0.08	0.45	0.2	1	109
703	256	1,213	927	0.8	1,771	868	7,200	1,758	0.36	2.27	0.9	5	110
88	32	151	115	0.1	221	108	900	219	0.04	0.28	0.1	1	111
146	232	1,409	1,035	1.5	2,117	836	1,710	419	0.61	2.78	0.9	6	112
18	29	176	129	0.2	265	105	210	52	0.08	0.35	0.1	1	113
13	38	274	202	0.3	412	163	175	44	0.12	0.54	0.2	1	114
113	469	827	594	2.5	1,585	706	1,480	308	0.26	0.71	1.0	31	115
14	59	103	74	0.3	198	88	190	39	0.03	0.09	0.1	4	116
10	43	345	271	0.2	442	133	100	25	0.08	0.40	0.2	1	117
14	16	415	326	0.2	531	159	150	36	0.10	0.49	0.3	2	118
4	17	452	355	0.2	579	174	20	5	0.11	0.53	0.3	2	119
29	11	274	215	0.1	351	105	280	68	0.07	0.32	0.2	1	120
213	1	25	89	0.7	60	63	320	95	0.03	0.25	Tr	0	121
0	Tr	2	4	Tr	48	55	0	0	Tr	0.15	Tr	0	122
213	Tr	23	81	0.6	16	7	320	97	0.03	0.11	Tr	0	123
211	1	25	89	0.7	61	162	390	114	0.03	0.24	Tr	0	124
213	1	25	86	0.6	63	62	280	84	0.03	0.26	Tr	0	125
212	1	25	89	0.7	60	140	320	95	0.02	0.22	Tr	0	126
215	1	44	104	0.7	84	171	420	119	0.03	0.27	Tr	Tr	127

Table 2. Nutritive Value of the Edible Part of Food (Continued)
(Tr indicates nutrient present in trace amount.)

Item No.	Foods, approximate measures, units, and weight (weight of edible portion only)		Water	Food energy	Pro-tein	Fat	Fatty acids Satu-rated	Fatty acids Mono-unsatu-rated	Fatty acids Poly-unsatu-rated
		Grams	Per-cent	Cal-ories	Grams	Grams	Grams	Grams	Grams
	Fats and Oils								
	Butter (4 sticks per lb):								
128	Stick-------------------------- 1/2 cup---------	113	16	810	1	92	57.1	26.4	3.4
129	Tablespoon (1/8 stick)--------- 1 tbsp----------	14	16	100	Tr	11	7.1	3.3	0.4
130	Pat (1 in square, 1/3 in high; 90 per lb)------------- 1 pat-----------	5	16	35	Tr	4	2.5	1.2	0.2
131	Fats, cooking (vegetable shortenings)------------------- 1 cup-----------	205	0	1,810	0	205	51.3	91.2	53.5
132	1 tbsp----------	13	0	115	0	13	3.3	5.8	3.4
133	Lard--------------------------- 1 cup-----------	205	0	1,850	0	205	80.4	92.5	23.0
134	1 tbsp----------	13	0	115	0	13	5.1	5.9	1.5
	Margarine:								
135	Imitation (about 40% fat), soft 8-oz container--	227	58	785	1	88	17.5	35.6	31.3
136	1 tbsp----------	14	58	50	Tr	5	1.1	2.2	1.9
	Regular (about 80% fat): Hard (4 sticks per lb):								
137	Stick-------------------------- 1/2 cup---------	113	16	810	1	91	17.9	40.5	28.7
138	Tablespoon (1/8 stick)----- 1 tbsp----------	14	16	100	Tr	11	2.2	5.0	3.6
139	Pat (1 in square, 1/3 in high; 90 per lb)--------- 1 pat-----------	5	16	35	Tr	4	0.8	1.8	1.3
140	Soft------------------------ 8-oz container--	227	16	1,625	2	183	31.3	64.7	78.5
141	1 tbsp----------	14	16	100	Tr	11	1.9	4.0	4.8
	Spread (about 60% fat): Hard (4 sticks per lb):								
142	Stick-------------------------- 1/2 cup---------	113	37	610	1	69	15.9	29.4	20.5
143	Tablespoon (1/8 stick)----- 1 tbsp----------	14	37	75	Tr	9	2.0	3.6	2.5
144	Pat (1 in square, 1/3 in high; 90 per lb)--------- 1 pat-----------	5	37	25	Tr	3	0.7	1.3	0.9
145	Soft------------------------ 8-oz container--	227	37	1,225	1	138	29.1	71.5	31.3
146	1 tbsp----------	14	37	75	Tr	9	1.8	4.4	1.9
	Oils, salad or cooking:								
147	Corn--------------------------- 1 cup-----------	218	0	1,925	0	218	27.7	52.8	128.0
148	1 tbsp----------	14	0	125	0	14	1.8	3.4	8.2
149	Olive-------------------------- 1 cup-----------	216	0	1,910	0	216	29.2	159.2	18.1
150	1 tbsp----------	14	0	125	0	14	1.9	10.3	1.2
151	Peanut------------------------- 1 cup-----------	216	0	1,910	0	216	36.5	99.8	69.1
152	1 tbsp----------	14	0	125	0	14	2.4	6.5	4.5
153	Safflower---------------------- 1 cup-----------	218	0	1,925	0	218	19.8	26.4	162.4
154	1 tbsp----------	14	0	125	0	14	1.3	1.7	10.4
155	Soybean oil, hydrogenated (partially hardened)--------- 1 cup-----------	218	0	1,925	0	218	32.5	93.7	82.0
156	1 tbsp----------	14	0	125	0	14	2.1	6.0	5.3
157	Soybean-cottonseed oil blend, hydrogenated----------------- 1 cup-----------	218	0	1,925	0	218	39.2	64.3	104.9
158	1 tbsp----------	14	0	125	0	14	2.5	4.1	6.7
159	Sunflower---------------------- 1 cup-----------	218	0	1,925	0	218	22.5	42.5	143.2
160	1 tbsp----------	14	0	125	0	14	1.4	2.7	9.2
	Salad dressings: Commercial:								
161	Blue cheese------------------- 1 tbsp----------	15	32	75	1	8	1.5	1.8	4.2
	French:								
162	Regular--------------------- 1 tbsp----------	16	35	85	Tr	9	1.4	4.0	3.5
163	Low calorie---------------- 1 tbsp----------	16	75	25	Tr	2	0.2	0.3	1.0
	Italian:								
164	Regular--------------------- 1 tbsp----------	15	34	80	Tr	9	1.3	3.7	3.2
165	Low calorie---------------- 1 tbsp----------	15	86	5	Tr	Tr	Tr	Tr	Tr
	Mayonnaise:								
166	Regular--------------------- 1 tbsp----------	14	15	100	Tr	11	1.7	3.2	5.8
167	Imitation------------------ 1 tbsp----------	15	63	35	Tr	3	0.5	0.7	1.6
168	Mayonnaise type------------- 1 tbsp----------	15	40	60	Tr	5	0.7	1.4	2.7
169	Tartar sauce---------------- 1 tbsp----------	14	34	75	Tr	8	1.2	2.6	3.9
	Thousand island:								
170	Regular--------------------- 1 tbsp----------	16	46	60	Tr	6	1.0	1.3	3.2
171	Low calorie---------------- 1 tbsp----------	15	69	25	Tr	2	0.2	0.4	0.9

[9] For salted butter; unsalted butter contains 12 mg sodium per stick, 2 mg per tbsp, or 1 mg per pat.
[10] Values for vitamin A are year-round average.

Nutrients in Indicated Quantity

Cholesterol	Carbohydrate	Calcium	Phosphorus	Iron	Potassium	Sodium	Vitamin A value (IU)	Vitamin A value (RE)	Thiamin	Riboflavin	Niacin	Ascorbic acid	Item No.
Milligrams	Grams	Milligrams	Milligrams	Milligrams	Milligrams	Milligrams	International units	Retinol equivalents	Milligrams	Milligrams	Milligrams	Milligrams	
247	Tr	27	26	0.2	29	[9]933	[10]3,460	[10]852	0.01	0.04	Tr	0	128
31	Tr	3	3	Tr	4	[9]116	[10]430	[10]106	Tr	Tr	Tr	0	129
11	Tr	1	1	Tr	1	[9]41	[10]150	[10]38	Tr	Tr	Tr	0	130
0	0	0	0	0.0	0	0	0	0	0.00	0.00	0.0	0	131
0	0	0	0	0.0	0	0	0	0	0.00	0.00	0.0	0	132
195	0	0	0	0.0	0	0	0	0	0.00	0.00	0.0	0	133
12	0	0	0	0.0	0	0	0	0	0.00	0.00	0.0	0	134
0	1	40	31	0.0	57	[11]2,178	[12]7,510	[12]2,254	0.01	0.05	Tr	Tr	135
0	Tr	2	2	0.0	4	[11]134	[12]460	[12]139	Tr	Tr	Tr	Tr	136
0	1	34	26	0.1	48	[11]1,066	[12]3,740	[12]1,122	0.01	0.04	Tr	Tr	137
0	Tr	4	3	Tr	6	[11]132	[12]460	[12]139	Tr	0.01	Tr	Tr	138
0	Tr	1	1	Tr	2	[11]47	[12]170	[12]50	Tr	Tr	Tr	Tr	139
0	1	60	46	0.0	86	[11]2,449	[12]7,510	[12]2,254	0.02	0.07	Tr	Tr	140
0	Tr	4	3	0.0	5	[11]151	[12]460	[12]139	Tr	Tr	Tr	Tr	141
0	0	24	18	0.0	34	[11]1,123	[12]3,740	[12]1,122	0.01	0.03	Tr	Tr	142
0	0	3	2	0.0	4	[11]139	[12]460	[12]139	Tr	Tr	Tr	Tr	143
0	0	1	1	0.0	1	[11]50	[12]170	[12]50	Tr	Tr	Tr	Tr	144
0	0	47	37	0.0	68	[11]2,256	[12]7,510	[12]2,254	0.02	0.06	Tr	Tr	145
0	0	3	2	0.0	4	[11]139	[12]460	[12]139	Tr	Tr	Tr	Tr	146
0	0	0	0	0.0	0	0	0	0	0.00	0.00	0.0	0	147
0	0	0	0	0.0	0	0	0	0	0.00	0.00	0.0	0	148
0	0	0	0	0.0	0	0	0	0	0.00	0.00	0.0	0	149
0	0	0	0	0.0	0	0	0	0	0.00	0.00	0.0	0	150
0	0	0	0	0.0	0	0	0	0	0.00	0.00	0.0	0	151
0	0	0	0	0.0	0	0	0	0	0.00	0.00	0.0	0	152
0	0	0	0	0.0	0	0	0	0	0.00	0.00	0.0	0	153
0	0	0	0	0.0	0	0	0	0	0.00	0.00	0.0	0	154
0	0	0	0	0.0	0	0	0	0	0.00	0.00	0.0	0	155
0	0	0	0	0.0	0	0	0	0	0.00	0.00	0.0	0	156
0	0	0	0	0.0	0	0	0	0	0.00	0.00	0.0	0	157
0	0	0	0	0.0	0	0	0	0	0.00	0.00	0.0	0	158
0	0	0	0	0.0	0	0	0	0	0.00	0.00	0.0	0	159
0	0	0	0	0.0	0	0	0	0	0.00	0.00	0.0	0	160
3	1	12	11	Tr	6	164	30	10	Tr	0.02	Tr	Tr	161
0	1	2	1	Tr	2	188	Tr	Tr	Tr	Tr	Tr	Tr	162
0	2	6	5	Tr	3	306	Tr	Tr	Tr	Tr	Tr	Tr	163
0	1	1	1	Tr	5	162	30	3	Tr	Tr	Tr	Tr	164
0	2	1	1	Tr	4	136	Tr	Tr	Tr	Tr	Tr	Tr	165
8	Tr	3	4	0.1	5	80	40	12	0.00	0.00	Tr	0	166
4	2	Tr	Tr	0.0	2	75	0	0	0.00	0.00	0.0	0	167
4	4	2	4	Tr	1	107	30	13	Tr	Tr	Tr	0	168
4	1	3	4	0.1	11	182	30	9	Tr	Tr	0.0	Tr	169
4	2	2	3	0.1	18	112	50	15	Tr	Tr	Tr	0	170
2	2	2	3	0.1	17	150	50	14	Tr	Tr	Tr	0	171

[11] For salted margarine.
[12] Based on average vitamin A content of fortified margarine. Federal specifications for fortified margarine require a minimum of 15,000 IU per pound.

Table 2. Nutritive Value of the Edible Part of Food (Continued)

(Tr indicates nutrient present in trace amount.)

Item No.	Foods, approximate measures, units, and weight (weight of edible portion only)		Water	Food energy	Pro-tein	Fat	Fatty acids Satu-rated	Mono-unsatu-rated	Poly-unsatu-rated
	Fats and Oils—Con.	Grams	Per-cent	Cal-ories	Grams	Grams	Grams	Grams	Grams
	Salad dressings:								
	Prepared from home recipe:								
172	Cooked type[13] -----------------	1 tbsp-----------	16	69	25	1	2	0.5	0.6	0.3
173	Vinegar and oil--------------	1 tbsp-----------	16	47	70	0	8	1.5	2.4	3.9
	Fish and Shellfish								
	Clams:								
174	Raw, meat only-----------------	3 oz------------	85	82	65	11	1	0.3	0.3	0.3
175	Canned, drained solids---------	3 oz------------	85	77	85	13	2	0.5	0.5	0.4
176	Crabmeat, canned-----------------	1 cup	135	77	135	23	3	0.5	0.8	1.4
177	Fish sticks, frozen, reheated, (stick, 4 by 1 by 1/2 in)------	1 fish stick----	28	52	70	6	3	0.8	1.4	0.8
	Flounder or Sole, baked, with lemon juice:								
178	With butter-------------------	3 oz------------	85	73	120	16	6	3.2	1.5	0.5
179	With margarine----------------	3 oz------------	85	73	120	16	6	1.2	2.3	1.9
180	Without added fat-------------	3 oz------------	85	78	80	17	1	0.3	0.2	0.4
181	Haddock, breaded, fried[14] --------	3 oz------------	85	61	175	17	9	2.4	3.9	2.4
182	Halibut, broiled, with butter and lemon juice---------------	3 oz------------	85	67	140	20	6	3.3	1.6	0.7
183	Herring, pickled-----------------	3 oz------------	85	59	190	17	13	4.3	4.6	3.1
184	Ocean perch, breaded, fried[14] ----	1 fillet--------	85	59	185	16	11	2.6	4.6	2.8
	Oysters:								
185	Raw, meat only (13-19 medium Selects)----------------------	1 cup	240	85	160	20	4	1.4	0.5	1.4
186	Breaded, fried[14] -----------------	1 oyster--------	45	65	90	5	5	1.4	2.1	1.4
	Salmon:								
187	Canned (pink), solids and liquid-------------------------	3 oz------------	85	71	120	17	5	0.9	1.5	2.1
188	Baked (red)--------------------	3 oz------------	85	67	140	21	5	1.2	2.4	1.4
189	Smoked------------------------	3 oz------------	85	59	150	18	8	2.6	3.9	0.7
190	Sardines, Atlantic, canned in oil, drained solids-----------	3 oz------------	85	62	175	20	9	2.1	3.7	2.9
191	Scallops, breaded, frozen, reheated-----------------------	6 scallops------	90	59	195	15	10	2.5	4.1	2.5
	Shrimp:								
192	Canned, drained solids---------	3 oz------------	85	70	100	21	1	0.2	0.2	0.4
193	French fried (7 medium)[16] ------	3 oz------------	85	55	200	16	10	2.5	4.1	2.6
194	Trout, broiled, with butter and lemon juice--------------------	3 oz------------	85	63	175	21	9	4.1	2.9	1.6
	Tuna, canned, drained solids:								
195	Oil pack, chunk light----------	3 oz------------	85	61	165	24	7	1.4	1.9	3.1
196	Water pack, solid white--------	3 oz------------	85	63	135	30	1	0.3	0.2	0.3
197	Tuna salad[17] ----------------------	1 cup	205	63	375	33	19	3.3	4.9	9.2
	Fruits and Fruit Juices								
	Apples:								
	Raw:								
	Unpeeled, without cores:								
198	2-3/4-in diam. (about 3 per lb with cores)-----------	1 apple---------	138	84	80	Tr	Tr	0.1	Tr	0.1
199	3-1/4-in diam. (about 2 per lb with cores)-----------	1 apple---------	212	84	125	Tr	1	0.1	Tr	0.2
200	Peeled, sliced----------------	1 cup	110	84	65	Tr	Tr	0.1	Tr	0.1
201	Dried, sulfured-----------------	10 rings--------	64	32	155	1	Tr	Tr	Tr	0.1
202	Apple juice, bottled or canned[19]	1 cup	248	88	115	Tr	Tr	Tr	Tr	0.1
	Applesauce, canned:								
203	Sweetened--------------------	1 cup	255	80	195	Tr	Tr	0.1	Tr	0.1
204	Unsweetened------------------	1 cup	244	88	105	Tr	Tr	Tr	Tr	Tr

[13] Fatty acid values apply to product made with regular margarine.
[14] Dipped in egg, milk, and breadcrumbs; fried in vegetable shortening.
[15] If bones are discarded, value for calcium will be greatly reduced.
[16] Dipped in egg, breadcrumbs, and flour; fried in vegetable shortening.

Cho-les-terol	Carbo-hydrate	Calcium	Phos-phorus	Iron	Potas-sium	Sodium	Vitamin A value		Thiamin	Ribo-flavin	Niacin	Ascorbic acid	Item No.
							(IU)	(RE)					
Milli-grams	Grams	Milli-grams	Milli-grams	Milli-grams	Milli-grams	Milli-grams	Inter-national units	Retinol equiva-lents	Milli-grams	Milli-grams	Milli-grams	Milli-grams	
9	2	13	14	0.1	19	117	70	20	0.01	0.02	Tr	Tr	172
0	Tr	0	0	0.0	1	Tr	0	0	0.00	0.00	0.0	0	173
43	2	59	138	2.6	154	102	90	26	0.09	0.15	1.1	9	174
54	2	47	116	3.5	119	102	90	26	0.01	0.09	0.9	3	175
135	1	61	246	1.1	149	1,350	50	14	0.11	0.11	2.6	0	176
26	4	11	58	0.3	94	53	20	5	0.03	0.05	0.6	0	177
68	Tr	13	187	0.3	272	145	210	54	0.05	0.08	1.6	1	178
55	Tr	14	187	0.3	273	151	230	69	0.05	0.08	1.6	1	179
59	Tr	13	197	0.3	286	101	30	10	0.05	0.08	1.7	1	180
75	7	34	183	1.0	270	123	70	20	0.06	0.10	2.9	0	181
62	Tr	14	206	0.7	441	103	610	174	0.06	0.07	7.7	1	182
85	0	29	128	0.9	85	850	110	33	0.04	0.18	2.8	0	183
66	7	31	191	1.2	241	138	70	20	0.10	0.11	2.0	0	184
120	8	226	343	15.6	290	175	740	223	0.34	0.43	6.0	24	185
35	5	49	73	3.0	64	70	150	44	0.07	0.10	1.3	4	186
34	0	[15]167	243	0.7	307	443	60	18	0.03	0.15	6.8	0	187
60	0	26	269	0.5	305	55	290	87	0.18	0.14	5.5	0	188
51	0	12	208	0.8	327	1,700	260	77	0.17	0.17	6.8	0	189
85	0	[15]371	424	2.6	349	425	190	56	0.03	0.17	4.6	0	190
70	10	39	203	2.0	369	298	70	21	0.11	0.11	1.6	0	191
128	1	98	224	1.4	104	1,955	50	15	0.01	0.03	1.5	0	192
168	11	61	154	2.0	189	384	90	26	0.06	0.09	2.8	0	193
71	Tr	26	259	1.0	297	122	230	60	0.07	0.07	2.3	1	194
55	0	7	199	1.6	298	303	70	20	0.04	0.09	10.1	0	195
48	0	17	202	0.6	255	468	110	32	0.03	0.10	13.4	0	196
80	19	31	281	2.5	531	877	230	53	0.06	0.14	13.3	6	197
0	21	10	10	0.2	159	Tr	70	7	0.02	0.02	0.1	8	198
0	32	15	15	0.4	244	Tr	110	11	0.04	0.03	0.2	12	199
0	16	4	8	0.1	124	Tr	50	5	0.02	0.01	0.1	4	200
0	42	9	24	0.9	288	[18]56	0	0	0.00	0.10	0.6	2	201
0	29	17	17	0.9	295	7	Tr	Tr	0.05	0.04	0.2	[20]2	202
0	51	10	18	0.9	156	8	30	3	0.03	0.07	0.5	[20]4	203
0	28	7	17	0.3	183	5	70	7	0.03	0.06	0.5	[20]3	204

[17] Made with drained chunk light tuna, celery, onion, pickle relish, and mayonnaise-type salad dressing.
[18] Sodium bisulfite used to preserve color; unsulfited product would contain less sodium.
[19] Also applies to pasteurized apple cider.
[20] Without added ascorbic acid. For value with added ascorbic acid, refer to label.

Item No.	Foods, approximate measures, units, and weight (weight of edible portion only)		Grams	Water	Food energy	Pro-tein	Fat	Fatty acids		
								Satu-rated	Mono-unsatu-rated	Poly-unsatu-rated
			Grams	Per-cent	Cal-ories	Grams	Grams	Grams	Grams	Grams
	Fruits and Fruit Juices—Con.									
	Apricots:									
205	Raw, without pits (about 12 per lb with pits)	3 apricots	106	86	50	1	Tr	Tr	0.2	0.1
	Canned (fruit and liquid):									
206	Heavy syrup pack	1 cup	258	78	215	1	Tr	Tr	0.1	Tr
207		3 halves	85	78	70	Tr	Tr	Tr	Tr	Tr
208	Juice pack	1 cup	248	87	120	2	Tr	Tr	Tr	Tr
209		3 halves	84	87	40	1	Tr	Tr	Tr	Tr
	Dried:									
210	Uncooked (28 large or 37 medium halves per cup)	1 cup	130	31	310	5	1	Tr	0.3	0.1
211	Cooked, unsweetened, fruit and liquid	1 cup	250	76	210	3	Tr	Tr	0.2	0.1
212	Apricot nectar, canned	1 cup	251	85	140	1	Tr	Tr	0.1	Tr
	Avocados, raw, whole, without skin and seed:									
213	California (about 2 per lb with skin and seed)	1 avocado	173	73	305	4	30	4.5	19.4	3.5
214	Florida (about 1 per lb with skin and seed)	1 avocado	304	80	340	5	27	5.3	14.8	4.5
	Bananas, raw, without peel:									
215	Whole (about 2-1/2 per lb with peel)	1 banana	114	74	105	1	1	0.2	Tr	0.1
216	Sliced	1 cup	150	74	140	2	1	0.3	0.1	0.1
217	Blackberries, raw	1 cup	144	86	75	1	1	0.2	0.1	0.1
	Blueberries:									
218	Raw	1 cup	145	85	80	1	1	Tr	0.1	0.3
219	Frozen, sweetened	10-oz container	284	77	230	1	Tr	Tr	0.1	0.2
220		1 cup	230	77	185	1	Tr	Tr	Tr	0.1
	Cantaloup. See Melons (item 251).									
	Cherries:									
221	Sour, red, pitted, canned, water pack	1 cup	244	90	90	2	Tr	0.1	0.1	0.1
222	Sweet, raw, without pits and stems	10 cherries	68	81	50	1	1	0.1	0.2	0.2
223	Cranberry juice cocktail, bottled, sweetened	1 cup	253	85	145	Tr	Tr	Tr	Tr	0.1
224	Cranberry sauce, sweetened, canned, strained	1 cup	277	61	420	1	Tr	Tr	0.1	0.2
	Dates:									
225	Whole, without pits	10 dates	83	23	230	2	Tr	0.1	0.1	Tr
226	Chopped	1 cup	178	23	490	4	1	0.3	0.2	Tr
227	Figs, dried	10 figs	187	28	475	6	2	0.4	0.5	1.0
	Fruit cocktail, canned, fruit and liquid:									
228	Heavy syrup pack	1 cup	255	80	185	1	Tr	Tr	Tr	0.1
229	Juice pack	1 cup	248	87	115	1	Tr	Tr	Tr	Tr
	Grapefruit:									
230	Raw, without peel, membrane and seeds (3-3/4-in diam., 1 lb 1 oz, whole, with refuse)	1/2 grapefruit	120	91	40	1	Tr	Tr	Tr	Tr
231	Canned, sections with syrup	1 cup	254	84	150	1	Tr	Tr	Tr	0.1
	Grapefruit juice:									
232	Raw	1 cup	247	90	95	1	Tr	Tr	Tr	0.1
	Canned:									
233	Unsweetened	1 cup	247	90	95	1	Tr	Tr	Tr	0.1
234	Sweetened	1 cup	250	87	115	1	Tr	Tr	Tr	0.1
	Frozen concentrate, unsweetened									
235	Undiluted	6-fl-oz can	207	62	300	4	1	0.1	0.1	0.2
236	Diluted with 3 parts water by volume	1 cup	247	89	100	1	Tr	Tr	Tr	0.1

[20] Without added ascorbic acid. For value with added ascorbic acid, refer to label.
[21] With added ascorbic acid.

Cho-les-terol	Carbo-hydrate	Calcium	Phos-phorus	Iron	Potas-sium	Sodium	Vitamin A value		Thiamin	Ribo-flavin	Niacin	Ascorbic acid	Item No.
							(IU)	(RE)					
Milli-grams	Grams	Milli-grams	Milli-grams	Milli-grams	Milli-grams	Milli-grams	Inter-national units	Retinol equiva-lents	Milli-grams	Milli-grams	Milli-grams	Milli-grams	
0	12	15	20	0.6	314	1	2,770	277	0.03	0.04	0.6	11	205
0	55	23	31	0.8	361	10	3,170	317	0.05	0.06	1.0	8	206
0	18	8	10	0.3	119	3	1,050	105	0.02	0.02	0.3	3	207
0	31	30	50	0.7	409	10	4,190	419	0.04	0.05	0.9	12	208
0	10	10	17	0.3	139	3	1,420	142	0.02	0.02	0.3	4	209
0	80	59	152	6.1	1,791	13	9,410	941	0.01	0.20	3.9	3	210
0	55	40	103	4.2	1,222	8	5,910	591	0.02	0.08	2.4	4	211
0	36	18	23	1.0	286	8	3,300	330	0.02	0.04	0.7	[20]2	212
0	12	19	73	2.0	1,097	21	1,060	106	0.19	0.21	3.3	14	213
0	27	33	119	1.6	1,484	15	1,860	186	0.33	0.37	5.8	24	214
0	27	7	23	0.4	451	1	90	9	0.05	0.11	0.6	10	215
0	35	9	30	0.5	594	2	120	12	0.07	0.15	0.8	14	216
0	18	46	30	0.8	282	Tr	240	24	0.04	0.06	0.6	30	217
0	20	9	15	0.2	129	9	150	15	0.07	0.07	0.5	19	218
0	62	17	20	1.1	170	3	120	12	0.06	0.15	0.7	3	219
0	50	14	16	0.9	138	2	100	10	0.05	0.12	0.6	2	220
0	22	27	24	3.3	239	17	1,840	184	0.04	0.10	0.4	5	221
0	11	10	13	0.3	152	Tr	150	15	0.03	0.04	0.3	5	222
0	38	8	3	0.4	61	10	10	1	0.01	0.04	0.1	[21]108	223
0	108	11	17	0.6	72	80	60	6	0.04	0.06	0.3	6	224
0	61	27	33	1.0	541	2	40	4	0.07	0.08	1.8	0	225
0	131	57	71	2.0	1,161	5	90	9	0.16	0.18	3.9	0	226
0	122	269	127	4.2	1,331	21	250	25	0.13	0.16	1.3	1	227
0	48	15	28	0.7	224	15	520	52	0.05	0.05	1.0	5	228
0	29	20	35	0.5	236	10	760	76	0.03	0.04	1.0	7	229
0	10	14	10	0.1	167	Tr	[22]10	[22]1	0.04	0.02	0.3	41	230
0	39	36	25	1.0	328	5	Tr	Tr	0.10	0.05	0.6	54	231
0	23	22	37	0.5	400	2	20	2	0.10	0.05	0.5	94	232
0	22	17	27	0.5	378	2	20	2	0.10	0.05	0.6	72	233
0	28	20	28	0.9	405	5	20	2	0.10	0.06	0.8	67	234
0	72	56	101	1.0	1,002	6	60	6	0.30	0.16	1.6	248	235
0	24	20	35	0.3	336	2	20	2	0.10	0.05	0.5	83	236

[22]For white grapefruit; pink grapefruit have about 310 IU or 31 RE.

Item No.	Foods, approximate measures, units, and weight (weight of edible portion only)		Water	Food energy	Pro-tein	Fat	Fatty acids		
							Satu-rated	Mono-unsatu-rated	Poly-unsatu-rated
		Grams	Per-cent	Cal-ories	Grams	Grams	Grams	Grams	Grams
	Fruits and Fruit Juices—Con.								
	Grapes, European type (adherent skin), raw:								
237	Thompson Seedless---------------- 10 grapes--------	50	81	35	Tr	Tr	0.1	Tr	0.1
238	Tokay and Emperor, seeded types 10 grapes--------	57	81	40	Tr	Tr	0.1	Tr	0.1
	Grape juice:								
239	Canned or bottled-------------- 1 cup------------	253	84	155	1	Tr	0.1	Tr	0.1
	Frozen concentrate, sweetened:								
240	Undiluted-------------------- 6-fl-oz can-----	216	54	385	1	1	0.2	Tr	0.2
241	Diluted with 3 parts water by volume-------------------- 1 cup------------	250	87	125	Tr	Tr	0.1	Tr	0.1
242	Kiwifruit, raw, without skin (about 5 per lb with skin)----- 1 kiwifruit-----	76	83	45	1	Tr	Tr	0.1	0.1
243	Lemons, raw, without peel and seeds (about 4 per lb with peel and seeds)---------------------- 1 lemon----------	58	89	15	1	Tr	Tr	Tr	0.1
	Lemon juice:								
244	Raw------------------------- 1 cup------------	244	91	60	1	Tr	Tr	Tr	Tr
245	Canned or bottled, unsweetened 1 cup------------	244	92	50	1	1	0.1	Tr	0.2
246	1 tbsp----------	15	92	5	Tr	Tr	Tr	Tr	Tr
247	Frozen, single-strength, unsweetened----------------- 6-fl-oz can-----	244	92	55	1	1	0.1	Tr	0.2
	Lime juice:								
248	Raw------------------------- 1 cup------------	246	90	65	1	Tr	Tr	Tr	0.1
249	Canned, unsweetened------------ 1 cup------------	246	93	50	1	1	0.1	0.1	0.2
250	Mangos, raw, without skin and seed (about 1-1/2 per lb with skin and seed)----------------- 1 mango----------	207	82	135	1	1	0.1	0.2	0.1
	Melons, raw, without rind and cavity contents:								
251	Cantaloup, orange-fleshed (5-in diam., 2-1/3 lb, whole, with rind and cavity contents)---- 1/2 melon-------	267	90	95	2	1	0.1	0.1	0.3
252	Honeydew (6-1/2-in diam., 5-1/4 lb, whole, with rind and cav-ity contents)----------------- 1/10 melon------	129	90	45	1	Tr	Tr	Tr	0.1
253	Nectarines, raw, without pits (about 3 per lb with pits)----- 1 nectarine-----	136	86	65	1	1	0.1	0.2	0.3
	Oranges, raw:								
254	Whole, without peel and seeds (2-5/8-in diam., about 2-1/2 per lb, with peel and seeds) 1 orange--------	131	87	60	1	Tr	Tr	Tr	Tr
255	Sections without membranes----- 1 cup------------	180	87	85	2	Tr	Tr	Tr	Tr
	Orange juice:								
256	Raw, all varieties------------- 1 cup------------	248	88	110	2	Tr	0.1	0.1	0.1
257	Canned, unsweetened------------ 1 cup------------	249	89	105	1	Tr	Tr	0.1	0.1
258	Chilled------------------------ 1 cup------------	249	88	110	2	1	0.1	0.1	0.2
	Frozen concentrate:								
259	Undiluted------------------- 6-fl-oz can-----	213	58	340	5	Tr	0.1	0.1	0.1
260	Diluted with 3 parts water by volume-------------------- 1 cup------------	249	88	110	2	Tr	Tr	Tr	Tr
261	Orange and grapefruit juice, canned------------------------- 1 cup------------	247	89	105	1	Tr	Tr	Tr	Tr
262	Papayas, raw, 1/2-in cubes------- 1 cup------------	140	86	65	1	Tr	0.1	0.1	Tr
	Peaches:								
	Raw:								
263	Whole, 2-1/2-in diam., peeled, pitted (about 4 per lb with peels and pits)---- 1 peach----------	87	88	35	1	Tr	Tr	Tr	Tr
264	Sliced------------------------- 1 cup------------	170	88	75	1	Tr	Tr	0.1	0.1
	Canned, fruit and liquid:								
265	Heavy syrup pack------------- 1 cup------------	256	79	190	1	Tr	Tr	0.1	0.1
266	1 half----------	81	79	60	Tr	Tr	Tr	Tr	Tr
267	Juice pack------------------- 1 cup------------	248	87	110	2	Tr	Tr	Tr	Tr
268	1 half----------	77	87	35	Tr	Tr	Tr	Tr	Tr

[20]Without added ascorbic acid. For value with added ascorbic acid, refer to label.
[21]With added ascorbic acid.

Cho-les-terol	Carbo-hydrate	Calcium	Phos-phorus	Iron	Potas-sium	Sodium	Vitamin A value		Thiamin	Ribo-flavin	Niacin	Ascorbic acid	Item No.
							(IU)	(RE)					
Milli-grams	Grams	Milli-grams	Milli-grams	Milli-grams	Milli-grams	Milli-grams	Inter-national units	Retinol equiva-lents	Milli-grams	Milli-grams	Milli-grams	Milli-grams	
0	9	6	7	0.1	93	1	40	4	0.05	0.03	0.2	5	237
0	10	6	7	0.1	105	1	40	4	0.05	0.03	0.2	6	238
0	38	23	28	0.6	334	8	20	2	0.07	0.09	0.7	[20]Tr	239
0	96	28	32	0.8	160	15	60	6	0.11	0.20	0.9	[21]179	240
0	32	10	10	0.3	53	5	20	2	0.04	0.07	0.3	[21]60	241
0	11	20	30	0.3	252	4	130	13	0.02	0.04	0.4	74	242
0	5	15	9	0.3	80	1	20	2	0.02	0.01	0.1	31	243
0	21	17	15	0.1	303	2	50	5	0.07	0.02	0.2	112	244
0	16	27	22	0.3	249	[23]51	40	4	0.10	0.02	0.5	61	245
0	1	2	1	Tr	15	[23]3	Tr	Tr	0.01	Tr	Tr	4	246
0	16	20	20	0.3	217	2	30	3	0.14	0.03	0.3	77	247
0	22	22	17	0.1	268	2	20	2	0.05	0.02	0.2	72	248
0	16	30	25	0.6	185	[23]39	40	4	0.08	0.01	0.4	16	249
0	35	21	23	0.3	323	4	8,060	806	0.12	0.12	1.2	57	250
0	22	29	45	0.6	825	24	8,610	861	0.10	0.06	1.5	113	251
0	12	8	13	0.1	350	13	50	5	0.10	0.02	0.8	32	252
0	16	7	22	0.2	288	Tr	1,000	100	0.02	0.06	1.3	7	253
0	15	52	18	0.1	237	Tr	270	27	0.11	0.05	0.4	70	254
0	21	72	25	0.2	326	Tr	370	37	0.16	0.07	0.5	96	255
0	26	27	42	0.5	496	2	500	50	0.22	0.07	1.0	124	256
0	25	20	35	1.1	436	5	440	44	0.15	0.07	0.8	86	257
0	25	25	27	0.4	473	2	190	19	0.28	0.05	0.7	82	258
0	81	68	121	0.7	1,436	6	590	59	0.60	0.14	1.5	294	259
0	27	22	40	0.2	473	2	190	19	0.20	0.04	0.5	97	260
0	25	20	35	1.1	390	7	290	29	0.14	0.07	0.8	72	261
0	17	35	12	0.3	247	9	400	40	0.04	0.04	0.5	92	262
0	10	4	10	0.1	171	Tr	470	47	0.01	0.04	0.9	6	263
0	19	9	20	0.2	335	Tr	910	91	0.03	0.07	1.7	11	264
0	51	8	28	0.7	236	15	850	85	0.03	0.06	1.6	7	265
0	16	2	9	0.2	75	5	270	27	0.01	0.02	0.5	2	266
0	29	15	42	0.7	317	10	940	94	0.02	0.04	1.4	9	267
0	9	5	13	0.2	99	3	290	29	0.01	0.01	0.4	3	268

[23]Sodium benzoate and sodium bisulfite added as preservatives.

Table 2. Nutritive Value of the Edible Part of Food (Continued)

(Tr indicates nutrient present in trace amount.)

Item No.	Foods, approximate measures, units, and weight (weight of edible portion only)			Water	Food energy	Pro-tein	Fat	Fatty acids		
								Satu-rated	Mono-unsatu-rated	Poly-unsatu-rated
	Fruits and Fruit Juices—Con.		Grams	Per-cent	Cal-ories	Grams	Grams	Grams	Grams	Grams
	Peaches:									
	Dried:									
269	Uncooked---------------------	1 cup------------	160	32	380	6	1	0.1	0.4	0.6
270	Cooked, unsweetened, fruit and liquid-----------------	1 cup----------	258	78	200	3	1	0.1	0.2	0.3
271	Frozen, sliced, sweetened------	10-oz container	284	75	265	2	Tr	Tr	0.1	0.2
272		1 cup----------	250	75	235	2	Tr	Tr	0.1	0.2
	Pears:									
	Raw, with skin, cored:									
273	Bartlett, 2-1/2-in diam. (about 2-1/2 per lb with cores and stems)-----------	1 pear----------	166	84	100	1	1	Tr	0.1	0.2
274	Bosc, 2-1/2-in diam. (about 3 per lb with cores and stems)---------------------	1 pear----------	141	84	85	1	1	Tr	0.1	0.1
275	D'Anjou, 3-in diam. (about 2 per lb with cores and stems)---------------------	1 pear----------	200	84	120	1	1	Tr	0.2	0.2
	Canned, fruit and liquid:									
276	Heavy syrup pack-------------	1 cup----------	255	80	190	1	Tr	Tr	0.1	0.1
277		1 half----------	79	80	60	Tr	Tr	Tr	Tr	Tr
278	Juice pack------------------	1 cup----------	248	86	125	1	Tr	Tr	Tr	Tr
279		1 half----------	77	86	40	Tr	Tr	Tr	Tr	Tr
	Pineapple:									
280	Raw, diced---------------------	1 cup----------	155	87	75	1	1	Tr	0.1	0.2
	Canned, fruit and liquid:									
	Heavy syrup pack:									
281	Crushed, chunks, tidbits---	1 cup----------	255	79	200	1	Tr	Tr	Tr	0.1
282	Slices-------------------	1 slice---------	58	79	45	Tr	Tr	Tr	Tr	Tr
	Juice pack:									
283	Chunks or tidbits----------	1 cup----------	250	84	150	1	Tr	Tr	Tr	0.1
284	Slices---------------------	1 slice---------	58	84	35	Tr	Tr	Tr	Tr	Tr
285	Pineapple juice, unsweetened, canned------------------------	1 cup----------	250	86	140	1	Tr	Tr	Tr	0.1
	Plantains, without peel:									
286	Raw---------------------------	1 plantain------	179	65	220	2	1	0.3	0.1	0.1
287	Cooked, boiled, sliced---------	1 cup----------	154	67	180	1	Tr	0.1	Tr	0.1
	Plums, without pits:									
	Raw:									
288	2-1/8-in diam. (about 6-1/2 per lb with pits)----------	1 plum----------	66	85	35	1	Tr	Tr	0.3	0.1
289	1-1/2-in diam. (about 15 per lb with pits)--------------	1 plum----------	28	85	15	Tr	Tr	Tr	0.1	Tr
	Canned, purple, fruit and liquid:									
290	Heavy syrup pack-------------	1 cup----------	258	76	230	1	Tr	Tr	0.2	0.1
291		3 plums---------	133	76	120	Tr	Tr	Tr	0.1	Tr
292	Juice pack------------------	1 cup----------	252	84	145	1	Tr	Tr	Tr	Tr
293		3 plums---------	95	84	55	Tr	Tr	Tr	Tr	Tr
	Prunes, dried:									
294	Uncooked----------------------	4 extra large or 5 large prunes	49	32	115	1	Tr	Tr	0.2	0.1
295	Cooked, unsweetened, fruit and liquid----------------------	1 cup----------	212	70	225	2	Tr	Tr	0.3	0.1
296	Prune juice, canned or bottled---	1 cup----------	256	81	180	2	Tr	Tr	0.1	Tr
	Raisins, seedless:									
297	Cup, not pressed down----------	1 cup----------	145	15	435	5	1	0.2	Tr	0.2
298	Packet, 1/2 oz (1-1/2 tbsp)----	1 packet--------	14	15	40	Tr	Tr	Tr	Tr	Tr
	Raspberries:									
299	Raw---------------------------	1 cup----------	123	87	60	1	1	Tr	0.1	0.4
300	Frozen, sweetened-------------	10-oz container	284	73	295	2	Tr	Tr	Tr	0.3
301		1 cup----------	250	73	255	2	Tr	Tr	Tr	0.2

[21] With added ascorbic acid.

182

Nutrients in Indicated Quantity

Cholesterol	Carbohydrate	Calcium	Phosphorus	Iron	Potassium	Sodium	Vitamin A value		Thiamin	Riboflavin	Niacin	Ascorbic acid	Item No.
							(IU)	(RE)					
Milligrams	Grams	Milligrams	Milligrams	Milligrams	Milligrams	Milligrams	International units	Retinol equivalents	Milligrams	Milligrams	Milligrams	Milligrams	
0	98	45	190	6.5	1,594	11	3,460	346	Tr	0.34	7.0	8	269
0	51	23	98	3.4	826	5	510	51	0.01	0.05	3.9	10	270
0	68	9	31	1.1	369	17	810	81	0.04	0.10	1.9	[21]268	271
0	60	8	28	0.9	325	15	710	71	0.03	0.09	1.6	[21]236	272
0	25	18	18	0.4	208	Tr	30	3	0.03	0.07	0.2	7	273
0	21	16	16	0.4	176	Tr	30	3	0.03	0.06	0.1	6	274
0	30	22	22	0.5	250	Tr	40	4	0.04	0.08	0.2	8	275
0	49	13	18	0.6	166	13	10	1	0.03	0.06	0.6	3	276
0	15	4	6	0.2	51	4	Tr	Tr	0.01	0.02	0.2	1	277
0	32	22	30	0.7	238	10	10	1	0.03	0.03	0.5	4	278
0	10	7	9	0.2	74	3	Tr	Tr	0.01	0.01	0.2	1	279
0	19	11	11	0.6	175	2	40	4	0.14	0.06	0.7	24	280
0	52	36	18	1.0	265	3	40	4	0.23	0.06	0.7	19	281
0	12	8	4	0.2	60	1	10	1	0.05	0.01	0.2	4	282
0	39	35	15	0.7	305	3	100	10	0.24	0.05	0.7	24	283
0	9	8	3	0.2	71	1	20	2	0.06	0.01	0.2	6	284
0	34	43	20	0.7	335	3	10	1	0.14	0.06	0.6	27	285
0	57	5	61	1.1	893	7	2,020	202	0.09	0.10	1.2	33	286
0	48	3	43	0.9	716	8	1,400	140	0.07	0.08	1.2	17	287
0	9	3	7	0.1	114	Tr	210	21	0.03	0.06	0.3	6	288
0	4	1	3	Tr	48	Tr	90	9	0.01	0.03	0.1	3	289
0	60	23	34	2.2	235	49	670	67	0.04	0.10	0.8	1	290
0	31	12	17	1.1	121	25	340	34	0.02	0.05	0.4	1	291
0	38	25	38	0.9	388	3	2,540	254	0.06	0.15	1.2	7	292
0	14	10	14	0.3	146	1	960	96	0.02	0.06	0.4	3	293
0	31	25	39	1.2	365	2	970	97	0.04	0.08	1.0	2	294
0	60	49	74	2.4	708	4	650	65	0.05	0.21	1.5	6	295
0	45	31	64	3.0	707	10	10	1	0.04	0.18	2.0	10	296
0	115	71	141	3.0	1,089	17	10	1	0.23	0.13	1.2	5	297
0	11	7	14	0.3	105	2	Tr	Tr	0.02	0.01	0.1	Tr	298
0	14	27	15	0.7	187	Tr	160	16	0.04	0.11	1.1	31	299
0	74	43	48	1.8	324	3	170	17	0.05	0.13	0.7	47	300
0	65	38	43	1.6	285	3	150	15	0.05	0.11	0.6	41	301

Table 2. Nutritive Value of the Edible Part of Food (Continued)
(Tr indicates nutrient present in trace amount.)

Item No.	Foods, approximate measures, units, and weight (weight of edible portion only)		Water	Food energy	Pro-tein	Fat	Fatty acids		
							Satu-rated	Mono-unsatu-rated	Poly-unsatu-rated
		Grams	Per-cent	Cal-ories	Grams	Grams	Grams	Grams	Grams
	Fruits and Fruit Juices—Con.								
302	Rhubarb, cooked, added sugar----- 1 cup-----------	240	68	280	1	Tr	Tr	Tr	0.1
	Strawberries:								
303	Raw, capped, whole-------------- 1 cup-----------	149	92	45	1	1	Tr	0.1	0.3
304	Frozen, sweetened, sliced------ 10-oz container	284	73	275	2	Tr	Tr	0.1	0.2
305	1 cup-----------	255	73	245	1	Tr	Tr	Tr	0.2
	Tangerines:								
306	Raw, without peel and seeds (2-3/8-in diam., about 4 per lb, with peel and seeds)----- 1 tangerine-----	84	88	35	1	Tr	Tr	Tr	Tr
307	Canned, light syrup, fruit and liquid---------------------- 1 cup-----------	252	83	155	1	Tr	Tr	Tr	0.1
308	Tangerine juice, canned, sweet-ened------------------------ 1 cup-----------	249	87	125	1	Tr	Tr	Tr	0.1
	Watermelon, raw, without rind and seeds:								
309	Piece (4 by 8 in wedge with rind and seeds; 1/16 of 32-2/3-lb melon, 10 by 16 in) 1 piece---------	482	92	155	3	2	0.3	0.2	1.0
310	Diced------------------------- 1 cup-----------	160	92	50	1	1	0.1	0.1	0.3
	Grain Products								
311	Bagels, plain or water, enriched, 3-1/2-in diam.[24] ---------------- 1 bagel---------	68	29	200	7	2	0.3	0.5	0.7
312	Barley, pearled, light, uncooked 1 cup-----------	200	11	700	16	2	0.3	0.2	0.9
	Biscuits, baking powder, 2-in diam. (enriched flour, vege-table shortening):								
313	From home recipe--------------- 1 biscuit-------	28	28	100	2	5	1.2	2.0	1.3
314	From mix----------------------- 1 biscuit-------	28	29	95	2	3	0.8	1.4	0.9
315	From refrigerated dough-------- 1 biscuit-------	20	30	65	1	2	0.6	0.9	0.6
	Breadcrumbs, enriched:								
316	Dry, grated-------------------- 1 cup-----------	100	7	390	13	5	1.5	1.6	1.0
	Soft. See White bread (item 351).								
	Breads:								
317	Boston brown bread, canned, slice, 3-1/4 in by 1/2 in[25]-- 1 slice---------	45	45	95	2	1	0.3	0.1	0.1
	Cracked-wheat bread (3/4 en-riched wheat flour, 1/4 cracked wheat flour):[25]								
318	Loaf, 1 lb-------------------- 1 loaf----------	454	35	1,190	42	16	3.1	4.3	5.7
319	Slice (18 per loaf)---------- 1 slice---------	25	35	65	2	1	0.2	0.2	0.3
320	Toasted--------------------- 1 slice---------	21	26	65	2	1	0.2	0.2	0.3
	French or vienna bread, en-riched:[25]								
321	Loaf, 1 lb-------------------- 1 loaf----------	454	34	1,270	43	18	3.8	5.7	5.9
	Slice:								
322	French, 5 by 2-1/2 by 1 in 1 slice---------	35	34	100	3	1	0.3	0.4	0.5
323	Vienna, 4-3/4 by 4 by 1/2 in---------------------- 1 slice---------	25	34	70	2	1	0.2	0.3	0.3
	Italian bread, enriched:								
324	Loaf, 1 lb-------------------- 1 loaf----------	454	32	1,255	41	4	0.6	0.3	1.6
325	Slice, 4-1/2 by 3-1/4 by 3/4 in---------------------- 1 slice---------	30	32	85	3	Tr	Tr	Tr	0.1
	Mixed grain bread, enriched:[25]								
326	Loaf, 1 lb-------------------- 1 loaf----------	454	37	1,165	45	17	3.2	4.1	6.5
327	Slice (18 per loaf)---------- 1 slice---------	25	37	65	2	1	0.2	0.2	0.4
328	Toasted--------------------- 1 slice---------	23	27	65	2	1	0.2	0.2	0.4

[24] Egg bagels have 44 mg cholesterol and 22 IU or 7 RE vitamin A per bagel.
[25] Made with vegetable shortening.

Cho-les-terol	Carbo-hydrate	Calcium	Phos-phorus	Iron	Potas-sium	Sodium	Vitamin A value		Thiamin	Ribo-flavin	Niacin	Ascorbic acid	Item No.
							(IU)	(RE)					
Milli-grams	Grams	Milli-grams	Milli-grams	Milli-grams	Milli-grams	Milli-grams	Inter-national units	Retinol equiva-lents	Milli-grams	Milli-grams	Milli-grams	Milli-grams	
0	75	348	19	0.5	230	2	170	17	0.04	0.06	0.5	8	302
0	10	21	28	0.6	247	1	40	4	0.03	0.10	0.3	84	303
0	74	31	37	1.7	278	9	70	7	0.05	0.14	1.1	118	304
0	66	28	33	1.5	250	8	60	6	0.04	0.13	1.0	106	305
0	9	12	8	0.1	132	1	770	77	0.09	0.02	0.1	26	306
0	41	18	25	0.9	197	15	2,120	212	0.13	0.11	1.1	50	307
0	30	45	35	0.5	443	2	1,050	105	0.15	0.05	0.2	55	308
0	35	39	43	0.8	559	10	1,760	176	0.39	0.10	1.0	46	309
0	11	13	14	0.3	186	3	590	59	0.13	0.03	0.3	15	310
0	38	29	46	1.8	50	245	0	0	0.26	0.20	2.4	0	311
0	158	32	378	4.2	320	6	0	0	0.24	0.10	6.2	0	312
Tr	13	47	36	0.7	32	195	10	3	0.08	0.08	0.8	Tr	313
Tr	14	58	128	0.7	56	262	20	4	0.12	0.11	0.8	Tr	314
1	10	4	79	0.5	18	249	0	0	0.08	0.05	0.7	0	315
5	73	122	141	4.1	152	736	0	0	0.35	0.35	4.8	0	316
3	21	41	72	0.9	131	113	[26]0	[26]0	0.06	0.04	0.7	0	317
0	227	295	581	12.1	608	1,966	Tr	Tr	1.73	1.73	15.3	Tr	318
0	12	16	32	0.7	34	106	Tr	Tr	0.10	0.09	0.8	Tr	319
0	12	16	32	0.7	34	106	Tr	Tr	0.07	0.09	0.8	Tr	320
0	230	499	386	14.0	409	2,633	Tr	Tr	2.09	1.59	18.2	Tr	321
0	18	39	30	1.1	32	203	Tr	Tr	0.16	0.12	1.4	Tr	322
0	13	28	21	0.8	23	145	Tr	Tr	0.12	0.09	1.0	Tr	323
0	256	77	350	12.7	336	2,656	0	0	1.80	1.10	15.0	0	324
0	17	5	23	0.8	22	176	0	0	0.12	0.07	1.0	0	325
0	212	472	962	14.8	990	1,870	Tr	Tr	1.77	1.73	18.9	Tr	326
0	12	27	55	0.8	56	106	Tr	Tr	0.10	0.10	1.1	Tr	327
0	12	27	55	0.8	56	106	Tr	Tr	0.08	0.10	1.1	Tr	328

[26]Made with white cornmeal. If made with yellow cornmeal, value is 32 IU or 3 RE.

Item No.	Foods, approximate measures, units, and weight (weight of edible portion only)			Water	Food energy	Pro-tein	Fat	Fatty acids		
								Satu-rated	Mono-unsatu-rated	Poly-unsatu-rated
			Grams	Per-cent	Cal-ories	Grams	Grams	Grams	Grams	Grams

Grain Products—Con.

Breads:
Oatmeal bread, enriched:[25]

329	Loaf, 1 lb	1 loaf	454	37	1,145	38	20	3.7	7.1	8.2
330	Slice (18 per loaf)	1 slice	25	37	65	2	1	0.2	0.4	0.5
331	Toasted	1 slice	23	30	65	2	1	0.2	0.4	0.5
332	Pita bread, enriched, white, 6-1/2-in diam.	1 pita	60	31	165	6	1	0.1	0.1	0.4
	Pumpernickel (2/3 rye flour, 1/3 enriched wheat flour):[25]									
333	Loaf, 1 lb	1 loaf	454	37	1,160	42	16	2.6	3.6	6.4
334	Slice, 5 by 4 by 3/8 in	1 slice	32	37	80	3	1	0.2	0.3	0.5
335	Toasted	1 slice	29	28	80	3	1	0.2	0.3	0.5
	Raisin bread, enriched:[25]									
336	Loaf, 1 lb	1 loaf	454	33	1,260	37	18	4.1	6.5	6.7
337	Slice (18 per loaf)	1 slice	25	33	65	2	1	0.2	0.3	0.4
338	Toasted	1 slice	21	24	65	2	1	0.2	0.3	0.4
	Rye bread, light (2/3 enriched wheat flour, 1/3 rye flour):[25]									
339	Loaf, 1 lb	1 loaf	454	37	1,190	38	17	3.3	5.2	5.5
340	Slice, 4-3/4 by 3-3/4 by 7/16 in	1 slice	25	37	65	2	1	0.2	0.3	0.3
341	Toasted	1 slice	22	28	65	2	1	0.2	0.3	0.3
	Wheat bread, enriched:[25]									
342	Loaf, 1 lb	1 loaf	454	37	1,160	43	19	3.9	7.3	4.5
343	Slice (18 per loaf)	1 slice	25	37	65	2	1	0.2	0.4	0.3
344	Toasted	1 slice	23	28	65	3	1	0.2	0.4	0.3
	White bread, enriched:[25]									
345	Loaf, 1 lb	1 loaf	454	37	1,210	38	18	5.6	6.5	4.2
346	Slice (18 per loaf)	1 slice	25	37	65	2	1	0.3	0.4	0.2
347	Toasted	1 slice	22	28	65	2	1	0.3	0.4	0.2
348	Slice (22 per loaf)	1 slice	20	37	55	2	1	0.2	0.3	0.2
349	Toasted	1 slice	17	28	55	2	1	0.2	0.3	0.2
350	Cubes	1 cup	30	37	80	2	1	0.4	0.4	0.3
351	Crumbs, soft	1 cup	45	37	120	4	2	0.6	0.6	0.4
	Whole-wheat bread:[25]									
352	Loaf, 1 lb	1 loaf	454	38	1,110	44	20	5.8	6.8	5.2
353	Slice (16 per loaf)	1 slice	28	38	70	3	1	0.4	0.4	0.3
354	Toasted	1 slice	25	29	70	3	1	0.4	0.4	0.3
	Bread stuffing (from enriched bread), prepared from mix:									
355	Dry type	1 cup	140	33	500	9	31	6.1	13.3	9.6
356	Moist type	1 cup	203	61	420	9	26	5.3	11.3	8.0
	Breakfast cereals:									
	Hot type, cooked:									
	Corn (hominy) grits:									
357	Regular and quick, enriched	1 cup	242	85	145	3	Tr	Tr	0.1	0.2
358	Instant, plain	1 pkt	137	85	80	2	Tr	Tr	Tr	0.1
	Cream of Wheat®:									
359	Regular, quick, instant	1 cup	244	86	140	4	Tr	0.1	Tr	0.2
360	Mix'n Eat, plain	1 pkt	142	82	100	3	Tr	Tr	Tr	0.1
361	Malt-O-Meal®	1 cup	240	88	120	4	Tr	Tr	Tr	0.1
	Oatmeal or rolled oats:									
362	Regular, quick, instant, nonfortified	1 cup	234	85	145	6	2	0.4	0.8	1.0
	Instant, fortified:									
363	Plain	1 pkt	177	86	105	4	2	0.3	0.6	0.7
364	Flavored	1 pkt	164	76	160	5	2	0.3	0.7	0.8

[25] Made with vegetable shortening.
[27] Nutrient added.
[28] Cooked without salt. If salt is added according to label recommendations, sodium content is 540 mg.
[29] For white corn grits. Cooked yellow grits contain 145 IU or 14 RE.
[30] Value based on label declaration for added nutrients.

Cholesterol	Carbohydrate	Calcium	Phosphorus	Iron	Potassium	Sodium	Vitamin A value		Thiamin	Riboflavin	Niacin	Ascorbic acid	Item No.
							(IU)	(RE)					
Milligrams	Grams	Milligrams	Milligrams	Milligrams	Milligrams	Milligrams	International units	Retinol equivalents	Milligrams	Milligrams	Milligrams	Milligrams	
0	212	267	563	12.0	707	2,231	0	0	2.09	1.20	15.4	0	329
0	12	15	31	0.7	39	124	0	0	0.12	0.07	0.9	0	330
0	12	15	31	0.7	39	124	0	0	0.09	0.07	0.9	0	331
0	33	49	60	1.4	71	339	0	0	0.27	0.12	2.2	0	332
0	218	322	990	12.4	1,966	2,461	0	0	1.54	2.36	15.0	0	333
0	16	23	71	0.9	141	177	0	0	0.11	0.17	1.1	0	334
0	16	23	71	0.9	141	177	0	0	0.09	0.17	1.1	0	335
0	239	463	395	14.1	1,058	1,657	Tr	Tr	1.50	2.81	18.6	Tr	336
0	13	25	22	0.8	59	92	Tr	Tr	0.08	0.15	1.0	Tr	337
0	13	25	22	0.8	59	92	Tr	Tr	0.06	0.15	1.0	Tr	338
0	218	363	658	12.3	926	3,164	0	0	1.86	1.45	15.0	0	339
0	12	20	36	0.7	51	175	0	0	0.10	0.08	0.8	0	340
0	12	20	36	0.7	51	175	0	0	0.08	0.08	0.8	0	341
0	213	572	835	15.8	627	2,447	Tr	Tr	2.09	1.45	20.5	Tr	342
0	12	32	47	0.9	35	138	Tr	Tr	0.12	0.08	1.2	Tr	343
0	12	32	47	0.9	35	138	Tr	Tr	0.10	0.08	1.2	Tr	344
0	222	572	490	12.9	508	2,334	Tr	Tr	2.13	1.41	17.0	Tr	345
0	12	32	27	0.7	28	129	Tr	Tr	0.12	0.08	0.9	Tr	346
0	12	32	27	0.7	28	129	Tr	Tr	0.09	0.08	0.9	Tr	347
0	10	25	21	0.6	22	101	Tr	Tr	0.09	0.06	0.7	Tr	348
0	10	25	21	0.6	22	101	Tr	Tr	0.07	0.06	0.7	Tr	349
0	15	38	32	0.9	34	154	Tr	Tr	0.14	0.09	1.1	Tr	350
0	22	57	49	1.3	50	231	Tr	Tr	0.21	0.14	1.7	Tr	351
0	206	327	1,180	15.5	799	2,887	Tr	Tr	1.59	0.95	17.4	Tr	352
0	13	20	74	1.0	50	180	Tr	Tr	0.10	0.06	1.1	Tr	353
0	13	20	74	1.0	50	180	Tr	Tr	0.08	0.06	1.1	Tr	354
0	50	92	136	2.2	126	1,254	910	273	0.17	0.20	2.5	0	355
67	40	81	134	2.0	118	1,023	850	256	0.10	0.18	1.6	0	356
0	31	0	29	[27]1.5	53	[28]0	[29]0	[29]0	[27]0.24	[27]0.15	[27]2.0	0	357
0	18	7	16	[27]1.0	29	343	0	0	[27]0.18	[27]0.08	[27]1.3	0	358
0	29	[30]54	[31]43	[30]10.9	46	[31,32]5	0	0	[30]0.24	[30]0.07	[30]1.5	0	359
0	21	[30]20	[30]20	[30]8.1	38	241	[30]1,250	[30]376	[30]0.43	[30]0.28	[30]5.0	0	360
0	26	5	[30]24	[30]9.6	31	[33]2	0	0	[30]0.48	[30]0.24	[30]5.8	0	361
0	25	19	178	1.6	131	[34]2	40	4	0.26	0.05	0.3	0	362
0	18	[27]163	133	[27]6.3	99	[27]285	[27]1,510	[27]453	[27]0.53	[27]0.28	[27]5.5	0	363
0	31	[27]168	148	[27]6.7	137	[27]254	[27]1,530	[27]460	[27]0.53	[27]0.38	[27]5.9	Tr	364

[31] For regular and instant cereal. For quick cereal, phosphorus is 102 mg and sodium is 142 mg.
[32] Cooked without salt. If salt is added according to label recommendations, sodium content is 390 mg.
[33] Cooked without salt. If salt is added according to label recommendations, sodium content is 324 mg.
[34] Cooked without salt. If salt is added according to label recommendations, sodium content is 374 mg.

Table 2. Nutritive Value of the Edible Part of Food (Continued)

(Tr indicates nutrient present in trace amount.)

Item No.	Foods, approximate measures, units, and weight (weight of edible portion only)			Water	Food energy	Pro-tein	Fat	Fatty acids		
								Satu-rated	Mono-unsatu-rated	Poly-unsatu-rated
	Grain Products—Con.		Grams	Per-cent	Cal-ories	Grams	Grams	Grams	Grams	Grams
	Breakfast cereals:									
	Ready to eat:									
365	All-Bran® (about 1/3 cup)----	1 oz------------	28	3	70	4	1	0.1	0.1	0.3
366	Cap'n Crunch® (about 3/4 cup)	1 oz------------	28	3	120	1	3	1.7	0.3	0.4
367	Cheerios® (about 1-1/4 cup)--	1 oz------------	28	5	110	4	2	0.3	0.6	0.7
	Corn Flakes (about 1-1/4 cup):									
368	Kellogg's® -----------------	1 oz------------	28	3	110	2	Tr	Tr	Tr	Tr
369	Toasties® ------------------	1 oz------------	28	3	110	2	Tr	Tr	Tr	Tr
	40% Bran Flakes:									
370	Kellogg's® (about 3/4 cup)	1 oz------------	28	3	90	4	1	0.1	0.1	0.3
371	Post® (about 2/3 cup)------	1 oz------------	28	3	90	3	Tr	0.1	0.1	0.2
372	Froot Loops® (about 1 cup)---	1 oz------------	28	3	110	2	1	0.2	0.1	0.1
373	Golden Grahams® (about 3/4 cup)----------------------	1 oz------------	28	2	110	2	1	0.7	0.1	0.2
374	Grape-Nuts® (about 1/4 cup)--	1 oz------------	28	3	100	3	Tr	Tr	Tr	0.1
375	Honey Nut Cheerios® (about 3/4 cup)-------------------	1 oz------------	28	3	105	3	1	0.1	0.3	0.3
376	Lucky Charms® (about 1 cup)--	1 oz------------	28	3	110	3	1	0.2	0.4	0.4
377	Nature Valley® Granola (about 1/3 cup)-------------------	1 oz------------	28	4	125	3	5	3.3	0.7	0.7
378	100% Natural Cereal (about 1/4 cup)-------------------	1 oz------------	28	2	135	3	6	4.1	1.2	0.5
379	Product 19® (about 3/4 cup)--	1 oz------------	28	3	110	3	Tr	Tr	Tr	0.1
	Raisin Bran:									
380	Kellogg's® (about 3/4 cup)	1 oz------------	28	8	90	3	1	0.1	0.1	0.3
381	Post® (about 1/2 cup)------	1 oz------------	28	9	85	3	1	0.1	0.1	0.3
382	Rice Krispies® (about 1 cup)	1 oz------------	28	2	110	2	Tr	Tr	Tr	0.1
383	Shredded Wheat (about 2/3 cup)----------------------	1 oz------------	28	5	100	3	1	0.1	0.1	0.3
384	Special K® (about 1-1/3 cup)	1 oz------------	28	2	110	6	Tr	Tr	Tr	Tr
385	Super Sugar Crisp® (about 7/8 cup)----------------------	1 oz------------	28	2	105	2	Tr	Tr	Tr	0.1
386	Sugar Frosted Flakes, Kellogg's® (about 3/4 cup)	1 oz------------	28	3	110	1	Tr	Tr	Tr	Tr
387	Sugar Smacks® (about 3/4 cup)	1 oz------------	28	3	105	2	1	0.1	0.1	0.2
388	Total® (about 1 cup)---------	1 oz------------	28	4	100	3	1	0.1	0.1	0.3
389	Trix® (about 1 cup)----------	1 oz------------	28	3	110	2	Tr	0.2	0.1	0.1
390	Wheaties® (about 1 cup)------	1 oz------------	28	5	100	3	Tr	0.1	Tr	0.2
391	Buckwheat flour, light, sifted---	1 cup----------	98	12	340	6	1	0.2	0.4	0.4
392	Bulgur, uncooked-----------------	1 cup----------	170	10	600	19	3	1.2	0.3	1.2
	Cakes prepared from cake mixes with enriched flour:[35]									
	Angelfood:									
393	Whole cake, 9-3/4-in diam. tube cake------------------	1 cake----------	635	38	1,510	38	2	0.4	0.2	1.0
394	Piece, 1/12 of cake----------	1 piece---------	53	38	125	3	Tr	Tr	Tr	0.1
	Coffeecake, crumb:									
395	Whole cake, 7-3/4 by 5-5/8 by 1-1/4 in----------------	1 cake----------	430	30	1,385	27	41	11.8	16.7	9.6
396	Piece, 1/6 of cake-----------	1 piece---------	72	30	230	5	7	2.0	2.8	1.6
	Devil's food with chocolate frosting:									
397	Whole, 2-layer cake, 8- or 9-in diam.-----------------	1 cake----------	1,107	24	3,755	49	136	55.6	51.4	19.7
398	Piece, 1/16 of cake----------	1 piece---------	69	24	235	3	8	3.5	3.2	1.2
399	Cupcake, 2-1/2-in diam.------	1 cupcake-------	35	24	120	2	4	1.8	1.6	0.6
	Gingerbread:									
400	Whole cake, 8 in square------	1 cake----------	570	37	1,575	18	39	9.6	16.4	10.5
401	Piece, 1/9 of cake-----------	1 piece---------	63	37	175	2	4	1.1	1.8	1.2

[27]Nutrient added.
[30]Value based on label declaration for added nutrients.

Nutrients in Indicated Quantity

Cholesterol	Carbohydrate	Calcium	Phosphorus	Iron	Potassium	Sodium	Vitamin A value (IU)	Vitamin A value (RE)	Thiamin	Riboflavin	Niacin	Ascorbic acid	Item No.
Milligrams	Grams	Milligrams	Milligrams	Milligrams	Milligrams	Milligrams	International units	Retinol equivalents	Milligrams	Milligrams	Milligrams	Milligrams	
0	21	23	264	[30]4.5	350	320	[30]1,250	[30]375	[30]0.37	[30]0.43	[30]5.0	[30]15	365
0	23	5	36	[27]7.5	37	213	40	[30]4	[27]0.50	[27]0.55	[27]6.6	0	366
0	20	48	134	[30]4.5	101	307	[30]1,250	[30]375	[30]0.37	[30]0.43	[30]5.0	[30]15	367
0	24	1	18	[30]1.8	26	351	[30]1,250	[30]375	[30]0.37	[30]0.43	[30]5.0	[30]15	368
0	24	1	12	[27]0.7	33	297	[30]1,250	[30]375	[30]0.37	[30]0.43	[30]5.0	0	369
0	22	14	139	[30]8.1	180	264	[30]1,250	[30]375	[30]0.37	[30]0.43	[30]5.0	0	370
0	22	12	179	[30]4.5	151	260	[30]1,250	[30]375	[30]0.37	[30]0.43	[30]5.0	0	371
0	25	3	24	[30]4.5	26	145	[30]1,250	[30]375	[30]0.37	[30]0.43	[30]5.0	[30]15	372
Tr	24	17	41	[30]4.5	63	346	[30]1,250	[30]375	[30]0.37	[30]0.43	[30]5.0	[30]15	373
0	23	11	71	1.2	95	197	[30]1,250	[30]375	[30]0.37	[30]0.43	[30]5.0	0	374
0	23	20	105	[30]4.5	99	257	[30]1,250	[30]375	[30]0.37	[30]0.43	[30]5.0	[30]15	375
0	23	32	79	[30]4.5	59	201	[30]1,250	[30]375	[30]0.37	[30]0.43	[30]5.0	[30]15	376
0	19	18	89	0.9	98	58	20	2	0.10	0.05	0.2	0	377
Tr	18	49	104	0.8	140	12	20	2	0.09	0.15	0.6	0	378
0	24	3	40	[30]18.0	44	325	[30]5,000	[30]1,501	[30]1.50	[30]1.70	[30]20.0	[30]60	379
0	21	10	105	[30]3.5	147	207	[30]960	[30]288	[30]0.28	[30]0.34	[30]3.9	0	380
0	21	13	119	[30]4.5	175	185	[30]1,250	[30]375	[30]0.37	[30]0.43	[30]5.0	0	381
0	25	4	34	[30]1.8	29	340	[30]1,250	[30]375	[30]0.37	[30]0.43	[30]5.0	[30]15	382
0	23	11	100	1.2	102	3	0	0	0.07	0.08	1.5	0	383
Tr	21	8	55	[30]4.5	49	265	[30]1,250	[30]375	[30]0.37	[30]0.43	[30]5.0	[30]15	384
0	26	6	52	[30]1.8	105	25	[30]1,250	[30]375	[30]0.37	[30]0.43	[30]5.0	0	385
0	26	1	21	[30]1.8	18	230	[30]1,250	[30]375	[30]0.37	[30]0.43	[30]5.0	[30]15	386
0	25	3	31	[30]1.8	42	75	[30]1,250	[30]375	[30]0.37	[30]0.43	[30]5.0	[30]15	387
0	22	48	118	[30]18.0	106	352	[30]5,000	[30]1,501	[30]1.50	[30]1.70	[30]20.0	[30]60	388
0	25	6	19	[30]4.5	27	181	[30]1,250	[30]375	[30]0.37	[30]0.43	[30]5.0	[30]15	389
0	23	43	98	[30]4.5	106	354	[30]1,250	[30]375	[30]0.37	[30]0.43	[30]5.0	[30]15	390
0	78	11	86	1.0	314	2	0	0	0.08	0.04	0.4	0	391
0	129	49	575	9.5	389	7	0	0	0.48	0.24	7.7	0	392
0	342	527	1,086	2.7	845	3,226	0	0	0.32	1.27	1.6	0	393
0	29	44	91	0.2	71	269	0	0	0.03	0.11	0.1	0	394
279	225	262	748	7.3	469	1,853	690	194	0.82	0.90	7.7	1	395
47	38	44	125	1.2	78	310	120	32	0.14	0.15	1.3	Tr	396
598	645	653	1,162	22.1	1,439	2,900	1,660	498	1.11	1.66	10.0	1	397
37	40	41	72	1.4	90	181	100	31	0.07	0.10	0.6	Tr	398
19	20	21	37	0.7	46	92	50	16	0.04	0.05	0.3	Tr	399
6	291	513	570	10.8	1,562	1,733	0	0	0.86	1.03	7.4	1	400
1	32	57	63	1.2	173	192	0	0	0.09	0.11	0.8	Tr	401

[35] Excepting angelfood cake, cakes were made from mixes containing vegetable shortening and frostings were made with margarine.

Item No.	Foods, approximate measures, units, and weight (weight of edible portion only)			Water	Food energy	Pro-tein	Fat	Fatty acids		
								Satu-rated	Mono-unsatu-rated	Poly-unsatu-rated
			Grams	Per-cent	Cal-ories	Grams	Grams	Grams	Grams	Grams
	Grain Products—Con.									
	Cakes prepared from cake mixes with enriched flour:[35]									
	Yellow with chocolate frosting:									
402	Whole, 2-layer cake, 8- or 9-in diam.-----------------	1 cake----------	1,108	26	3,735	45	125	47.8	48.8	21.8
403	Piece, 1/16 of cake----------	1 piece---------	69	26	235	3	8	3.0	3.0	1.4
	Cakes prepared from home recipes using enriched flour:									
	Carrot, with cream cheese frosting:[36]									
404	Whole cake, 10-in diam. tube cake------------------------	1 cake----------	1,536	23	6,175	63	328	66.0	135.2	107.5
405	Piece, 1/16 of cake----------	1 piece---------	96	23	385	4	21	4.1	8.4	6.7
	Fruitcake, dark:[36]									
406	Whole cake, 7-1/2-in diam., 2-1/4-in high tube cake----	1 cake----------	1,361	18	5,185	74	228	47.6	113.0	51.7
407	Piece, 1/32 of cake, 2/3-in arc--------------------------	1 piece---------	43	18	165	2	7	1.5	3.6	1.6
	Plain sheet cake:[37]									
	Without frosting:									
408	Whole cake, 9-in square----	1 cake----------	777	25	2,830	35	108	29.5	45.1	25.6
409	Piece, 1/9 of cake---------	1 piece---------	86	25	315	4	12	3.3	5.0	2.8
	With uncooked white frosting:									
410	Whole cake, 9-in square----	1 cake----------	1,096	21	4,020	37	129	41.6	50.4	26.3
411	Piece, 1/9 of cake---------	1 piece---------	121	21	445	4	14	4.6	5.6	2.9
	Pound:[38]									
412	Loaf, 8-1/2 by 3-1/2 by 3-1/4 in-------------------------	1 loaf----------	514	22	2,025	33	94	21.1	40.9	26.7
413	Slice, 1/17 of loaf----------	1 slice---------	30	22	120	2	5	1.2	2.4	1.6
	Cakes, commercial, made with en-riched flour:									
	Pound:									
414	Loaf, 8-1/2 by 3-1/2 by 3 in	1 loaf----------	500	24	1,935	26	94	52.0	30.0	4.0
415	Slice, 1/17 of loaf----------	1 slice---------	29	24	110	2	5	3.0	1.7	0.2
	Snack cakes:									
416	Devil's food with creme filling (2 small cakes per pkg)----------------------	1 small cake----	28	20	105	1	4	1.7	1.5	0.6
417	Sponge with creme filling (2 small cakes per pkg)-------	1 small cake----	42	19	155	1	5	2.3	2.1	0.5
	White with white frosting:									
418	Whole, 2-layer cake, 8- or 9-in diam.-----------------	1 cake----------	1,140	24	4,170	43	148	33.1	61.6	42.2
419	Piece, 1/16 of cake----------	1 piece---------	71	24	260	3	9	2.1	3.8	2.6
	Yellow with chocolate frosting:									
420	Whole, 2-layer cake, 8- or 9-in diam.-----------------	1 cake----------	1,108	23	3,895	40	175	92.0	58.7	10.0
421	Piece, 1/16 of cake----------	1 piece---------	69	23	245	2	11	5.7	3.7	0.6
	Cheesecake:									
422	Whole cake, 9-in diam.----------	1 cake----------	1,110	46	3,350	60	213	119.9	65.5	14.4
423	Piece, 1/12 of cake------------	1 piece---------	92	46	280	5	18	9.9	5.4	1.2
	Cookies made with enriched flour:									
	Brownies with nuts:									
424	Commercial, with frosting, 1-1/2 by 1-3/4 by 7/8 in---	1 brownie-------	25	13	100	1	4	1.6	2.0	0.6
425	From home recipe, 1-3/4 by 1-3/4 by 7/8 in[36]----------	1 brownie-------	20	10	95	1	6	1.4	2.8	1.2
	Chocolate chip:									
426	Commercial, 2-1/4-in diam., 3/8 in thick--------------	4 cookies-------	42	4	180	2	9	2.9	3.1	2.6

[35] Excepting angelfood cake, cakes were made from mixes containing vegetable shortening and frostings were made with margarine.
[36] Made with vegetable oil.

Cho-les-terol	Carbo-hydrate	Calcium	Phos-phorus	Iron	Potas-sium	Sodium	Vitamin A value		Thiamin	Ribo-flavin	Niacin	Ascorbic acid	Item No.
							(IU)	(RE)					
Milli-grams	Grams	Milli-grams	Milli-grams	Milli-grams	Milli-grams	Milli-grams	Inter-national units	Retinol equiva-lents	Milli-grams	Milli-grams	Milli-grams	Milli-grams	
576	638	1,008	2,017	15.5	1,208	2,515	1,550	465	1.22	1.66	11.1	1	402
36	40	63	126	1.0	75	157	100	29	0.08	0.10	0.7	Tr	403
1183	775	707	998	21.0	1,720	4,470	2,240	246	1.83	1.97	14.7	23	404
74	48	44	62	1.3	108	279	140	15	0.11	0.12	0.9	1	405
640	783	1,293	1,592	37.6	6,138	2,123	1,720	422	2.41	2.55	17.0	504	406
20	25	41	50	1.2	194	67	50	13	0.08	0.08	0.5	16	407
552	434	497	793	11.7	614	2,331	1,320	373	1.24	1.40	10.1	2	408
61	48	55	88	1.3	68	258	150	41	0.14	0.15	1.1	Tr	409
636	694	548	822	11.0	669	2,488	2,190	647	1.21	1.42	9.9	2	410
70	77	61	91	1.2	74	275	240	71	0.13	0.16	1.1	Tr	411
555	265	339	473	9.3	483	1,645	3,470	1,033	0.93	1.08	7.8	1	412
32	15	20	28	0.5	28	96	200	60	0.05	0.06	0.5	Tr	413
1100	257	146	517	8.0	443	1,857	2,820	715	0.96	1.12	8.1	0	414
64	15	8	30	0.5	26	108	160	41	0.06	0.06	0.5	0	415
15	17	21	26	1.0	34	105	20	4	0.06	0.09	0.7	0	416
7	27	14	44	0.6	37	155	30	9	0.07	0.06	0.6	0	417
46	670	536	1,585	15.5	832	2,827	640	194	3.19	2.05	27.6	0	418
3	42	33	99	1.0	52	176	40	12	0.20	0.13	1.7	0	419
609	620	366	1,884	19.9	1,972	3,080	1,850	488	0.78	2.22	10.0	0	420
38	39	23	117	1.2	123	192	120	30	0.05	0.14	0.6	0	421
2053	317	622	977	5.3	1,088	2,464	2,820	833	0.33	1.44	5.1	56	422
170	26	52	81	0.4	90	204	230	69	0.03	0.12	0.4	5	423
14	16	13	26	0.6	50	59	70	18	0.08	0.07	0.3	Tr	424
18	11	9	26	0.4	35	51	20	6	0.05	0.05	0.3	Tr	425
5	28	13	41	0.8	68	140	50	15	0.10	0.23	1.0	Tr	426

[37]Cake made with vegetable shortening; frosting with margarine.
[38]Made with margarine.

191

Item No.	Foods, approximate measures, units, and weight (weight of edible portion only)			Water	Food energy	Pro-tein	Fat	Fatty acids		
								Satu-rated	Mono-unsatu-rated	Poly-unsatu-rated
	Grain Products—Con.		Grams	Per-cent	Cal-ories	Grams	Grams	Grams	Grams	Grams
	Cookies made with enriched flour:									
	Chocolate chip:									
427	From home recipe, 2-1/3-in diam.[25]	4 cookies	40	3	185	2	11	3.9	4.3	2.0
428	From refrigerated dough, 2-1/4-in diam., 3/8 in thick	4 cookies	48	5	225	2	11	4.0	4.4	2.0
429	Fig bars, square, 1-5/8 by 1-5/8 by 3/8 in or rectangular, 1-1/2 by 1-3/4 by 1/2 in	4 cookies	56	12	210	2	4	1.0	1.5	1.0
430	Oatmeal with raisins, 2-5/8-in diam., 1/4 in thick	4 cookies	52	4	245	3	10	2.5	4.5	2.8
431	Peanut butter cookie, from home recipe, 2-5/8-in diam.[25]	4 cookies	48	3	245	4	14	4.0	5.8	2.8
432	Sandwich type (chocolate or vanilla), 1-3/4-in diam., 3/8 in thick	4 cookies	40	2	195	2	8	2.0	3.6	2.2
	Shortbread:									
433	Commercial	4 small cookies	32	6	155	2	8	2.9	3.0	1.1
434	From home recipe[38]	2 large cookies	28	3	145	2	8	1.3	2.7	3.4
435	Sugar cookie, from refrigerated dough, 2-1/2-in diam., 1/4 in thick	4 cookies	48	4	235	2	12	2.3	5.0	3.6
436	Vanilla wafers, 1-3/4-in diam., 1/4 in thick	10 cookies	40	4	185	2	7	1.8	3.0	1.8
437	Corn chips	1-oz package	28	1	155	2	9	1.4	2.4	3.7
	Cornmeal:									
438	Whole-ground, unbolted, dry form	1 cup	122	12	435	11	5	0.5	1.1	2.5
439	Bolted (nearly whole-grain), dry form	1 cup	122	12	440	11	4	0.5	0.9	2.2
	Degermed, enriched:									
440	Dry form	1 cup	138	12	500	11	2	0.2	0.4	0.9
441	Cooked	1 cup	240	88	120	3	Tr	Tr	0.1	0.2
	Crackers:[39]									
	Cheese:									
442	Plain, 1 in square	10 crackers	10	4	50	1	3	0.9	1.2	0.3
443	Sandwich type (peanut butter)	1 sandwich	8	3	40	1	2	0.4	0.8	0.3
444	Graham, plain, 2-1/2 in square	2 crackers	14	5	60	1	1	0.4	0.6	0.4
445	Melba toast, plain	1 piece	5	4	20	1	Tr	0.1	0.1	0.1
446	Rye wafers, whole-grain, 1-7/8 by 3-1/2 in	2 wafers	14	5	55	1	1	0.3	0.4	0.3
447	Saltines[40]	4 crackers	12	4	50	1	1	0.5	0.4	0.2
448	Snack-type, standard	1 round cracker	3	3	15	Tr	1	0.2	0.4	0.1
449	Wheat, thin	4 crackers	8	3	35	1	1	0.5	0.5	0.4
450	Whole-wheat wafers	2 crackers	8	4	35	1	2	0.5	0.6	0.4
451	Croissants, made with enriched flour, 4-1/2 by 4 by 1-3/4 in	1 croissant	57	22	235	5	12	3.5	6.7	1.4
	Danish pastry, made with enriched flour:									
	Plain without fruit or nuts:									
452	Packaged ring, 12 oz	1 ring	340	27	1,305	21	71	21.8	28.6	15.6
453	Round piece, about 4-1/4-in diam., 1 in high	1 pastry	57	27	220	4	12	3.6	4.8	2.6
454	Ounce	1 oz	28	27	110	2	6	1.8	2.4	1.3
455	Fruit, round piece	1 pastry	65	30	235	4	13	3.9	5.2	2.9
	Doughnuts, made with enriched flour:									
456	Cake type, plain, 3-1/4-in diam., 1 in high	1 doughnut	50	21	210	3	12	2.8	5.0	3.0
457	Yeast-leavened, glazed, 3-3/4-in diam., 1-1/4 in high	1 doughnut	60	27	235	4	13	5.2	5.5	0.9
458	English muffins, plain, enriched	1 muffin	57	42	140	5	1	0.3	0.2	0.3
459	Toasted	1 muffin	50	29	140	5	1	0.3	0.2	0.3

[25]Made with vegetable shortening.
[38]Made with margarine.

Cho-les-terol	Carbo-hydrate	Calcium	Phos-phorus	Iron	Potas-sium	Sodium	Vitamin A value		Thiamin	Ribo-flavin	Niacin	Ascorbic acid	Item No.
							(IU)	(RE)					
Milli-grams	Grams	Milli-grams	Milli-grams	Milli-grams	Milli-grams	Milli-grams	Inter-national units	Retinol equiva-lents	Milli-grams	Milli-grams	Milli-grams	Milli-grams	
18	26	13	34	1.0	82	82	20	5	0.06	0.06	0.6	0	427
22	32	13	34	1.0	62	173	30	8	0.06	0.10	0.9	0	428
27	42	40	34	1.4	162	180	60	6	0.08	0.07	0.7	Tr	429
2	36	18	58	1.1	90	148	40	12	0.09	0.08	1.0	0	430
22	28	21	60	1.1	110	142	20	5	0.07	0.07	1.9	0	431
0	29	12	40	1.4	66	189	0	0	0.09	0.07	0.8	0	432
27	20	13	39	0.8	38	123	30	8	0.10	0.09	0.9	0	433
0	17	6	31	0.6	18	125	300	89	0.08	0.06	0.7	Tr	434
29	31	50	91	0.9	33	261	40	11	0.09	0.06	1.1	0	435
25	29	16	36	0.8	50	150	50	14	0.07	0.10	1.0	0	436
0	16	35	52	0.5	52	233	110	11	0.04	0.05	0.4	1	437
0	90	24	312	2.2	346	1	620	62	0.46	0.13	2.4	0	438
0	91	21	272	2.2	303	1	590	59	0.37	0.10	2.3	0	439
0	108	8	137	5.9	166	1	610	61	0.61	0.36	4.8	0	440
0	26	2	34	1.4	38	0	140	14	0.14	0.10	1.2	0	441
6	6	11	17	0.3	17	112	20	5	0.05	0.04	0.4	0	442
1	5	7	25	0.3	17	90	Tr	Tr	0.04	0.03	0.6	0	443
0	11	6	20	0.4	36	86	0	0	0.02	0.03	0.6	0	444
0	4	6	10	0.1	11	44	0	0	0.01	0.01	0.1	0	445
0	10	7	44	0.5	65	115	0	0	0.06	0.03	0.5	0	446
4	9	3	12	0.5	17	165	0	0	0.06	0.05	0.6	0	447
0	2	3	6	0.1	4	30	Tr	Tr	0.01	0.01	0.1	0	448
0	5	3	15	0.3	17	69	Tr	Tr	0.04	0.03	0.4	0	449
0	5	3	22	0.2	31	59	0	0	0.02	0.03	0.4	0	450
13	27	20	64	2.1	68	452	50	13	0.17	0.13	1.3	0	451
292	152	360	347	6.5	316	1,302	360	99	0.95	1.02	8.5	Tr	452
49	26	60	58	1.1	53	218	60	17	0.16	0.17	1.4	Tr	453
24	13	30	29	0.5	26	109	30	8	0.08	0.09	0.7	Tr	454
56	28	17	80	1.3	57	233	40	11	0.16	0.14	1.4	Tr	455
20	24	22	111	1.0	58	192	20	5	0.12	0.12	1.1	Tr	456
21	26	17	55	1.4	64	222	Tr	Tr	0.28	0.12	1.8	0	457
0	27	96	67	1.7	331	378	0	0	0.26	0.19	2.2	0	458
0	27	96	67	1.7	331	378	0	0	0.23	0.19	2.2	0	459

[39] Crackers made with enriched flour except for rye wafers and whole-wheat wafers.
[40] Made with lard.

Item No.	Foods, approximate measures, units, and weight (weight of edible portion only)		Water	Food energy	Pro-tein	Fat	Fatty acids Satu-rated	Mono-unsatu-rated	Poly-unsatu-rated
		Grams	Per-cent	Cal-ories	Grams	Grams	Grams	Grams	Grams
	Grain Products—Con.								
460	French toast, from home recipe---	1 slice---------	65	53	155	6	7	1.6	2.0	1.6
	Macaroni, enriched, cooked (cut lengths, elbows, shells):									
461	Firm stage (hot)---------------	1 cup-----------	130	64	190	7	1	0.1	0.1	0.3
	Tender stage:									
462	Cold------------------------	1 cup-----------	105	72	115	4	Tr	0.1	0.1	0.2
463	Hot-------------------------	1 cup-----------	140	72	155	5	1	0.1	0.1	0.2
	Muffins made with enriched flour, 2-1/2-in diam., 1-1/2 in high:									
	From home recipe:									
464	Blueberry [25] -------------------	1 muffin--------	45	37	135	3	5	1.5	2.1	1.2
465	Bran [36] -----------------------	1 muffin--------	45	35	125	3	6	1.4	1.6	2.3
466	Corn (enriched, degermed cornmeal and flour) [25] ------	1 muffin--------	45	33	145	3	5	1.5	2.2	1.4
	From commercial mix (egg and water added):									
467	Blueberry--------------------	1 muffin--------	45	33	140	3	5	1.4	2.0	1.2
468	Bran-------------------------	1 muffin--------	45	28	140	3	4	1.3	1.6	1.0
469	Corn-------------------------	1 muffin--------	45	30	145	3	6	1.7	2.3	1.4
470	Noodles (egg noodles), enriched, cooked------------------------	1 cup-----------	160	70	200	7	2	0.5	0.6	0.6
471	Noodles, chow mein, canned-------	1 cup-----------	45	11	220	6	11	2.1	7.3	0.4
	Pancakes, 4-in diam.:									
472	Buckwheat, from mix (with buckwheat and enriched flours), egg and milk added-----------	1 pancake-------	27	58	55	2	2	0.9	0.9	0.5
	Plain:									
473	From home recipe using enriched flour-------------	1 pancake-------	27	50	60	2	2	0.5	0.8	0.5
474	From mix (with enriched flour), egg, milk, and oil added---------------------	1 pancake-------	27	54	60	2	2	0.5	0.9	0.5
	Piecrust, made with enriched flour and vegetable shortening, baked:									
475	From home recipe, 9-in diam.---	1 pie shell-----	180	15	900	11	60	14.8	25.9	15.7
476	From mix, 9-in diam.-----------	Piecrust for 2-crust pie-----	320	19	1,485	20	93	22.7	41.0	25.0
	Pies, piecrust made with enriched flour, vegetable shortening, 9-in diam.:									
	Apple:									
477	Whole-----------------------	1 pie-----------	945	48	2,420	21	105	27.4	44.4	26.5
478	Piece, 1/6 of pie------------	1 piece---------	158	48	405	3	18	4.6	7.4	4.4
	Blueberry:									
479	Whole-----------------------	1 pie-----------	945	51	2,285	23	102	25.5	44.4	27.4
480	Piece, 1/6 of pie------------	1 piece---------	158	51	380	4	17	4.3	7.4	4.6
	Cherry:									
481	Whole-----------------------	1 pie-----------	945	47	2,465	25	107	28.4	46.3	27.4
482	Piece, 1/6 of pie------------	1 piece---------	158	47	410	4	18	4.7	7.7	4.6
	Creme:									
483	Whole-----------------------	1 pie-----------	910	43	2,710	20	139	90.1	23.7	6.4
484	Piece, 1/6 of pie------------	1 piece---------	152	43	455	3	23	15.0	4.0	1.1
	Custard:									
485	Whole-----------------------	1 pie-----------	910	58	1,985	56	101	33.7	40.0	19.1
486	Piece, 1/6 of pie------------	1 piece---------	152	58	330	9	17	5.6	6.7	3.2
	Lemon meringue:									
487	Whole-----------------------	1 pie-----------	840	47	2,140	31	86	26.0	34.4	17.6
488	Piece, 1/6 of pie------------	1 piece---------	140	47	355	5	14	4.3	5.7	2.9
	Peach:									
489	Whole-----------------------	1 pie-----------	945	48	2,410	24	101	24.6	43.5	26.5
490	Piece, 1/6 of pie------------	1 piece---------	158	48	405	4	17	4.1	7.3	4.4

[25] Made with vegetable shortening.

							Vitamin A value						
Cho-les-terol	Carbo-hydrate	Calcium	Phos-phorus	Iron	Potas-sium	Sodium	(IU)	(RE)	Thiamin	Ribo-flavin	Niacin	Ascorbic acid	Item No.
Milli-grams	Grams	Milli-grams	Milli-grams	Milli-grams	Milli-grams	Milli-grams	Inter-national units	Retinol equiva-lents	Milli-grams	Milli-grams	Milli-grams	Milli-grams	
112	17	72	85	1.3	86	257	110	32	0.12	0.16	1.0	Tr	460
0	39	14	85	2.1	103	1	0	0	0.23	0.13	1.8	0	461
0	24	8	53	1.3	64	1	0	0	0.15	0.08	1.2	0	462
0	32	11	70	1.7	85	1	0	0	0.20	0.11	1.5	0	463
19	20	54	46	0.9	47	198	40	9	0.10	0.11	0.9	1	464
24	19	60	125	1.4	99	189	230	30	0.11	0.13	1.3	3	465
23	21	66	59	0.9	57	169	80	15	0.11	0.11	0.9	Tr	466
45	22	15	90	0.9	54	225	50	11	0.10	0.17	1.1	Tr	467
28	24	27	182	1.7	50	385	100	14	0.08	0.12	1.9	0	468
42	22	30	128	1.3	31	291	90	16	0.09	0.09	0.8	Tr	469
50	37	16	94	2.6	70	3	110	34	0.22	0.13	1.9	0	470
5	26	14	41	0.4	33	450	0	0	0.05	0.03	0.6	0	471
20	6	59	91	0.4	66	125	60	17	0.04	0.05	0.2	Tr	472
16	9	27	38	0.5	33	115	30	10	0.06	0.07	0.5	Tr	473
16	8	36	71	0.7	43	160	30	7	0.09	0.12	0.8	Tr	474
0	79	25	90	4.5	90	1,100	0	0	0.54	0.40	5.0	0	475
0	141	131	272	9.3	179	2,602	0	0	1.06	0.80	9.9	0	476
0	360	76	208	9.5	756	2,844	280	28	1.04	0.76	9.5	9	477
0	60	13	35	1.6	126	476	50	5	0.17	0.13	1.6	2	478
0	330	104	217	12.3	945	2,533	850	85	1.04	0.85	10.4	38	479
0	55	17	36	2.1	158	423	140	14	0.17	0.14	1.7	6	480
0	363	132	236	9.5	992	2,873	4,160	416	1.13	0.85	9.5	0	481
0	61	22	40	1.6	166	480	700	70	0.19	0.14	1.6	0	482
46	351	273	919	6.8	796	2,207	1,250	391	0.36	0.89	6.4	0	483
8	59	46	154	1.1	133	369	210	65	0.06	0.15	1.1	0	484
1010	213	874	1,028	9.1	1,247	2,612	2,090	573	0.82	1.91	5.5	0	485
169	36	146	172	1.5	208	436	350	96	0.14	0.32	0.9	0	486
857	317	118	412	8.4	420	2,369	1,430	395	0.59	0.84	5.0	25	487
143	53	20	69	1.4	70	395	240	66	0.10	0.14	0.8	4	488
0	361	95	274	11.3	1,408	2,533	6,900	690	1.04	0.95	14.2	28	489
0	60	16	46	1.9	235	423	1,150	115	0.17	0.16	2.4	5	490

[36] Made with vegetable oil.

195

Item No.	Foods, approximate measures, units, and weight (weight of edible portion only)			Water	Food energy	Pro-tein	Fat	Fatty acids		
								Satu-rated	Mono-unsatu-rated	Poly-unsatu-rated
			Grams	Per-cent	Cal-ories	Grams	Grams	Grams	Grams	Grams

Grain Products—Con.

Pies, piecrust made with enriched flour, vegetable shortening, 9-inch diam.:

Pecan:

| 491 | Whole------------------------ | 1 pie---------- | 825 | 20 | 3,450 | 42 | 189 | 28.1 | 101.5 | 47.0 |
| 492 | Piece, 1/6 of pie------------ | 1 piece--------- | 138 | 20 | 575 | 7 | 32 | 4.7 | 17.0 | 7.9 |

Pumpkin:

| 493 | Whole------------------------ | 1 pie---------- | 910 | 59 | 1,920 | 36 | 102 | 38.2 | 40.0 | 18.2 |
| 494 | Piece, 1/6 of pie------------ | 1 piece--------- | 152 | 59 | 320 | 6 | 17 | 6.4 | 6.7 | 3.0 |

Pies, fried:

| 495 | Apple------------------------ | 1 pie---------- | 85 | 43 | 255 | 2 | 14 | 5.8 | 6.6 | 0.6 |
| 496 | Cherry----------------------- | 1 pie---------- | 85 | 42 | 250 | 2 | 14 | 5.8 | 6.7 | 0.6 |

Popcorn, popped:

497	Air-popped, unsalted-----------	1 cup----------	8	4	30	1	Tr	Tr	0.1	0.2
498	Popped in vegetable oil, salted	1 cup----------	11	3	55	1	3	0.5	1.4	1.2
499	Sugar syrup coated------------	1 cup----------	35	4	135	2	1	0.1	0.3	0.6

Pretzels, made with enriched flour:

500	Stick, 2-1/4 in long-----------	10 pretzels-----	3	3	10	Tr	Tr	Tr	Tr	Tr
501	Twisted, dutch, 2-3/4 by 2-5/8 in----------------------------	1 pretzel-------	16	3	65	2	1	0.1	0.2	0.2
502	Twisted, thin, 3-1/4 by 2-1/4 by 1/4 in--------------------	10 pretzels-----	60	3	240	6	2	0.4	0.8	0.6

Rice:

| 503 | Brown, cooked, served hot------ | 1 cup---------- | 195 | 70 | 230 | 5 | 1 | 0.3 | 0.3 | 0.4 |

White, enriched:

Commercial varieties, all types:

504	Raw--------------------------	1 cup----------	185	12	670	12	1	0.2	0.2	0.3
505	Cooked, served hot---------	1 cup----------	205	73	225	4	Tr	0.1	0.1	0.1
506	Instant, ready-to-serve, hot	1 cup----------	165	73	180	4	0	0.1	0.1	0.1

Parboiled:

| 507 | Raw-------------------------- | 1 cup---------- | 185 | 10 | 685 | 14 | 1 | 0.1 | 0.1 | 0.2 |
| 508 | Cooked, served hot--------- | 1 cup---------- | 175 | 73 | 185 | 4 | Tr | Tr | Tr | 0.1 |

Rolls, enriched:

Commercial:

509	Dinner, 2-1/2-in diam., 2 in high----------------------	1 roll----------	28	32	85	2	2	0.5	0.8	0.6
510	Frankfurter and hamburger (8 per 11-1/2-oz pkg.)--------	1 roll----------	40	34	115	3	2	0.5	0.8	0.6
511	Hard, 3-3/4-in diam., 2 in high----------------------	1 roll----------	50	25	155	5	2	0.4	0.5	0.6
512	Hoagie or submarine, 11-1/2 by 3 by 2-1/2 in-----------	1 roll----------	135	31	400	11	8	1.8	3.0	2.2

From home recipe:

| 513 | Dinner, 2-1/2-in diam., 2 in high---------------------- | 1 roll---------- | 35 | 26 | 120 | 3 | 3 | 0.8 | 1.2 | 0.9 |

Spaghetti, enriched, cooked:

514	Firm stage, "al dente," served hot-------------------------	1 cup----------	130	64	190	7	1	0.1	0.1	0.3
515	Tender stage, served hot-------	1 cup----------	140	73	155	5	1	0.1	0.1	0.2
516	Toaster pastries-----------------	1 pastry--------	54	13	210	2	6	1.7	3.6	0.4
517	Tortillas, corn-------------------	1 tortilla------	30	45	65	2	1	0.1	0.3	0.6

Waffles, made with enriched flour, 7-in diam.:

| 518 | From home recipe-------------- | 1 waffle-------- | 75 | 37 | 245 | 7 | 13 | 4.0 | 4.9 | 2.6 |
| 519 | From mix, egg and milk added--- | 1 waffle-------- | 75 | 42 | 205 | 7 | 8 | 2.7 | 2.9 | 1.5 |

Wheat flours:

All-purpose or family flour, enriched:

520	Sifted, spooned---------------	1 cup----------	115	12	420	12	1	0.2	0.1	0.5
521	Unsifted, spooned-------------	1 cup----------	125	12	455	13	1	0.2	0.1	0.5
522	Cake or pastry flour, enriched, sifted, spooned--------------	1 cup----------	96	12	350	7	1	0.1	0.1	0.3
523	Self-rising, enriched, unsifted, spooned-------------	1 cup----------	125	12	440	12	1	0.2	0.1	0.5
524	Whole-wheat, from hard wheats, stirred-----------------------	1 cup----------	120	12	400	16	2	0.3	0.3	1.1

							Nutrients in Indicated Quantity						

Cho-les-terol	Carbo-hydrate	Calcium	Phos-phorus	Iron	Potas-sium	Sodium	Vitamin A value		Thiamin	Ribo-flavin	Niacin	Ascorbic acid	Item No.
							(IU)	(RE)					
Milli-grams	Grams	Milli-grams	Milli-grams	Milli-grams	Milli-grams	Milli-grams	Inter-national units	Retinol equiva-lents	Milli-grams	Milli-grams	Milli-grams	Milli-grams	
569	423	388	850	27.2	1,015	1,823	1,320	322	1.82	0.99	6.6	0	491
95	71	65	142	4.6	170	305	220	54	0.30	0.17	1.1	0	492
655	223	464	628	8.2	1,456	1,947	22,480	2,493	0.82	1.27	7.3	0	493
109	37	78	105	1.4	243	325	3,750	416	0.14	0.21	1.2	0	494
14	31	12	34	0.9	42	326	30	3	0.09	0.06	1.0	1	495
13	32	11	41	0.7	61	371	190	19	0.06	0.06	0.6	1	496
0	6	1	22	0.2	20	Tr	10	1	0.03	0.01	0.2	0	497
0	6	3	31	0.3	19	86	20	2	0.01	0.02	0.1	0	498
0	30	2	47	0.5	90	Tr	30	3	0.13	0.02	0.4	0	499
0	2	1	3	0.1	3	48	0	0	0.01	0.01	0.1	0	500
0	13	4	15	0.3	16	258	0	0	0.05	0.04	0.7	0	501
0	48	16	55	1.2	61	966	0	0	0.19	0.15	2.6	0	502
0	50	23	142	1.0	137	0	0	0	0.18	0.04	2.7	0	503
0	149	44	174	5.4	170	9	0	0	0.81	0.06	6.5	0	504
0	50	21	57	1.8	57	0	0	0	0.23	0.02	2.1	0	505
0	40	5	31	1.3	0	0	0	0	0.21	0.02	1.7	0	506
0	150	111	370	5.4	278	17	0	0	0.81	0.07	6.5	0	507
0	41	33	100	1.4	75	0	0	0	0.19	0.02	2.1	0	508
Tr	14	33	44	0.8	36	155	Tr	Tr	0.14	0.09	1.1	Tr	509
Tr	20	54	44	1.2	56	241	Tr	Tr	0.20	0.13	1.6	Tr	510
Tr	30	24	46	1.4	49	313	0	0	0.20	0.12	1.7	0	511
Tr	72	100	115	3.8	128	683	0	0	0.54	0.33	4.5	0	512
12	20	16	36	1.1	41	98	30	8	0.12	0.12	1.2	0	513
0	39	14	85	2.0	103	1	0	0	0.23	0.13	1.8	0	514
0	32	11	70	1.7	85	1	0	0	0.20	0.11	1.5	0	515
0	38	104	104	2.2	91	248	520	52	0.17	0.18	2.3	4	516
0	13	42	55	0.6	43	1	80	8	0.05	0.03	0.4	0	517
102	26	154	135	1.5	129	445	140	39	0.18	0.24	1.5	Tr	518
59	27	179	257	1.2	146	515	170	49	0.14	0.23	0.9	Tr	519
0	88	18	100	5.1	109	2	0	0	0.73	0.46	6.1	0	520
0	95	20	109	5.5	119	3	0	0	0.80	0.50	6.6	0	521
0	76	16	70	4.2	91	2	0	0	0.58	0.38	5.1	0	522
0	93	331	583	5.5	113	1,349	0	0	0.80	0.50	6.6	0	523
0	85	49	446	5.2	444	4	0	0	0.66	0.14	5.2	0	524

Item No.	Foods, approximate measures, units, and weight (weight of edible portion only)			Water	Food energy	Pro-tein	Fat	Fatty acids		
								Satu-rated	Mono-unsatu-rated	Poly-unsatu-rated
			Grams	Per-cent	Cal-ories	Grams	Grams	Grams	Grams	Grams
	Legumes, Nuts, and Seeds									
	Almonds, shelled:									
525	Slivered, packed	1 cup	135	4	795	27	70	6.7	45.8	14.8
526	Whole	1 oz	28	4	165	6	15	1.4	9.6	3.1
	Beans, dry:									
	Cooked, drained:									
527	Black	1 cup	171	66	225	15	1	0.1	0.1	0.5
528	Great Northern	1 cup	180	69	210	14	1	0.1	0.1	0.6
529	Lima	1 cup	190	64	260	16	1	0.2	0.1	0.5
530	Pea (navy)	1 cup	190	69	225	15	1	0.1	0.1	0.7
531	Pinto	1 cup	180	65	265	15	1	0.1	0.1	0.5
	Canned, solids and liquid:									
	White with:									
532	Frankfurters (sliced)	1 cup	255	71	365	19	18	7.4	8.8	0.7
533	Pork and tomato sauce	1 cup	255	71	310	16	7	2.4	2.7	0.7
534	Pork and sweet sauce	1 cup	255	66	385	16	12	4.3	4.9	1.2
535	Red kidney	1 cup	255	76	230	15	1	0.1	0.1	0.6
536	Black-eyed peas, dry, cooked (with residual cooking liquid)	1 cup	250	80	190	13	1	0.2	Tr	0.3
537	Brazil nuts, shelled	1 oz	28	3	185	4	19	4.6	6.5	6.8
538	Carob flour	1 cup	140	3	255	6	Tr	Tr	0.1	0.1
	Cashew nuts, salted:									
539	Dry roasted	1 cup	137	2	785	21	63	12.5	37.4	10.7
540		1 oz	28	2	165	4	13	2.6	7.7	2.2
541	Roasted in oil	1 cup	130	4	750	21	63	12.4	36.9	10.6
542		1 oz	28	4	165	5	14	2.7	8.1	2.3
543	Chestnuts, European (Italian), roasted, shelled	1 cup	143	40	350	5	3	0.6	1.1	1.2
544	Chickpeas, cooked, drained	1 cup	163	60	270	15	4	0.4	0.9	1.9
	Coconut:									
	Raw:									
545	Piece, about 2 by 2 by 1/2 in	1 piece	45	47	160	1	15	13.4	0.6	0.2
546	Shredded or grated	1 cup	80	47	285	3	27	23.8	1.1	0.3
547	Dried, sweetened, shredded	1 cup	93	13	470	3	33	29.3	1.4	0.4
548	Filberts (hazelnuts), chopped	1 cup	115	5	725	15	72	5.3	56.5	6.9
549		1 oz	28	5	180	4	18	1.3	13.9	1.7
550	Lentils, dry, cooked	1 cup	200	72	215	16	1	0.1	0.2	0.5
551	Macadamia nuts, roasted in oil, salted	1 cup	134	2	960	10	103	15.4	80.9	1.8
552		1 oz	28	2	205	2	22	3.2	17.1	0.4
	Mixed nuts, with peanuts, salted:									
553	Dry roasted	1 oz	28	2	170	5	15	2.0	8.9	3.1
554	Roasted in oil	1 oz	28	2	175	5	16	2.5	9.0	3.8
555	Peanuts, roasted in oil, salted	1 cup	145	2	840	39	71	9.9	35.5	22.6
556		1 oz	28	2	165	8	14	1.9	6.9	4.4
557	Peanut butter	1 tbsp	16	1	95	5	8	1.4	4.0	2.5
558	Peas, split, dry, cooked	1 cup	200	70	230	16	1	0.1	0.1	0.3
559	Pecans, halves	1 cup	108	5	720	8	73	5.9	45.5	18.1
560		1 oz	28	5	190	2	19	1.5	12.0	4.7
561	Pine nuts (pinyons), shelled	1 oz	28	6	160	3	17	2.7	6.5	7.3
562	Pistachio nuts, dried, shelled	1 oz	28	4	165	6	14	1.7	9.3	2.1
563	Pumpkin and squash kernels, dry, hulled	1 oz	28	7	155	7	13	2.5	4.0	5.9
564	Refried beans, canned	1 cup	290	72	295	18	3	0.4	0.6	1.4
565	Sesame seeds, dry, hulled	1 tbsp	8	5	45	2	4	0.6	1.7	1.9
566	Soybeans, dry, cooked, drained	1 cup	180	71	235	20	10	1.3	1.9	5.3
	Soy products:									
567	Miso	1 cup	276	53	470	29	13	1.8	2.6	7.3
568	Tofu, piece 2-1/2 by 2-3/4 by 1 in	1 piece	120	85	85	9	5	0.7	1.0	2.9
569	Sunflower seeds, dry, hulled	1 oz	28	5	160	6	14	1.5	2.7	9.3
570	Tahini	1 tbsp	15	3	90	3	8	1.1	3.0	3.5

[41] Cashews without salt contain 21 mg sodium per cup or 4 mg per oz.
[42] Cashews without salt contain 22 mg sodium per cup or 5 mg per oz.
[43] Macadamia nuts without salt contain 9 mg sodium per cup or 2 mg per oz.

Cho-les-terol	Carbo-hydrate	Calcium	Phos-phorus	Iron	Potas-sium	Sodium	Vitamin A value		Thiamin	Ribo-flavin	Niacin	Ascorbic acid	Item No.
							(IU)	(RE)					
Milli-grams	Grams	Milli-grams	Milli-grams	Milli-grams	Milli-grams	Milli-grams	Inter-national units	Retinol equiva-lents	Milli-grams	Milli-grams	Milli-grams	Milli-grams	
0	28	359	702	4.9	988	15	0	0	0.28	1.05	4.5	1	525
0	6	75	147	1.0	208	3	0	0	0.06	0.22	1.0	Tr	526
0	41	47	239	2.9	608	1	Tr	Tr	0.43	0.05	0.9	0	527
0	38	90	266	4.9	749	13	0	0	0.25	0.13	1.3	0	528
0	49	55	293	5.9	1,163	4	0	0	0.25	0.11	1.3	0	529
0	40	95	281	5.1	790	13	0	0	0.27	0.13	1.3	0	530
0	49	86	296	5.4	882	3	Tr	Tr	0.33	0.16	0.7	0	531
30	32	94	303	4.8	668	1,374	330	33	0.18	0.15	3.3	Tr	532
10	48	138	235	4.6	536	1,181	330	33	0.20	0.08	1.5	5	533
10	54	161	291	5.9	536	969	330	33	0.15	0.10	1.3	5	534
0	42	74	278	4.6	673	968	10	1	0.13	0.10	1.5	0	535
0	35	43	238	3.3	573	20	30	3	0.40	0.10	1.0	0	536
0	4	50	170	1.0	170	1	Tr	Tr	0.28	0.03	0.5	Tr	537
0	126	390	102	5.7	1,275	24	Tr	Tr	0.07	0.07	2.2	Tr	538
0	45	62	671	8.2	774	[41]877	0	0	0.27	0.27	1.9	0	539
0	9	13	139	1.7	160	[41]181	0	0	0.06	0.06	0.4	0	540
0	37	53	554	5.3	689	[42]814	0	0	0.55	0.23	2.3	0	541
0	8	12	121	1.2	150	[42]177	0	0	0.12	0.05	0.5	0	542
0	76	41	153	1.3	847	3	30	3	0.35	0.25	1.9	37	543
0	45	80	273	4.9	475	11	Tr	Tr	0.18	0.09	0.9	0	544
0	7	6	51	1.1	160	9	0	0	0.03	0.01	0.2	1	545
0	12	11	90	1.9	285	16	0	0	0.05	0.02	0.4	3	546
0	44	14	99	1.8	313	244	0	0	0.03	0.02	0.4	1	547
0	18	216	359	3.8	512	3	80	8	0.58	0.13	1.3	1	548
0	4	53	88	0.9	126	1	20	2	0.14	0.03	0.3	Tr	549
0	38	50	238	4.2	498	26	40	4	0.14	0.12	1.2	0	550
0	17	60	268	2.4	441	[43]348	10	1	0.29	0.15	2.7	0	551
0	4	13	57	0.5	93	[43]74	Tr	Tr	0.06	0.03	0.6	0	552
0	7	20	123	1.0	169	[44]190	Tr	Tr	0.06	0.06	1.3	0	553
0	6	31	131	0.9	165	[44]185	10	1	0.14	0.06	1.4	Tr	554
0	27	125	734	2.8	1,019	[45]626	0	0	0.42	0.15	21.5	0	555
0	5	24	143	0.5	199	[45]122	0	0	0.08	0.03	4.2	0	556
0	3	5	60	0.3	110	75	0	0	0.02	0.02	2.2	0	557
0	42	22	178	3.4	592	26	80	8	0.30	0.18	1.8	0	558
0	20	39	314	2.3	423	1	140	14	0.92	0.14	1.0	2	559
0	5	10	83	0.6	111	Tr	40	4	0.24	0.04	0.3	1	560
0	5	2	10	0.9	178	20	10	1	0.35	0.06	1.2	1	561
0	7	38	143	1.9	310	2	70	7	0.23	0.05	0.3	Tr	562
0	5	12	333	4.2	229	5	110	11	0.06	0.09	0.5	Tr	563
0	51	141	245	5.1	1,141	1,228	0	0	0.14	0.16	1.4	17	564
0	1	11	62	0.6	33	3	10	1	0.06	0.01	0.4	0	565
0	19	131	322	4.9	972	4	50	5	0.38	0.16	1.1	0	566
0	65	188	853	4.7	922	8,142	110	11	0.17	0.28	0.8	0	567
0	3	108	151	2.3	50	8	0	0	0.07	0.04	0.1	0	568
0	5	33	200	1.9	195	1	10	1	0.65	0.07	1.3	Tr	569
0	3	21	119	0.7	69	5	10	1	0.24	0.02	0.8	1	570

[44]Mixed nuts without salt contain 3 mg sodium per oz.
[45]Peanuts without salt contain 22 mg sodium per cup or 4 mg per oz.

Item No.	Foods, approximate measures, units, and weight (weight of edible portion only)		Water	Food energy	Pro-tein	Fat	Fatty acids		
							Satu-rated	Mono-unsatu-rated	Poly-unsatu-rated
		Grams	Per-cent	Cal-ories	Grams	Grams	Grams	Grams	Grams
	Legumes, Nuts, and Seeds—Con.								
	Walnuts:								
571	Black, chopped------------------ 1 cup-----------	125	4	760	30	71	4.5	15.9	46.9
572	1 oz------------	28	4	170	7	16	1.0	3.6	10.6
573	English or Persian, pieces or chips----------------------- 1 cup-----------	120	4	770	17	74	6.7	17.0	47.0
574	1 oz------------	28	4	180	4	18	1.6	4.0	11.1
	Meat and Meat Products								
	Beef, cooked: [46]								
	Cuts braised, simmered, or pot roasted:								
	Relatively fat such as chuck blade:								
575	Lean and fat, piece, 2-1/2 by 2-1/2 by 3/4 in------- 3 oz------------	85	43	325	22	26	10.8	11.7	0.9
576	Lean only from item 575---- 2.2 oz----------	62	53	170	19	9	3.9	4.2	0.3
	Relatively lean, such as bottom round:								
577	Lean and fat, piece, 4-1/8 by 2-1/4 by 1/2 in-------- 3 oz------------	85	54	220	25	13	4.8	5.7	0.5
578	Lean only from item 577---- 2.8 oz----------	78	57	175	25	8	2.7	3.4	0.3
	Ground beef, broiled, patty, 3 by 5/8 in:								
579	Lean----------------------- 3 oz------------	85	56	230	21	16	6.2	6.9	0.6
580	Regular--------------------- 3 oz------------	85	54	245	20	18	6.9	7.7	0.7
581	Heart, lean, braised----------- 3 oz------------	85	65	150	24	5	1.2	0.8	1.6
582	Liver, fried, slice, 6-1/2 by 2-3/8 by 3/8 in [47] ------------ 3 oz------------	85	56	185	23	7	2.5	3.6	1.3
	Roast, oven cooked, no liquid added:								
	Relatively fat, such as rib:								
583	Lean and fat, 2 pieces, 4-1/8 by 2-1/4 by 1/4 in 3 oz------------	85	46	315	19	26	10.8	11.4	0.9
584	Lean only from item 583---- 2.2 oz----------	61	57	150	17	9	3.6	3.7	0.3
	Relatively lean, such as eye of round:								
585	Lean and fat, 2 pieces, 2-1/2 by 2-1/2 by 3/8 in 3 oz------------	85	57	205	23	12	4.9	5.4	0.5
586	Lean only from item 585---- 2.6 oz----------	75	63	135	22	5	1.9	2.1	0.2
	Steak:								
	Sirloin, broiled:								
587	Lean and fat, piece, 2-1/2 by 2-1/2 by 3/4 in------- 3 oz------------	85	53	240	23	15	6.4	6.9	0.6
588	Lean only from item 587---- 2.5 oz----------	72	59	150	22	6	2.6	2.8	0.3
589	Beef, canned, corned------------- 3 oz------------	85	59	185	22	10	4.2	4.9	0.4
590	Beef, dried, chipped------------- 2.5 oz----------	72	48	145	24	4	1.8	2.0	0.2
	Lamb, cooked:								
	Chops, (3 per lb with bone):								
	Arm, braised:								
591	Lean and fat--------------- 2.2 oz----------	63	44	220	20	15	6.9	6.0	0.9
592	Lean only from item 591----- 1.7 oz----------	48	49	135	17	7	2.9	2.6	0.4
	Loin, broiled:								
593	Lean and fat--------------- 2.8 oz----------	80	54	235	22	16	7.3	6.4	1.0
594	Lean only from item 593---- 2.3 oz----------	64	61	140	19	6	2.6	2.4	0.4
	Leg, roasted:								
595	Lean and fat, 2 pieces, 4-1/8 by 2-1/4 by 1/4 in--------- 3 oz------------	85	59	205	22	13	5.6	4.9	0.8
596	Lean only from item 595------ 2.6 oz----------	73	64	140	20	6	2.4	2.2	0.4
	Rib, roasted:								
597	Lean and fat, 3 pieces, 2-1/2 by 2-1/2 by 1/4 in--------- 3 oz------------	85	47	315	18	26	12.1	10.6	1.5
598	Lean only from item 597------ 2 oz------------	57	60	130	15	7	3.2	3.0	0.5

[46] Outer layer of fat was removed to within approximately 1/2 inch of the lean. Deposits of fat within the cut were not removed.
[47] Fried in vegetable shortening.

Cho-les-terol	Carbo-hydrate	Calcium	Phos-phorus	Iron	Potas-sium	Sodium	Vitamin A value		Thiamin	Ribo-flavin	Niacin	Ascorbic acid	Item No.
							(IU)	(RE)					
Milli-grams	Grams	Milli-grams	Milli-grams	Milli-grams	Milli-grams	Milli-grams	Inter-national units	Retinol equiva-lents	Milli-grams	Milli-grams	Milli-grams	Milli-grams	
0	15	73	580	3.8	655	1	370	37	0.27	0.14	0.9	Tr	571
0	3	16	132	0.9	149	Tr	80	8	0.06	0.03	0.2	Tr	572
0	22	113	380	2.9	602	12	150	15	0.46	0.18	1.3	4	573
0	5	27	90	0.7	142	3	40	4	0.11	0.04	0.3	1	574
87	0	11	163	2.5	163	53	Tr	Tr	0.06	0.19	2.0	0	575
66	0	8	146	2.3	163	44	Tr	Tr	0.05	0.17	1.7	0	576
81	0	5	217	2.8	248	43	Tr	Tr	0.06	0.21	3.3	0	577
75	0	4	212	2.7	240	40	Tr	Tr	0.06	0.20	3.0	0	578
74	0	9	134	1.8	256	65	Tr	Tr	0.04	0.18	4.4	0	579
76	0	9	144	2.1	248	70	Tr	Tr	0.03	0.16	4.9	0	580
164	0	5	213	6.4	198	54	Tr	Tr	0.12	1.31	3.4	5	581
410	7	9	392	5.3	309	90	[48]30,690	[48]9,120	0.18	3.52	12.3	23	582
72	0	8	145	2.0	246	54	Tr	Tr	0.06	0.16	3.1	0	583
49	0	5	127	1.7	218	45	Tr	Tr	0.05	0.13	2.7	0	584
62	0	5	177	1.6	308	50	Tr	Tr	0.07	0.14	3.0	0	585
52	0	3	170	1.5	297	46	Tr	Tr	0.07	0.13	2.8	0	586
77	0	9	186	2.6	306	53	Tr	Tr	0.10	0.23	3.3	0	587
64	0	8	176	2.4	290	48	Tr	Tr	0.09	0.22	3.1	0	588
80	0	17	90	3.7	51	802	Tr	Tr	0.02	0.20	2.9	0	589
46	0	14	287	2.3	142	3,053	Tr	Tr	0.05	0.23	2.7	0	590
77	0	16	132	1.5	195	46	Tr	Tr	0.04	0.16	4.4	0	591
59	0	12	111	1.3	162	36	Tr	Tr	0.03	0.13	3.0	0	592
78	0	16	162	1.4	272	62	Tr	Tr	0.09	0.21	5.5	0	593
60	0	12	145	1.3	241	54	Tr	Tr	0.08	0.18	4.4	0	594
78	0	8	162	1.7	273	57	Tr	Tr	0.09	0.24	5.5	0	595
65	0	6	150	1.5	247	50	Tr	Tr	0.08	0.20	4.6	0	596
77	0	19	139	1.4	224	60	Tr	Tr	0.08	0.18	5.5	0	597
50	0	12	111	1.0	179	46	Tr	Tr	0.05	0.13	3.5	0	598

[48] Value varies widely.

Table 2. Nutritive Value of the Edible Part of Food (Continued)

(Tr indicates nutrient present in trace amount.)

Item No.	Foods, approximate measures, units, and weight (weight of edible portion only)		Water	Food energy	Pro-tein	Fat	Fatty acids Satu-rated	Mono-unsatu-rated	Poly-unsatu-rated
		Grams	Per-cent	Cal-ories	Grams	Grams	Grams	Grams	Grams
	Meat and Meat Products—Con.								
	Pork, cured, cooked:								
	Bacon:								
599	Regular-----------------------	3 medium slices	19	13	110	6	9	3.3	4.5	1.1
600	Canadian-style----------------	2 slices--------	46	62	85	11	4	1.3	1.9	0.4
	Ham, light cure, roasted:								
601	Lean and fat, 2 pieces, 4-1/8 by 2-1/4 by 1/4 in----	3 oz------------	85	58	205	18	14	5.1	6.7	1.5
602	Lean only from item 601------	2.4 oz----------	68	66	105	17	4	1.3	1.7	0.4
603	Ham, canned, roasted, 2 pieces, 4-1/8 by 2-1/4 by 1/4 in-----	3 oz------------	85	67	140	18	7	2.4	3.5	0.8
	Luncheon meat:								
604	Canned, spiced or unspiced, slice, 3 by 2 by 1/2 in----	2 slices--------	42	52	140	5	13	4.5	6.0	1.5
605	Chopped ham (8 slices per 6 oz pkg)---------------------	2 slices--------	42	64	95	7	7	2.4	3.4	0.9
	Cooked ham (8 slices per 8-oz pkg):								
606	Regular------------------	2 slices--------	57	65	105	10	6	1.9	2.8	0.7
607	Extra lean---------------	2 slices--------	57	71	75	11	3	0.9	1.3	0.3
	Pork, fresh, cooked:								
	Chop, loin (cut 3 per lb with bone):								
	Broiled:								
608	Lean and fat----------------	3.1 oz----------	87	50	275	24	19	7.0	8.8	2.2
609	Lean only from item 608----	2.5 oz----------	72	57	165	23	8	2.6	3.4	0.9
	Pan fried:								
610	Lean and fat----------------	3.1 oz----------	89	45	335	21	27	9.8	12.5	3.1
611	Lean only from item 610----	2.4 oz----------	67	54	180	19	11	3.7	4.8	1.3
	Ham (leg), roasted:								
612	Lean and fat, piece, 2-1/2 by 2-1/2 by 3/4 in------------	3 oz------------	85	53	250	21	18	6.4	8.1	2.0
613	Lean only from item 612------	2.5 oz----------	72	60	160	20	8	2.7	3.6	1.0
	Rib, roasted:								
614	Lean and fat, piece, 2-1/2 by 3/4 in--------------------	3 oz------------	85	51	270	21	20	7.2	9.2	2.3
615	Lean only from item 614------	2.5 oz----------	71	57	175	20	10	3.4	4.4	1.2
	Shoulder cut, braised:								
616	Lean and fat, 3 pieces, 2-1/2 by 2-1/2 by 1/4 in---------	3 oz------------	85	47	295	23	22	7.9	10.0	2.4
617	Lean only from item 616------	2.4 oz----------	67	54	165	22	8	2.8	3.7	1.0
	Sausages (See also Luncheon meats, items 604-607):								
618	Bologna, slice (8 per 8-oz pkg)	2 slices--------	57	54	180	7	16	6.1	7.6	1.4
619	Braunschweiger, slice (6 per 6-oz pkg)---------------------	2 slices--------	57	48	205	8	18	6.2	8.5	2.1
620	Brown and serve (10-11 per 8-oz pkg), browned------------	1 link----------	13	45	50	2	5	1.7	2.2	0.5
621	Frankfurter (10 per 1-lb pkg), cooked (reheated)------------	1 frankfurter---	45	54	145	5	13	4.8	6.2	1.2
622	Pork link (16 per 1-lb pkg), cooked[50] ---------------------	1 link----------	13	45	50	3	4	1.4	1.8	0.5
	Salami:								
623	Cooked type, slice (8 per 8-oz pkg)-------------------	2 slices--------	57	60	145	8	11	4.6	5.2	1.2
624	Dry type, slice (12 per 4-oz pkg)---------------------	2 slices--------	20	35	85	5	7	2.4	3.4	0.6
625	Sandwich spread (pork, beef)---	1 tbsp----------	15	60	35	1	3	0.9	1.1	0.4
626	Vienna sausage (7 per 4-oz can)	1 sausage-------	16	60	45	2	4	1.5	2.0	0.3
	Veal, medium fat, cooked, bone removed:								
627	Cutlet, 4-1/8 by 2-1/4 by 1/2 in, braised or broiled-------	3 oz------------	85	60	185	23	9	4.1	4.1	0.6
628	Rib, 2 pieces, 4-1/8 by 2-1/4 by 1/4 in, roasted-----------	3 oz------------	85	55	230	23	14	6.0	6.0	1.0

[49] Contains added sodium ascorbate. If sodium ascorbate is not added, ascorbic acid content is negligible.

202

Cho-les-terol	Carbo-hydrate	Calcium	Phos-phorus	Iron	Potas-sium	Sodium	Vitamin A value (IU)	Vitamin A value (RE)	Thiamin	Ribo-flavin	Niacin	Ascorbic acid	Item No.
Milli-grams	Grams	Milli-grams	Milli-grams	Milli-grams	Milli-grams	Milli-grams	Inter-national units	Retinol equiva-lents	Milli-grams	Milli-grams	Milli-grams	Milli-grams	
16	Tr	2	64	0.3	92	303	0	0	0.13	0.05	1.4	6	599
27	1	5	136	0.4	179	711	0	0	0.38	0.09	3.2	10	600
53	0	6	182	0.7	243	1,009	0	0	0.51	0.19	3.8	0	601
37	0	5	154	0.6	215	902	0	0	0.46	0.17	3.4	0	602
35	Tr	6	188	0.9	298	908	0	0	0.82	0.21	4.3	[49]19	603
26	1	3	34	0.3	90	541	0	0	0.15	0.08	1.3	Tr	604
21	0	3	65	0.3	134	576	0	0	0.27	0.09	1.6	[49]8	605
32	2	4	141	0.6	189	751	0	0	0.49	0.14	3.0	[49]16	606
27	1	4	124	0.4	200	815	0	0	0.53	0.13	2.8	[49]15	607
84	0	3	184	0.7	312	61	10	3	0.87	0.24	4.3	Tr	608
71	0	4	176	0.7	302	56	10	1	0.83	0.22	4.0	Tr	609
92	0	4	190	0.7	323	64	10	3	0.91	0.24	4.6	Tr	610
72	0	3	178	0.7	305	57	10	1	0.84	0.22	4.0	Tr	611
79	0	5	210	0.9	280	50	10	2	0.54	0.27	3.9	Tr	612
68	0	5	202	0.8	269	46	10	1	0.50	0.25	3.6	Tr	613
69	0	9	190	0.8	313	37	10	3	0.50	0.24	4.2	Tr	614
56	0	8	182	0.7	300	33	10	2	0.45	0.22	3.8	Tr	615
93	0	6	162	1.4	286	75	10	3	0.46	0.26	4.4	Tr	616
76	0	5	151	1.3	271	68	10	1	0.40	0.24	4.0	Tr	617
31	2	7	52	0.9	103	581	0	0	0.10	0.08	1.5	[49]12	618
89	2	5	96	5.3	113	652	8,010	2,405	0.14	0.87	4.8	[49]6	619
9	Tr	1	14	0.1	25	105	0	0	0.05	0.02	0.4	0	620
23	1	5	39	0.5	75	504	0	0	0.09	0.05	1.2	[49]12	621
11	Tr	4	24	0.2	47	168	0	0	0.10	0.03	0.6	Tr	622
37	1	7	66	1.5	113	607	0	0	0.14	0.21	2.0	[49]7	623
16	1	2	28	0.3	76	372	0	0	0.12	0.06	1.0	[49]5	624
6	2	2	9	0.1	17	152	10	1	0.03	0.02	0.3	0	625
8	Tr	2	8	0.1	16	152	0	0	0.01	0.02	0.3	0	626
109	0	9	196	0.8	258	56	Tr	Tr	0.06	0.21	4.6	0	627
109	0	10	211	0.7	259	57	Tr	Tr	0.11	0.26	6.6	0	628

[50] One patty (8 per pound) of bulk sausage is equivalent to 2 links.

Table 2. Nutritive Value of the Edible Part of Food (Continued)
(Tr indicates nutrient present in trace amount.)

Item No.	Foods, approximate measures, units, and weight (weight of edible portion only)			Water	Food energy	Pro-tein	Fat	Fatty acids		
								Satu-rated	Mono-unsatu-rated	Poly-unsatu-rated
	Mixed Dishes and Fast Foods		Grams	Per-cent	Cal-ories	Grams	Grams	Grams	Grams	Grams
	Mixed dishes:									
629	Beef and vegetable stew, from home recipe	1 cup	245	82	220	16	11	4.4	4.5	0.5
630	Beef potpie, from home recipe, baked, piece, 1/3 of 9-in diam. pie[51]	1 piece	210	55	515	21	30	7.9	12.9	7.4
631	Chicken a la king, cooked, from home recipe	1 cup	245	68	470	27	34	12.9	13.4	6.2
632	Chicken and noodles, cooked, from home recipe	1 cup	240	71	365	22	18	5.1	7.1	3.9
	Chicken chow mein:									
633	Canned	1 cup	250	89	95	7	Tr	0.1	0.1	0.8
634	From home recipe	1 cup	250	78	255	31	10	4.1	4.9	3.5
635	Chicken potpie, from home recipe, baked, piece, 1/3 of 9-in diam. pie[51]	1 piece	232	57	545	23	31	10.3	15.5	6.6
636	Chili con carne with beans, canned	1 cup	255	72	340	19	16	5.8	7.2	1.0
637	Chop suey with beef and pork, from home recipe	1 cup	250	75	300	26	17	4.3	7.4	4.2
	Macaroni (enriched) and cheese:									
638	Canned[52]	1 cup	240	80	230	9	10	4.7	2.9	1.3
639	From home recipe[38]	1 cup	200	58	430	17	22	9.8	7.4	3.6
640	Quiche Lorraine, 1/8 of 8-in diam. quiche[51]	1 slice	176	47	600	13	48	23.2	17.8	4.1
	Spaghetti (enriched) in tomato sauce with cheese:									
641	Canned	1 cup	250	80	190	6	2	0.4	0.4	0.5
642	From home recipe	1 cup	250	77	260	9	9	3.0	3.6	1.2
	Spaghetti (enriched) with meat-balls and tomato sauce:									
643	Canned	1 cup	250	78	260	12	10	2.4	3.9	3.1
644	From home recipe	1 cup	248	70	330	19	12	3.9	4.4	2.2
	Fast food entrees:									
	Cheeseburger:									
645	Regular	1 sandwich	112	46	300	15	15	7.3	5.6	1.0
646	4 oz patty	1 sandwich	194	46	525	30	31	15.1	12.2	1.4
	Chicken, fried. See Poultry and Poultry Products (items 656-659).									
647	Enchilada	1 enchilada	230	72	235	20	16	7.7	6.7	0.6
648	English muffin, egg, cheese, and bacon	1 sandwich	138	49	360	18	18	8.0	8.0	0.7
	Fish sandwich:									
649	Regular, with cheese	1 sandwich	140	43	420	16	23	6.3	6.9	7.7
650	Large, without cheese	1 sandwich	170	48	470	18	27	6.3	8.7	9.5
	Hamburger:									
651	Regular	1 sandwich	98	46	245	12	11	4.4	5.3	0.5
652	4 oz patty	1 sandwich	174	50	445	25	21	7.1	11.7	0.6
653	Pizza, cheese, 1/8 of 15-in diam. pizza[51]	1 slice	120	46	290	15	9	4.1	2.6	1.3
654	Roast beef sandwich	1 sandwich	150	52	345	22	13	3.5	6.9	1.8
655	Taco	1 taco	81	55	195	9	11	4.1	5.5	0.8

[38] Made with margarine.
[51] Crust made with vegetable shortening and enriched flour.

Cho-les-terol	Carbo-hydrate	Calcium	Phos-phorus	Iron	Potas-sium	Sodium	Vitamin A value		Thiamin	Ribo-flavin	Niacin	Ascorbic acid	Item No.
							(IU)	(RE)					
Milli-grams	Grams	Milli-grams	Milli-grams	Milli-grams	Milli-grams	Milli-grams	Inter-national units	Retinol equiva-lents	Milli-grams	Milli-grams	Milli-grams	Milli-grams	
71	15	29	184	2.9	613	292	5,690	568	0.15	0.17	4.7	17	629
42	39	29	149	3.8	334	596	4,220	517	0.29	0.29	4.8	6	630
221	12	127	358	2.5	404	760	1,130	272	0.10	0.42	5.4	12	631
103	26	26	247	2.2	149	600	430	130	0.05	0.17	4.3	Tr	632
8	18	45	85	1.3	418	725	150	28	0.05	0.10	1.0	13	633
75	10	58	293	2.5	473	718	280	50	0.08	0.23	4.3	10	634
56	42	70	232	3.0	343	594	7,220	735	0.32	0.32	4.9	5	635
28	31	82	321	4.3	594	1,354	150	15	0.08	0.18	3.3	8	636
68	13	60	248	4.8	425	1,053	600	60	0.28	0.38	5.0	33	637
24	26	199	182	1.0	139	730	260	72	0.12	0.24	1.0	Tr	638
44	40	362	322	1.8	240	1,086	860	232	0.20	0.40	1.8	1	639
285	29	211	276	1.0	283	653	1,640	454	0.11	0.32	Tr	Tr	640
3	39	40	88	2.8	303	955	930	120	0.35	0.28	4.5	10	641
8	37	80	135	2.3	408	955	1,080	140	0.25	0.18	2.3	13	642
23	29	53	113	3.3	245	1,220	1,000	100	0.15	0.18	2.3	5	643
89	39	124	236	3.7	665	1,009	1,590	159	0.25	0.30	4.0	22	644
44	28	135	174	2.3	219	672	340	65	0.26	0.24	3.7	1	645
104	40	236	320	4.5	407	1,224	670	128	0.33	0.48	7.4	3	646
19	24	97	198	3.3	653	1,332	2,720	352	0.18	0.26	Tr	Tr	647
213	31	197	290	3.1	201	832	650	160	0.46	0.50	3.7	1	648
56	39	132	223	1.8	274	667	160	25	0.32	0.26	3.3	2	649
91	41	61	246	2.2	375	621	110	15	0.35	0.23	3.5	1	650
32	28	56	107	2.2	202	463	80	14	0.23	0.24	3.8	1	651
71	38	75	225	4.8	404	763	160	28	0.38	0.38	7.8	1	652
56	39	220	216	1.6	230	699	750	106	0.34	0.29	4.2	2	653
55	34	60	222	4.0	338	757	240	32	0.40	0.33	6.0	2	654
21	15	109	134	1.2	263	456	420	57	0.09	0.07	1.4	1	655

[52]Made with corn oil.

Item No.	Foods, approximate measures, units, and weight (weight of edible portion only)		Water	Food energy	Pro-tein	Fat	Fatty acids		
							Satu-rated	Mono-unsatu-rated	Poly-unsatu-rated
		Grams	Per-cent	Cal-ories	Grams	Grams	Grams	Grams	Grams

Poultry and Poultry Products

	Chicken:								
	Fried, flesh, with skin:[53]								
	Batter dipped:								
656	Breast, 1/2 breast (5.6 oz with bones)-------------- 4.9 oz----------	140	52	365	35	18	4.9	7.6	4.3
657	Drumstick (3.4 oz with bones)-------------------- 2.5 oz----------	72	53	195	16	11	3.0	4.6	2.7
	Flour coated:								
658	Breast, 1/2 breast (4.2 oz with bones)-------------- 3.5 oz----------	98	57	220	31	9	2.4	3.4	1.9
659	Drumstick (2.6 oz with bones)-------------------- 1.7 oz----------	49	57	120	13	7	1.8	2.7	1.6
	Roasted, flesh only:								
660	Breast, 1/2 breast (4.2 oz with bones and skin)------- 3.0 oz----------	86	65	140	27	3	0.9	1.1	0.7
661	Drumstick, (2.9 oz with bones and skin)-------------------- 1.6 oz----------	44	67	75	12	2	0.7	0.8	0.6
662	Stewed, flesh only, light and dark meat, chopped or diced-- 1 cup-----------	140	67	250	38	9	2.6	3.3	2.2
663	Chicken liver, cooked------------ 1 liver---------	20	68	30	5	1	0.4	0.3	0.2
664	Duck, roasted, flesh only-------- 1/2 duck----------	221	64	445	52	25	9.2	8.2	3.2
	Turkey, roasted, flesh only:								
665	Dark meat, piece, 2-1/2 by 1-5/8 by 1/4 in-------------- 4 pieces--------	85	63	160	24	6	2.1	1.4	1.8
666	Light meat, piece, 4 by 2 by 1/4 in----------------------- 2 pieces--------	85	66	135	25	3	0.9	0.5	0.7
	Light and dark meat:								
667	Chopped or diced------------- 1 cup-----------	140	65	240	41	7	2.3	1.4	2.0
668	Pieces (1 slice white meat, 4 by 2 by 1/4 in and 2 slices dark meat, 2-1/2 by 1-5/8 by 1/4 in)-------- 3 pieces--------	85	65	145	25	4	1.4	0.9	1.2
	Poultry food products:								
	Chicken:								
669	Canned, boneless------------- 5 oz-------------	142	69	235	31	11	3.1	4.5	2.5
670	Frankfurter (10 per 1-lb pkg) 1 frankfurter---	45	58	115	6	9	2.5	3.8	1.8
671	Roll, light (6 slices per 6 oz pkg)--------------------- 2 slices--------	57	69	90	11	4	1.1	1.7	0.9
	Turkey:								
672	Gravy and turkey, frozen----- 5-oz package----	142	85	95	8	4	1.2	1.4	0.7
673	Ham, cured turkey thigh meat (8 slices per 8-oz pkg)---- 2 slices--------	57	71	75	11	3	1.0	0.7	0.9
674	Loaf, breast meat (8 slices per 6-oz pkg)-------------- 2 slices--------	42	72	45	10	1	0.2	0.2	0.1
675	Patties, breaded, battered, fried (2.25 oz)------------ 1 patty---------	64	50	180	9	12	3.0	4.8	3.0
676	Roast, boneless, frozen, sea-soned, light and dark meat, cooked-------------------- 3 oz-------------	85	68	130	18	5	1.6	1.0	1.4

Soups, Sauces, and Gravies

	Soups:								
	Canned, condensed:								
	Prepared with equal volume of milk:								
677	Clam chowder, New England-- 1 cup-----------	248	85	165	9	7	3.0	2.3	1.1
678	Cream of chicken----------- 1 cup-----------	248	85	190	7	11	4.6	4.5	1.6
679	Cream of mushroom---------- 1 cup-----------	248	85	205	6	14	5.1	3.0	4.6
680	Tomato--------------------- 1 cup-----------	248	85	160	6	6	2.9	1.6	1.1

[53] Fried in vegetable shortening.

Cho-les-terol	Carbo-hydrate	Calcium	Phos-phorus	Iron	Potas-sium	Sodium	Vitamin A value		Thiamin	Ribo-flavin	Niacin	Ascorbic acid	Item No.
							(IU)	(RE)					
Milli-grams	Grams	Milli-grams	Milli-grams	Milli-grams	Milli-grams	Milli-grams	Inter-national units	Retinol equiva-lents	Milli-grams	Milli-grams	Milli-grams	Milli-grams	
119	13	28	259	1.8	281	385	90	28	0.16	0.20	14.7	0	656
62	6	12	106	1.0	134	194	60	19	0.08	0.15	3.7	0	657
87	2	16	228	1.2	254	74	50	15	0.08	0.13	13.5	0	658
44	1	6	86	0.7	112	44	40	12	0.04	0.11	3.0	0	659
73	0	13	196	0.9	220	64	20	5	0.06	0.10	11.8	0	660
41	0	5	81	0.6	108	42	30	8	0.03	0.10	2.7	0	661
116	0	20	210	1.6	252	98	70	21	0.07	0.23	8.6	0	662
126	Tr	3	62	1.7	28	10	3,270	983	0.03	0.35	0.9	3	663
197	0	27	449	6.0	557	144	170	51	0.57	1.04	11.3	0	664
72	0	27	173	2.0	246	67	0	0	0.05	0.21	3.1	0	665
59	0	16	186	1.1	259	54	0	0	0.05	0.11	5.8	0	666
106	0	35	298	2.5	417	98	0	0	0.09	0.25	7.6	0	667
65	0	21	181	1.5	253	60	0	0	0.05	0.15	4.6	0	668
88	0	20	158	2.2	196	714	170	48	0.02	0.18	9.0	3	669
45	3	43	48	0.9	38	616	60	17	0.03	0.05	1.4	0	670
28	1	24	89	0.6	129	331	50	14	0.04	0.07	3.0	0	671
26	7	20	115	1.3	87	787	60	18	0.03	0.18	2.6	0	672
32	Tr	6	108	1.6	184	565	0	0	0.03	0.14	2.0	0	673
17	0	3	97	0.2	118	608	0	0	0.02	0.05	3.5	[54]0	674
40	10	9	173	1.4	176	512	20	7	0.06	0.12	1.5	0	675
45	3	4	207	1.4	253	578	0	0	0.04	0.14	5.3	0	676
22	17	186	156	1.5	300	992	160	40	0.07	0.24	1.0	3	677
27	15	181	151	0.7	273	1,047	710	94	0.07	0.26	0.9	1	678
20	15	179	156	0.6	270	1,076	150	37	0.08	0.28	0.9	2	679
17	22	159	149	1.8	449	932	850	109	0.13	0.25	1.5	68	680

[54]If sodium ascorbate is added, product contains 11 mg ascorbic acid.

Table 2. Nutritive Value of the Edible Part of Food (Continued)

(Tr indicates nutrient present in trace amount.)

Item No.	Foods, approximate measures, units, and weight (weight of edible portion only)		Water	Food energy	Pro-tein	Fat	Fatty acids		
							Satu-rated	Mono-unsatu-rated	Poly-unsatu-rated
		Grams	Per-cent	Cal-ories	Grams	Grams	Grams	Grams	Grams

Soups, Sauces, and Gravies—Con.

Soups:
  Canned, condensed:
    Prepared with equal volume of water:

Item No.	Food	Measure	Grams	Percent	Calories	Protein g	Fat g	Sat g	Mono g	Poly g
681	Bean with bacon	1 cup	253	84	170	8	6	1.5	2.2	1.8
682	Beef broth, bouillon, consomme	1 cup	240	98	15	3	1	0.3	0.2	Tr
683	Beef noodle	1 cup	244	92	85	5	3	1.1	1.2	0.5
684	Chicken noodle	1 cup	241	92	75	4	2	0.7	1.1	0.6
685	Chicken rice	1 cup	241	94	60	4	2	0.5	0.9	0.4
686	Clam chowder, Manhattan	1 cup	244	90	80	4	2	0.4	0.4	1.3
687	Cream of chicken	1 cup	244	91	115	3	7	2.1	3.3	1.5
688	Cream of mushroom	1 cup	244	90	130	2	9	2.4	1.7	4.2
689	Minestrone	1 cup	241	91	80	4	3	0.6	0.7	1.1
690	Pea, green	1 cup	250	83	165	9	3	1.4	1.0	0.4
691	Tomato	1 cup	244	90	85	2	2	0.4	0.4	1.0
692	Vegetable beef	1 cup	244	92	80	6	2	0.9	0.8	0.1
693	Vegetarian	1 cup	241	92	70	2	2	0.3	0.8	0.7
	Dehydrated: Unprepared:									
694	Bouillon	1 pkt	6	3	15	1	1	0.3	0.2	Tr
695	Onion	1 pkt	7	4	20	1	Tr	0.1	0.2	Tr
	Prepared with water:									
696	Chicken noodle	1 pkt (6-fl-oz)	188	94	40	2	1	0.2	0.4	0.3
697	Onion	1 pkt (6-fl-oz)	184	96	20	1	Tr	0.1	0.2	0.1
698	Tomato vegetable	1 pkt (6-fl-oz)	189	94	40	1	1	0.3	0.2	0.1
	Sauces: From dry mix:									
699	Cheese, prepared with milk	1 cup	279	77	305	16	17	9.3	5.3	1.6
700	Hollandaise, prepared with water	1 cup	259	84	240	5	20	11.6	5.9	0.9
701	White sauce, prepared with milk	1 cup	264	81	240	10	13	6.4	4.7	1.7
	From home recipe:									
702	White sauce, medium[55]	1 cup	250	73	395	10	30	9.1	11.9	7.2
	Ready to serve:									
703	Barbecue	1 tbsp	16	81	10	Tr	Tr	Tr	0.1	0.1
704	Soy	1 tbsp	18	68	10	2	0	0.0	0.0	0.0
	Gravies: Canned:									
705	Beef	1 cup	233	87	125	9	5	2.7	2.3	0.2
706	Chicken	1 cup	238	85	190	5	14	3.4	6.1	3.6
707	Mushroom	1 cup	238	89	120	3	6	1.0	2.8	2.4
	From dry mix:									
708	Brown	1 cup	261	91	80	3	2	0.9	0.8	0.1
709	Chicken	1 cup	260	91	85	3	2	0.5	0.9	0.4

Sugars and Sweets

Item No.	Food	Measure	Grams	Percent	Calories	Protein g	Fat g	Sat g	Mono g	Poly g
	Candy:									
710	Caramels, plain or chocolate	1 oz	28	8	115	1	3	2.2	0.3	0.1
	Chocolate:									
711	Milk, plain	1 oz	28	1	145	2	9	5.4	3.0	0.3
712	Milk, with almonds	1 oz	28	2	150	3	10	4.8	4.1	0.7
713	Milk, with peanuts	1 oz	28	1	155	4	11	4.2	3.5	1.5
714	Milk, with rice cereal	1 oz	28	2	140	2	7	4.4	2.5	0.2
715	Semisweet, small pieces (60 per oz)	1 cup or 6 oz	170	1	860	7	61	36.2	19.9	1.9
716	Sweet (dark)	1 oz	28	1	150	1	10	5.9	3.3	0.3
717	Fondant, uncoated (mints, candy corn, other)	1 oz	28	3	105	Tr	0	0.0	0.0	0.0
718	Fudge, chocolate, plain	1 oz	28	8	115	1	3	2.1	1.0	0.1
719	Gum drops	1 oz	28	12	100	Tr	Tr	Tr	Tr	0.1

[55] Made with enriched flour, margarine, and whole milk.

Cholesterol	Carbohydrate	Calcium	Phosphorus	Iron	Potassium	Sodium	Vitamin A value (IU)	Vitamin A value (RE)	Thiamin	Riboflavin	Niacin	Ascorbic acid	Item No.
Milligrams	Grams	Milligrams	Milligrams	Milligrams	Milligrams	Milligrams	International units	Retinol equivalents	Milligrams	Milligrams	Milligrams	Milligrams	
3	23	81	132	2.0	402	951	890	89	0.09	0.03	0.6	2	681
Tr	Tr	14	31	0.4	130	782	0	0	Tr	0.05	1.9	0	682
5	9	15	46	1.1	100	952	630	63	0.07	0.06	1.1	Tr	683
7	9	17	36	0.8	55	1,106	710	71	0.05	0.06	1.4	Tr	684
7	7	17	22	0.7	101	815	660	66	0.02	0.02	1.1	Tr	685
2	12	34	59	1.9	261	1,808	920	92	0.06	0.05	1.3	3	686
10	9	34	37	0.6	88	986	560	56	0.03	0.06	0.8	Tr	687
2	9	46	49	0.5	100	1,032	0	0	0.05	0.09	0.7	1	688
2	11	34	55	0.9	313	911	2,340	234	0.05	0.04	0.9	1	689
0	27	28	125	2.0	190	988	200	20	0.11	0.07	1.2	2	690
0	17	12	34	1.8	264	871	690	69	0.09	0.05	1.4	66	691
5	10	17	41	1.1	173	956	1,890	189	0.04	0.05	1.0	2	692
0	12	22	34	1.1	210	822	3,010	301	0.05	0.05	0.9	1	693
1	1	4	19	0.1	27	1,019	Tr	Tr	Tr	0.01	0.3	0	694
Tr	4	10	23	0.1	47	627	Tr	Tr	0.02	0.04	0.4	Tr	695
2	6	24	24	0.4	23	957	50	5	0.05	0.04	0.7	Tr	696
0	4	9	22	0.1	48	635	Tr	Tr	0.02	0.04	0.4	Tr	697
0	8	6	23	0.5	78	856	140	14	0.04	0.03	0.6	5	698
53	23	569	438	0.3	552	1,565	390	117	0.15	0.56	0.3	2	699
52	14	124	127	0.9	124	1,564	730	220	0.05	0.18	0.1	Tr	700
34	21	425	256	0.3	444	797	310	92	0.08	0.45	0.5	3	701
32	24	292	238	0.9	381	888	1,190	340	0.15	0.43	0.8	2	702
0	2	3	3	0.1	28	130	140	14	Tr	Tr	0.1	1	703
0	2	3	38	0.5	64	1,029	0	0	0.01	0.02	0.6	0	704
7	11	14	70	1.6	189	1,305	0	0	0.07	0.08	1.5	0	705
5	13	48	69	1.1	259	1,373	880	264	0.04	0.10	1.1	0	706
0	13	17	36	1.6	252	1,357	0	0	0.08	0.15	1.6	0	707
2	14	66	47	0.2	61	1,147	0	0	0.04	0.09	0.9	0	708
3	14	39	47	0.3	62	1,134	0	0	0.05	0.15	0.8	3	709
1	22	42	35	0.4	54	64	Tr	Tr	0.01	0.05	0.1	Tr	710
6	16	50	61	0.4	96	23	30	10	0.02	0.10	0.1	Tr	711
5	15	65	77	0.5	125	23	30	8	0.02	0.12	0.2	Tr	712
5	13	49	83	0.4	138	19	30	8	0.07	0.07	1.4	Tr	713
6	18	48	57	0.2	100	46	30	8	0.01	0.08	0.1	Tr	714
0	97	51	178	5.8	593	24	30	3	0.10	0.14	0.9	Tr	715
0	16	7	41	0.6	86	5	10	1	0.01	0.04	0.1	Tr	716
0	27	2	Tr	0.1	1	57	0	0	Tr	Tr	Tr	0	717
1	21	22	24	0.3	42	54	Tr	Tr	0.01	0.03	0.1	Tr	718
0	25	2	Tr	0.1	1	10	0	0	0.00	Tr	Tr	0	719

Item No.	Foods, approximate measures, units, and weight (weight of edible portion only)		Grams	Water Per-cent	Food energy Cal-ories	Pro-tein Grams	Fat Grams	Fatty acids Satu-rated Grams	Mono-unsatu-rated Grams	Poly-unsatu-rated Grams
	Sugars and Sweets—Con.									
	Candy:									
720	Hard	1 oz	28	1	110	0	0	0.0	0.0	0.0
721	Jelly beans	1 oz	28	6	105	Tr	Tr	Tr	Tr	0.1
722	Marshmallows	1 oz	28	17	90	1	0	0.0	0.0	0.0
723	Custard, baked	1 cup	265	77	305	14	15	6.8	5.4	0.7
724	Gelatin dessert prepared with gelatin dessert powder and water	1/2 cup	120	84	70	2	0	0.0	0.0	0.0
725	Honey, strained or extracted	1 cup	339	17	1,030	1	0	0.0	0.0	0.0
726		1 tbsp	21	17	65	Tr	0	0.0	0.0	0.0
727	Jams and preserves	1 tbsp	20	29	55	Tr	Tr	0.0	Tr	Tr
728		1 packet	14	29	40	Tr	Tr	0.0	Tr	Tr
729	Jellies	1 tbsp	18	28	50	Tr	Tr	Tr	Tr	Tr
730		1 packet	14	28	40	Tr	Tr	Tr	Tr	Tr
731	Popsicle, 3-fl-oz size	1 popsicle	95	80	70	0	0	0.0	0.0	0.0
	Puddings:									
	Canned:									
732	Chocolate	5-oz can	142	68	205	3	11	9.5	0.5	0.1
733	Tapioca	5-oz can	142	74	160	3	5	4.8	Tr	Tr
734	Vanilla	5-oz can	142	69	220	2	10	9.5	0.2	0.1
	Dry mix, prepared with whole milk:									
	Chocolate:									
735	Instant	1/2 cup	130	71	155	4	4	2.3	1.1	0.2
736	Regular (cooked)	1/2 cup	130	73	150	4	4	2.4	1.1	0.1
737	Rice	1/2 cup	132	73	155	4	4	2.3	1.1	0.1
738	Tapioca	1/2 cup	130	75	145	4	4	2.3	1.1	0.1
	Vanilla:									
739	Instant	1/2 cup	130	73	150	4	4	2.2	1.1	0.2
740	Regular (cooked)	1/2 cup	130	74	145	4	4	2.3	1.0	0.1
	Sugars:									
741	Brown, pressed down	1 cup	220	2	820	0	0	0.0	0.0	0.0
	White:									
742	Granulated	1 cup	200	1	770	0	0	0.0	0.0	0.0
743		1 tbsp	12	1	45	0	0	0.0	0.0	0.0
744		1 packet	6	1	25	0	0	0.0	0.0	0.0
745	Powdered, sifted, spooned into cup	1 cup	100	1	385	0	0	0.0	0.0	0.0
	Syrups:									
	Chocolate-flavored syrup or topping:									
746	Thin type	2 tbsp	38	37	85	1	Tr	0.2	0.1	0.1
747	Fudge type	2 tbsp	38	25	125	2	5	3.1	1.7	0.2
748	Molasses, cane, blackstrap	2 tbsp	40	24	85	0	0	0.0	0.0	0.0
749	Table syrup (corn and maple)	2 tbsp	42	25	122	0	0	0.0	0.0	0.0
	Vegetables and Vegetable Products									
750	Alfalfa seeds, sprouted, raw	1 cup	33	91	10	1	Tr	Tr	Tr	0.1
751	Artichokes, globe or French, cooked, drained	1 artichoke	120	87	55	3	Tr	Tr	Tr	0.1
	Asparagus, green:									
	Cooked, drained:									
	From raw:									
752	Cuts and tips	1 cup	180	92	45	5	1	0.1	Tr	0.2
753	Spears, 1/2-in diam. at base	4 spears	60	92	15	2	Tr	Tr	Tr	0.1
	From frozen:									
754	Cuts and tips	1 cup	180	91	50	5	1	0.2	Tr	0.3
755	Spears, 1/2-in diam. at base	4 spears	60	91	15	2	Tr	0.1	Tr	0.1
756	Canned, spears, 1/2-in diam. at base	4 spears	80	95	10	1	Tr	Tr	Tr	0.1
757	Bamboo shoots, canned, drained	1 cup	131	94	25	2	1	0.1	Tr	0.2

[56] For regular pack; special dietary pack contains 3 mg sodium.

Nutrients in Indicated Quantity

Cholesterol	Carbohydrate	Calcium	Phosphorus	Iron	Potassium	Sodium	Vitamin A value (IU)	Vitamin A value (RE)	Thiamin	Riboflavin	Niacin	Ascorbic acid	Item No.
Milligrams	Grams	Milligrams	Milligrams	Milligrams	Milligrams	Milligrams	International units	Retinol equivalents	Milligrams	Milligrams	Milligrams	Milligrams	
0	28	Tr	2	0.1	1	7	0	0	0.10	0.00	0.0	0	720
0	26	1	1	0.3	11	7	0	0	0.00	Tr	Tr	0	721
0	23	1	2	0.5	2	25	0	0	0.00	Tr	Tr	0	722
278	29	297	310	1.1	387	209	530	146	0.11	0.50	0.3	1	723
0	17	2	23	Tr	Tr	55	0	0	0.00	0.00	0.0	0	724
0	279	17	20	1.7	173	17	0	0	0.02	0.14	1.0	3	725
0	17	1	1	0.1	11	1	0	0	Tr	0.01	0.1	Tr	726
0	14	4	2	0.2	18	2	Tr	Tr	Tr	0.01	Tr	Tr	727
0	10	3	1	0.1	12	2	Tr	Tr	Tr	Tr	Tr	Tr	728
0	13	2	Tr	0.1	16	5	Tr	Tr	Tr	0.01	Tr	1	729
0	10	1	Tr	Tr	13	4	Tr	Tr	Tr	Tr	Tr	1	730
0	18	0	0	Tr	4	11	0	0	0.00	0.00	0.0	0	731
1	30	74	117	1.2	254	285	100	31	0.04	0.17	0.6	Tr	732
Tr	28	119	113	0.3	212	252	Tr	Tr	0.03	0.14	0.4	Tr	733
1	33	79	94	0.2	155	305	Tr	Tr	0.03	0.12	0.6	Tr	734
14	27	130	329	0.3	176	440	130	33	0.04	0.18	0.1	1	735
15	25	146	120	0.2	190	167	140	34	0.05	0.20	0.1	1	736
15	27	133	110	0.5	165	140	140	33	0.10	0.18	0.6	1	737
15	25	131	103	0.1	167	152	140	34	0.04	0.18	0.1	1	738
15	27	129	273	0.1	164	375	140	33	0.04	0.17	0.1	1	739
15	25	132	102	0.1	166	178	140	34	0.04	0.18	0.1	1	740
0	212	187	56	4.8	757	97	0	0	0.02	0.07	0.2	0	741
0	199	3	Tr	0.1	7	5	0	0	0.00	0.00	0.0	0	742
0	12	Tr	Tr	Tr	Tr	Tr	0	0	0.00	0.00	0.0	0	743
0	6	Tr	Tr	Tr	Tr	Tr	0	0	0.00	0.00	0.0	0	744
0	100	1	Tr	Tr	4	2	0	0	0.00	0.00	0.0	0	745
0	22	6	49	0.8	85	36	Tr	Tr	Tr	0.02	0.1	0	746
0	21	38	60	0.5	82	42	40	13	0.02	0.08	0.1	0	747
0	22	274	34	10.1	1,171	38	0	0	0.04	0.08	0.8	0	748
0	32	1	4	Tr	7	19	0	0	0.00	0.00	0.0	0	749
0	1	11	23	0.3	26	2	50	5	0.03	0.04	0.2	3	750
0	12	47	72	1.6	316	79	170	17	0.07	0.06	0.7	9	751
0	8	43	110	1.2	558	7	1,490	149	0.18	0.22	1.9	49	752
0	3	14	37	0.4	186	2	500	50	0.06	0.07	0.6	16	753
0	9	41	99	1.2	392	7	1,470	147	0.12	0.19	1.9	44	754
0	3	14	33	0.4	131	2	490	49	0.04	0.06	0.6	15	755
0	2	11	30	0.5	122	[56]278	380	38	0.04	0.07	0.7	13	756
0	4	10	33	0.4	105	9	10	1	0.03	0.03	0.2	1	757

Item No.	Foods, approximate measures, units, and weight (weight of edible portion only)		Water	Food energy	Pro-tein	Fat	Fatty acids		
							Satu-rated	Mono-unsatu-rated	Poly-unsatu-rated
	Vegetables and Vegetable Products—Con.	Grams	Per-cent	Cal-ories	Grams	Grams	Grams	Grams	Grams
	Beans:								
	Lima, immature seeds, frozen, cooked, drained:								
758	Thick-seeded types (Ford-hooks)--------------------- 1 cup-----------	170	74	170	10	1	0.1	Tr	0.3
759	Thin-seeded types (baby limas)--------------------- 1 cup-----------	180	72	190	12	1	0.1	Tr	0.3
	Snap:								
	Cooked, drained:								
760	From raw (cut and French style)-------------------- 1 cup-----------	125	89	45	2	Tr	0.1	Tr	0.2
761	From frozen (cut)---------- 1 cup-----------	135	92	35	2	Tr	Tr	Tr	0.1
762	Canned, drained solids (cut) 1 cup-----------	135	93	25	2	Tr	Tr	Tr	0.1
	Beans, mature. See Beans, dry (items 527-535) and Black-eyed peas, dry (item 536).								
	Bean sprouts (mung):								
763	Raw--------------------------- 1 cup-----------	104	90	30	3	Tr	Tr	Tr	0.1
764	Cooked, drained---------------- 1 cup-----------	124	93	25	3	Tr	Tr	Tr	Tr
	Beets:								
	Cooked, drained:								
765	Diced or sliced-------------- 1 cup-----------	170	91	55	2	Tr	Tr	Tr	Tr
766	Whole beets, 2-in diam.------ 2 beets---------	100	91	30	1	Tr	Tr	Tr	Tr
767	Canned, drained solids, diced or sliced-------------------- 1 cup-----------	170	91	55	2	Tr	Tr	Tr	0.1
768	Beet greens, leaves and stems, cooked, drained--------------- 1 cup-----------	144	89	40	4	Tr	Tr	0.1	0.1
	Black-eyed peas, immature seeds, cooked and drained:								
769	From raw----------------------- 1 cup-----------	165	72	180	13	1	0.3	0.1	0.6
770	From frozen-------------------- 1 cup-----------	170	66	225	14	1	0.3	0.1	0.5
	Broccoli:								
771	Raw-------------------------- 1 spear---------	151	91	40	4	1	0.1	Tr	0.3
	Cooked, drained:								
	From raw:								
772	Spear, medium--------------- 1 spear---------	180	90	50	5	1	0.1	Tr	0.2
773	Spears, cut into 1/2-in pieces-------------------- 1 cup-----------	155	90	45	5	Tr	0.1	Tr	0.2
	From frozen:								
774	Piece, 4-1/2 to 5 in long-- 1 piece---------	30	91	10	1	Tr	Tr	Tr	Tr
775	Chopped-------------------- 1 cup-----------	185	91	50	6	Tr	Tr	Tr	0.1
	Brussels sprouts, cooked, drained:								
776	From raw, 7-8 sprouts, 1-1/4 to 1-1/2-in diam.------------ 1 cup-----------	155	87	60	4	1	0.2	0.1	0.4
777	From frozen-------------------- 1 cup-----------	155	87	65	6	1	0.1	Tr	0.3
	Cabbage, common varieties:								
778	Raw, coarsely shredded or sliced----------------------- 1 cup-----------	70	93	15	1	Tr	Tr	Tr	0.1
779	Cooked, drained---------------- 1 cup-----------	150	94	30	1	Tr	Tr	Tr	0.2
	Cabbage, Chinese:								
780	Pak-choi, cooked, drained------ 1 cup-----------	170	96	20	3	Tr	Tr	Tr	0.1
781	Pe-tsai, raw, 1-in pieces------ 1 cup-----------	76	94	10	1	Tr	Tr	Tr	0.1
782	Cabbage, red, raw, coarsely shredded or sliced------------ 1 cup-----------	70	92	20	1	Tr	Tr	Tr	0.1
783	Cabbage, savoy, raw, coarsely shredded or sliced------------ 1 cup-----------	70	91	20	1	Tr	Tr	Tr	Tr

[57] For green varieties; yellow varieties contain 101 IU or 10 RE.
[58] For green varieties; yellow varieties contain 151 IU or 15 RE.
[59] For regular pack; special dietary pack contains 3 mg sodium.

Cho-les-terol	Carbo-hydrate	Calcium	Phos-phorus	Iron	Potas-sium	Sodium	Vitamin A value		Thiamin	Ribo-flavin	Niacin	Ascorbic acid	Item No.
							(IU)	(RE)					
Milli-grams	Grams	Milli-grams	Milli-grams	Milli-grams	Milli-grams	Milli-grams	Inter-national units	Retinol equiva-lents	Milli-grams	Milli-grams	Milli-grams	Milli-grams	
0	32	37	107	2.3	694	90	320	32	0.13	0.10	1.8	22	758
0	35	50	202	3.5	740	52	300	30	0.13	0.10	1.4	10	759
0	10	58	49	1.6	374	4	[57]830	[57]83	0.09	0.12	0.8	12	760
0	8	61	32	1.1	151	18	[58]710	[58]71	0.06	0.10	0.6	11	761
0	6	35	26	1.2	147	[59]339	[60]470	[60]47	0.02	0.08	0.3	6	762
0	6	14	56	0.9	155	6	20	2	0.09	0.13	0.8	14	763
0	5	15	35	0.8	125	12	20	2	0.06	0.13	1.0	14	764
0	11	19	53	1.1	530	83	20	2	0.05	0.02	0.5	9	765
0	7	11	31	0.6	312	49	10	1	0.03	0.01	0.3	6	766
0	12	26	29	3.1	252	[61]466	20	2	0.02	0.07	0.3	7	767
0	8	164	59	2.7	1,309	347	7,340	734	0.17	0.42	0.7	36	768
0	30	46	196	2.4	693	7	1,050	105	0.11	0.18	1.8	3	769
0	40	39	207	3.6	638	9	130	13	0.44	0.11	1.2	4	770
0	8	72	100	1.3	491	41	2,330	233	0.10	0.18	1.0	141	771
0	10	82	86	2.1	293	20	2,540	254	0.15	0.37	1.4	113	772
0	9	71	74	1.8	253	17	2,180	218	0.13	0.32	1.2	97	773
0	2	15	17	0.2	54	7	570	57	0.02	0.02	0.1	12	774
0	10	94	102	1.1	333	44	3,500	350	0.10	0.15	0.8	74	775
0	13	56	87	1.9	491	33	1,110	111	0.17	0.12	0.9	96	776
0	13	37	84	1.1	504	36	910	91	0.16	0.18	0.8	71	777
0	4	33	16	0.4	172	13	90	9	0.04	0.02	0.2	33	778
0	7	50	38	0.6	308	29	130	13	0.09	0.08	0.3	36	779
0	3	158	49	1.8	631	58	4,370	437	0.05	0.11	0.7	44	780
0	2	59	22	0.2	181	7	910	91	0.03	0.04	0.3	21	781
0	4	36	29	0.3	144	8	30	3	0.04	0.02	0.2	40	782
0	4	25	29	0.3	161	20	700	70	0.05	0.02	0.2	22	783

[60] For green varieties; yellow varieties contain 142 IU or 14 RE.
[61] For regular pack; special dietary pack contains 78 mg sodium.

Item No.	Foods, approximate measures, units, and weight (weight of edible portion only)		Water	Food energy	Pro-tein	Fat	Fatty acids		
							Satu-rated	Mono-unsatu-rated	Poly-unsatu-rated
		Grams	Per-cent	Cal-ories	Grams	Grams	Grams	Grams	Grams

Vegetables and Vegetable Products—Con.

	Carrots:								
	Raw, without crowns and tips, scraped:								
784	Whole, 7-1/2 by 1-1/8 in, or strips, 2-1/2 to 3 in long	1 carrot or 18 strips	72	88	30	1	Tr	Tr	Tr	0.1
785	Grated	1 cup	110	88	45	1	Tr	Tr	Tr	0.1
	Cooked, sliced, drained:								
786	From raw	1 cup	156	87	70	2	Tr	0.1	Tr	0.1
787	From frozen	1 cup	146	90	55	2	Tr	Tr	Tr	0.1
788	Canned, sliced, drained solids	1 cup	146	93	35	1	Tr	0.1	Tr	0.1
	Cauliflower:								
789	Raw, (flowerets)	1 cup	100	92	25	2	Tr	Tr	Tr	0.1
	Cooked, drained:								
790	From raw (flowerets)	1 cup	125	93	30	2	Tr	Tr	Tr	0.1
791	From frozen (flowerets)	1 cup	180	94	35	3	Tr	0.1	Tr	0.2
	Celery, pascal type, raw:								
792	Stalk, large outer, 8 by 1-1/2 in (at root end)	1 stalk	40	95	5	Tr	Tr	Tr	Tr	Tr
793	Pieces, diced	1 cup	120	95	20	1	Tr	Tr	Tr	0.1
	Collards, cooked, drained:								
794	From raw (leaves without stems)	1 cup	190	96	25	2	Tr	0.1	Tr	0.2
795	From frozen (chopped)	1 cup	170	88	60	5	1	0.1	0.1	0.4
	Corn, sweet:								
	Cooked, drained:								
796	From raw, ear 5 by 1-3/4 in	1 ear	77	70	85	3	1	0.2	0.3	0.5
	From frozen:								
797	Ear, trimmed to about 3-1/2 in long	1 ear	63	73	60	2	Tr	0.1	0.1	0.2
798	Kernels	1 cup	165	76	135	5	Tr	Tr	Tr	0.1
	Canned:								
799	Cream style	1 cup	256	79	185	4	1	0.2	0.3	0.5
800	Whole kernel, vacuum pack	1 cup	210	77	165	5	1	0.2	0.3	0.5
	Cowpeas. See Black-eyed peas, immature (items 769,770), mature (item 536).								
801	Cucumber, with peel, slices, 1/8 in thick (large, 2-1/8-in diam.; small, 1-3/4-in diam.)	6 large or 8 small slices	28	96	5	Tr	Tr	Tr	Tr	Tr
802	Dandelion greens, cooked, drained	1 cup	105	90	35	2	1	0.1	Tr	0.3
803	Eggplant, cooked, steamed	1 cup	96	92	25	1	Tr	Tr	Tr	0.1
804	Endive, curly (including escarole), raw, small pieces	1 cup	50	94	10	1	Tr	Tr	Tr	Tr
805	Jerusalem-artichoke, raw, sliced	1 cup	150	78	115	3	Tr	0.0	Tr	Tr
	Kale, cooked, drained:								
806	From raw, chopped	1 cup	130	91	40	2	1	0.1	Tr	0.3
807	From frozen, chopped	1 cup	130	91	40	4	1	0.1	Tr	0.3
808	Kohlrabi, thickened bulb-like stems, cooked, drained, diced	1 cup	165	90	50	3	Tr	Tr	Tr	0.1
	Lettuce, raw:								
	Butterhead, as Boston types:								
809	Head, 5-in diam	1 head	163	96	20	2	Tr	Tr	Tr	0.2
810	Leaves	1 outer or 2 inner leaves	15	96	Tr	Tr	Tr	Tr	Tr	Tr
	Crisphead, as iceberg:								
811	Head, 6-in diam	1 head	539	96	70	5	1	0.1	Tr	0.5
812	Wedge, 1/4 of head	1 wedge	135	96	20	1	Tr	Tr	Tr	0.1
813	Pieces, chopped or shredded	1 cup	55	96	5	1	Tr	Tr	Tr	0.1
814	Looseleaf (bunching varieties including romaine or cos), chopped or shredded pieces	1 cup	56	94	10	1	Tr	Tr	Tr	0.1

[62]For regular pack; special dietary pack contains 61 mg sodium.
[63]For yellow varieties; white varieties contain only a trace of vitamin A.

Cho-les-terol	Carbo-hydrate	Calcium	Phos-phorus	Iron	Potas-sium	Sodium	Vitamin A value		Thiamin	Ribo-flavin	Niacin	Ascorbic acid	Item No.
							(IU)	(RE)					
Milli-grams	Grams	Milli-grams	Milli-grams	Milli-grams	Milli-grams	Milli-grams	Inter-national units	Retinol equiva-lents	Milli-grams	Milli-grams	Milli-grams	Milli-grams	
0	7	19	32	0.4	233	25	20,250	2,025	0.07	0.04	0.7	7	784
0	11	30	48	0.6	355	39	30,940	3,094	0.11	0.06	1.0	10	785
0	16	48	47	1.0	354	103	38,300	3,830	0.05	0.09	0.8	4	786
0	12	41	38	0.7	231	86	25,850	2,585	0.04	0.05	0.6	4	787
0	8	37	35	0.9	261	[62]352	20,110	2,011	0.03	0.04	0.8	4	788
0	5	29	46	0.6	355	15	20	2	0.08	0.06	0.6	72	789
0	6	34	44	0.5	404	8	20	2	0.08	0.07	0.7	69	790
0	7	31	43	0.7	250	32	40	4	0.07	0.10	0.6	56	791
0	1	14	10	0.2	114	35	50	5	0.01	0.01	0.1	3	792
0	4	43	31	0.6	341	106	150	15	0.04	0.04	0.4	8	793
0	5	148	19	0.8	177	36	4,220	422	0.03	0.08	0.4	19	794
0	12	357	46	1.9	427	85	10,170	1,017	0.08	0.20	1.1	45	795
0	19	2	79	0.5	192	13	[63]170	[63]17	0.17	0.06	1.2	5	796
0	14	2	47	0.4	158	3	[63]130	[63]13	0.11	0.04	1.0	3	797
0	34	3	78	0.5	229	8	[63]410	[63]41	0.11	0.12	2.1	4	798
0	46	8	131	1.0	343	[64]730	[63]250	[63]25	0.06	0.14	2.5	12	799
0	41	11	134	0.9	391	[65]571	[63]510	[63]51	0.09	0.15	2.5	17	800
0	1	4	5	0.1	42	1	10	1	0.01	0.01	0.1	1	801
0	7	147	44	1.9	244	46	12,290	1,229	0.14	0.18	0.5	19	802
0	6	6	21	0.3	238	3	60	6	0.07	0.02	0.6	1	803
0	2	26	14	0.4	157	11	1,030	103	0.04	0.04	0.2	3	804
0	26	21	117	5.1	644	6	30	3	0.30	0.09	2.0	6	805
0	7	94	36	1.2	296	30	9,620	962	0.07	0.09	0.7	53	806
0	7	179	36	1.2	417	20	8,260	826	0.06	0.15	0.9	33	807
0	11	41	74	0.7	561	35	60	6	0.07	0.03	0.6	89	808
0	4	52	38	0.5	419	8	1,580	158	0.10	0.10	0.5	13	809
0	Tr	5	3	Tr	39	1	150	15	0.01	0.01	Tr	1	810
0	11	102	108	2.7	852	49	1,780	178	0.25	0.16	1.0	21	811
0	3	26	27	0.7	213	12	450	45	0.06	0.04	0.3	5	812
0	1	10	11	0.3	87	5	180	18	0.03	0.02	0.1	2	813
0	2	38	14	0.8	148	5	1,060	106	0.03	0.04	0.2	10	814

[64] For regular pack; special dietary pack contains 8 mg sodium.
[65] For regular pack; special dietary pack contains 6 mg sodium.

Item No.	Foods, approximate measures, units, and weight (weight of edible portion only)			Water	Food energy	Pro-tein	Fat	Fatty acids		
								Satu-rated	Mono-unsatu-rated	Poly-unsatu-rated
			Grams	Per-cent	Cal-ories	Grams	Grams	Grams	Grams	Grams
	Vegetables and Vegetable Products—Con.									
	Mushrooms:									
815	Raw, sliced or chopped---------	1 cup-----------	70	92	20	1	Tr	Tr	Tr	0.1
816	Cooked, drained-----------------	1 cup-----------	156	91	40	3	1	0.1	Tr	0.3
817	Canned, drained solids---------	1 cup-----------	156	91	35	3	Tr	0.1	Tr	0.2
818	Mustard greens, without stems and midribs, cooked, drained-------	1 cup-----------	140	94	20	3	Tr	Tr	0.2	0.1
819	Okra pods, 3 by 5/8 in, cooked---	8 pods-----------	85	90	25	2	Tr	Tr	Tr	Tr
	Onions:									
	Raw:									
820	Chopped----------------------	1 cup-----------	160	91	55	2	Tr	0.1	0.1	0.2
821	Sliced-----------------------	1 cup-----------	115	91	40	1	Tr	0.1	Tr	0.1
822	Cooked (whole or sliced), drained----------------------	1 cup-----------	210	92	60	2	Tr	0.1	Tr	0.1
823	Onions, spring, raw, bulb (3/8-in diam.) and white portion of top	6 onions--------	30	92	10	1	Tr	Tr	Tr	Tr
824	Onion rings, breaded, par-fried, frozen, prepared---------------	2 rings---------	20	29	80	1	5	1.7	2.2	1.0
	Parsley:									
825	Raw--------------------------	10 sprigs-------	10	88	5	Tr	Tr	Tr	Tr	Tr
826	Freeze-dried-----------------	1 tbsp---------	0.4	2	Tr	Tr	Tr	Tr	Tr	Tr
827	Parsnips, cooked (diced or 2 in lengths), drained--------------	1 cup-----------	156	78	125	2	Tr	0.1	0.2	0.1
828	Peas, edible pod, cooked, drained	1 cup-----------	160	89	65	5	Tr	0.1	Tr	0.2
	Peas, green:									
829	Canned, drained solids---------	1 cup-----------	170	82	115	8	1	0.1	0.1	0.3
830	Frozen, cooked, drained--------	1 cup-----------	160	80	125	8	Tr	0.1	Tr	0.2
	Peppers:									
831	Hot chili, raw------------------	1 pepper--------	45	88	20	1	Tr	Tr	Tr	Tr
	Sweet (about 5 per lb, whole), stem and seeds removed:									
832	Raw--------------------------	1 pepper--------	74	93	20	1	Tr	Tr	Tr	0.2
833	Cooked, drained--------------	1 pepper--------	73	95	15	Tr	Tr	Tr	Tr	0.1
	Potatoes, cooked:									
	Baked (about 2 per lb, raw):									
834	With skin--------------------	1 potato--------	202	71	220	5	Tr	0.1	Tr	0.1
835	Flesh only-------------------	1 potato--------	156	75	145	3	Tr	Tr	Tr	0.1
	Boiled (about 3 per lb, raw):									
836	Peeled after boiling---------	1 potato--------	136	77	120	3	Tr	Tr	Tr	0.1
837	Peeled before boiling--------	1 potato--------	135	77	115	2	Tr	Tr	Tr	0.1
	French fried, strip, 2 to 3-1/2 in long, frozen:									
838	Oven heated------------------	10 strips-------	50	53	110	2	4	2.1	1.8	0.3
839	Fried in vegetable oil-------	10 strips-------	50	38	160	2	8	2.5	1.6	3.8
	Potato products, prepared:									
	Au gratin:									
840	From dry mix-----------------	1 cup-----------	245	79	230	6	10	6.3	2.9	0.3
841	From home recipe-------------	1 cup-----------	245	74	325	12	19	11.6	5.3	0.7
842	Hashed brown, from frozen------	1 cup-----------	156	56	340	5	18	7.0	8.0	2.1
	Mashed:									
	From home recipe:									
843	Milk added-------------------	1 cup-----------	210	78	160	4	1	0.7	0.3	0.1
844	Milk and margarine added---	1 cup-----------	210	76	225	4	9	2.2	3.7	2.5
845	From dehydrated flakes (without milk), water, milk, butter, and salt added----------------------	1 cup-----------	210	76	235	4	12	7.2	3.3	0.5
846	Potato salad, made with mayonnaise-------------------	1 cup-----------	250	76	360	7	21	3.6	6.2	9.3
	Scalloped:									
847	From dry mix-----------------	1 cup-----------	245	79	230	5	11	6.5	3.0	0.5
848	From home recipe-------------	1 cup-----------	245	81	210	7	9	5.5	2.5	0.4

[66] For regular pack; special dietary pack contains 3 mg sodium.
[67] For red peppers; green peppers contain 350 IU or 35 RE.
[68] For green peppers; red peppers contain 4,220 IU or 422 RE.

Cho-les-terol	Carbo-hydrate	Calcium	Phos-phorus	Iron	Potas-sium	Sodium	Vitamin A value		Thiamin	Ribo-flavin	Niacin	Ascorbic acid	Item No.
							(IU)	(RE)					
Milli-grams	Grams	Milli-grams	Milli-grams	Milli-grams	Milli-grams	Milli-grams	Inter-national units	Retinol equiva-lents	Milli-grams	Milli-grams	Milli-grams	Milli-grams	
0	3	4	73	0.9	259	3	0	0	0.07	0.31	2.9	2	815
0	8	9	136	2.7	555	3	0	0	0.11	0.47	7.0	6	816
0	8	17	103	1.2	201	663	0	0	0.13	0.03	2.5	0	817
0	3	104	57	1.0	283	22	4,240	424	0.06	0.09	0.6	35	818
0	6	54	48	0.4	274	4	490	49	0.11	0.05	0.7	14	819
0	12	40	46	0.6	248	3	0	0	0.10	0.02	0.2	13	820
0	8	29	33	0.4	178	2	0	0	0.07	0.01	0.1	10	821
0	13	57	48	0.4	319	17	0	0	0.09	0.02	0.2	12	822
0	2	18	10	0.6	77	1	1,500	150	0.02	0.04	0.1	14	823
0	8	6	16	0.3	26	75	50	5	0.06	0.03	0.7	Tr	824
0	1	13	4	0.6	54	4	520	52	0.01	0.01	0.1	9	825
0	Tr	1	2	0.2	25	2	250	25	Tr	0.01	Tr	1	826
0	30	58	108	0.9	573	16	0	0	0.13	0.08	1.1	20	827
0	11	67	88	3.2	384	6	210	21	0.20	0.12	0.9	77	828
0	21	34	114	1.6	294	[66]372	1,310	131	0.21	0.13	1.2	16	829
0	23	38	144	2.5	269	139	1,070	107	0.45	0.16	2.4	16	830
0	4	8	21	0.5	153	3	[67]4,840	[67]484	0.04	0.04	0.4	109	831
0	4	4	16	0.9	144	2	[68]390	[68]39	0.06	0.04	0.4	[69]95	832
0	3	3	11	0.6	94	1	[70]280	[70]28	0.04	0.03	0.3	[71]81	833
0	51	20	115	2.7	844	16	0	0	0.22	0.07	3.3	26	834
0	34	8	78	0.5	610	8	0	0	0.16	0.03	2.2	20	835
0	27	7	60	0.4	515	5	0	0	0.14	0.03	2.0	18	836
0	27	11	54	0.4	443	7	0	0	0.13	0.03	1.8	10	837
0	17	5	43	0.7	229	16	0	0	0.06	0.02	1.2	5	838
0	20	10	47	0.4	366	108	0	0	0.09	0.01	1.6	5	839
12	31	203	233	0.8	537	1,076	520	76	0.05	0.20	2.3	8	840
56	28	292	277	1.6	970	1,061	650	93	0.16	0.28	2.4	24	841
0	44	23	112	2.4	680	53	0	0	0.17	0.03	3.8	10	842
4	37	55	101	0.6	628	636	40	12	0.18	0.08	2.3	14	843
4	35	55	97	0.5	607	620	360	42	0.18	0.08	2.3	13	844
29	32	103	118	0.5	489	697	380	44	0.23	0.11	1.4	20	845
170	28	48	130	1.6	635	1,323	520	83	0.19	0.15	2.2	25	846
27	31	88	137	0.9	497	835	360	51	0.05	0.14	2.5	8	847
29	26	140	154	1.4	926	821	330	47	0.17	0.23	2.6	26	848

[69]For green peppers; red peppers contain 141 mg ascorbic acid.
[70]For green peppers; red peppers contain 2,740 IU or 274 RE.
[71]For green peppers; red peppers contain 121 mg ascorbic acid.

Item No.	Foods, approximate measures, units, and weight (weight of edible portion only)			Water	Food energy	Pro-tein	Fat	Fatty acids		
								Satu-rated	Mono-unsatu-rated	Poly-unsatu-rated
	Vegetables and Vegetable Products—Con.		Grams	Per-cent	Cal-ories	Grams	Grams	Grams	Grams	Grams
849	Potato chips----------------------	10 chips--------	20	3	105	1	7	1.8	1.2	3.6
	Pumpkin:									
850	Cooked from raw, mashed--------	1 cup-----------	245	94	50	2	Tr	0.1	Tr	Tr
851	Canned-------------------------	1 cup-----------	245	90	85	3	1	0.4	0.1	Tr
852	Radishes, raw, stem ends, rootlets cut off--	4 radishes------	18	95	5	Tr	Tr	Tr	Tr	Tr
853	Sauerkraut, canned, solids and liquid--------------------------	1 cup-----------	236	93	45	2	Tr	0.1	Tr	0.1
	Seaweed:									
854	Kelp, raw----------------------	1 oz-----------	28	82	10	Tr	Tr	0.1	Tr	Tr
855	Spirulina, dried---------------	1 oz-----------	28	5	80	16	2	0.8	0.2	0.6
	Southern peas. See Black-eyed peas, immature (items 769,770), mature (item 536).									
	Spinach:									
856	Raw, chopped-------------------	1 cup-----------	55	92	10	2	Tr	Tr	Tr	0.1
	Cooked, drained:									
857	From raw-----------------------	1 cup-----------	180	91	40	5	Tr	0.1	Tr	0.2
858	From frozen (leaf)-------------	1 cup-----------	190	90	55	6	Tr	0.1	Tr	0.2
859	Canned, drained solids---------	1 cup-----------	214	92	50	6	1	0.2	Tr	0.4
860	Spinach souffle-----------------	1 cup-----------	136	74	220	11	18	7.1	6.8	3.1
	Squash, cooked:									
861	Summer (all varieties), sliced, drained--------------------	1 cup-----------	180	94	35	2	1	0.1	Tr	0.2
862	Winter (all varieties), baked, cubes-----------------------	1 cup-----------	205	89	80	2	1	0.3	0.1	0.5
	Sunchoke. See Jerusalem-arti-choke (item 805).									
	Sweetpotatoes:									
	Cooked (raw, 5 by 2 in; about 2-1/2 per lb):									
863	Baked in skin, peeled--------	1 potato--------	114	73	115	2	Tr	Tr	Tr	0.1
864	Boiled, without skin---------	1 potato--------	151	73	160	2	Tr	0.1	Tr	0.2
865	Candied, 2-1/2 by 2-in piece---	1 piece--------	105	67	145	1	3	1.4	0.7	0.2
	Canned:									
866	Solid pack (mashed)----------	1 cup-----------	255	74	260	5	1	0.1	Tr	0.2
867	Vacuum pack, piece 2-3/4 by 1 in---------------------	1 piece--------	40	76	35	1	Tr	Tr	Tr	Tr
	Tomatoes:									
868	Raw, 2-3/5-in diam. (3 per 12 oz pkg.)-------------------	1 tomato--------	123	94	25	1	Tr	Tr	Tr	0.1
869	Canned, solids and liquid------	1 cup-----------	240	94	50	2	1	0.1	0.1	0.2
870	Tomato juice, canned------------	1 cup-----------	244	94	40	2	Tr	Tr	Tr	0.1
	Tomato products, canned:									
871	Paste-------------------------	1 cup-----------	262	74	220	10	2	0.3	0.4	0.9
872	Puree-------------------------	1 cup-----------	250	87	105	4	Tr	Tr	Tr	0.1
873	Sauce-------------------------	1 cup-----------	245	89	75	3	Tr	0.1	0.1	0.2
874	Turnips, cooked, diced----------	1 cup-----------	156	94	30	1	Tr	Tr	Tr	0.1
	Turnip greens, cooked, drained:									
875	From raw (leaves and stems)----	1 cup-----------	144	93	30	2	Tr	0.1	Tr	0.1
876	From frozen (chopped)----------	1 cup-----------	164	90	50	5	1	0.2	Tr	0.3
877	Vegetable juice cocktail, canned	1 cup-----------	242	94	45	2	Tr	Tr	Tr	0.1
	Vegetables, mixed:									
878	Canned, drained solids---------	1 cup-----------	163	87	75	4	Tr	0.1	Tr	0.2
879	Frozen, cooked, drained--------	1 cup-----------	182	83	105	5	Tr	0.1	Tr	0.1
880	Waterchestnuts, canned----------	1 cup-----------	140	86	70	1	Tr	Tr	Tr	Tr

[1] Value not determined.
[72] With added salt; if none is added, sodium content is 58 mg.
[73] For regular pack; special dietary pack contains 31 mg sodium.
[74] With added salt; if none is added, sodium content is 24 mg.

Nutrients in Indicated Quantity

Cho-les-terol	Carbo-hydrate	Calcium	Phos-phorus	Iron	Potas-sium	Sodium	Vitamin A value		Thiamin	Ribo-flavin	Niacin	Ascorbic acid	Item No.
							(IU)	(RE)					
Milli-grams	Grams	Milli-grams	Milli-grams	Milli-grams	Milli-grams	Milli-grams	Inter-national units	Retinol equiva-lents	Milli-grams	Milli-grams	Milli-grams	Milli-grams	
0	10	5	31	0.2	260	94	0	0	0.03	Tr	0.8	8	849
0	12	37	74	1.4	564	2	2,650	265	0.08	0.19	1.0	12	850
0	20	64	86	3.4	505	12	54,040	5,404	0.06	0.13	0.9	10	851
0	1	4	3	0.1	42	4	Tr	Tr	Tr	0.01	0.1	4	852
0	10	71	47	3.5	401	1,560	40	4	0.05	0.05	0.3	35	853
0	3	48	12	0.8	25	66	30	3	0.01	0.04	0.1	(¹)	854
0	7	34	33	8.1	386	297	160	16	0.67	1.04	3.6	3	855
0	2	54	27	1.5	307	43	3,690	369	0.04	0.10	0.4	15	856
0	7	245	101	6.4	839	126	14,740	1,474	0.17	0.42	0.9	18	857
0	10	277	91	2.9	566	72163	14,790	1,479	0.11	0.32	0.8	23	858
0	7	272	94	4.9	740	72683	18,780	1,878	0.03	0.30	0.8	31	859
184	3	230	231	1.3	201	763	3,460	675	0.09	0.30	0.5	3	860
0	8	49	70	0.6	346	2	520	52	0.08	0.07	0.9	10	861
0	18	29	41	0.7	896	2	7,290	729	0.17	0.05	1.4	20	862
0	28	32	63	0.5	397	11	24,880	2,488	0.08	0.14	0.7	28	863
0	37	32	41	0.8	278	20	25,750	2,575	0.08	0.21	1.0	26	864
8	29	27	27	1.2	198	74	4,400	440	0.02	0.04	0.4	7	865
0	59	77	133	3.4	536	191	38,570	3,857	0.07	0.23	2.4	13	866
0	8	9	20	0.4	125	21	3,190	319	0.01	0.02	0.3	11	867
0	5	9	28	0.6	255	10	1,390	139	0.07	0.06	0.7	22	868
0	10	62	46	1.5	530	73391	1,450	145	0.11	0.07	1.8	36	869
0	10	22	46	1.4	537	74881	1,360	136	0.11	0.08	1.6	45	870
0	49	92	207	7.8	2,442	75170	6,470	647	0.41	0.50	8.4	111	871
0	25	38	100	2.3	1,050	7650	3,400	340	0.18	0.14	4.3	88	872
0	18	34	78	1.9	909	771,482	2,400	240	0.16	0.14	2.8	32	873
0	8	34	30	0.3	211	78	0	0	0.04	0.04	0.5	18	874
0	6	197	42	1.2	292	42	7,920	792	0.06	0.10	0.6	39	875
0	8	249	56	3.2	367	25	13,080	1,308	0.09	0.12	0.8	36	876
0	11	27	41	1.0	467	883	2,830	283	0.10	0.07	1.8	67	877
0	15	44	68	1.7	474	243	18,990	1,899	0.08	0.08	0.9	8	878
0	24	46	93	1.5	308	64	7,780	778	0.13	0.22	1.5	6	879
0	17	6	27	1.2	165	11	10	1	0.02	0.03	0.5	2	880

[75] With no added salt; if salt is added, sodium content is 2,070 mg.
[76] With no added salt; if salt is added, sodium content is 998 mg.
[77] With salt added.

Table 2. Nutritive Value of the Edible Part of Food (Continued)

(Tr indicates nutrient present in trace amount.)

Item No.	Foods, approximate measures, units, and weight (weight of edible portion only)		Water	Food energy	Pro-tein	Fat	Fatty acids		
							Satu-rated	Mono-unsatu-rated	Poly-unsatu-rated
		Grams	Per-cent	Cal-ories	Grams	Grams	Grams	Grams	Grams

Miscellaneous Items

Item No.	Food	Measure	Grams	Percent	Calories	Protein g	Fat g	Sat g	Mono g	Poly g
	Baking powders for home use:									
	Sodium aluminum sulfate:									
881	With monocalcium phosphate monohydrate	1 tsp	3	2	5	Tr	0	0.0	0.0	0.0
882	With monocalcium phosphate monohydrate, calcium sulfate	1 tsp	2.9	1	5	Tr	0	0.0	0.0	0.0
883	Straight phosphate	1 tsp	3.8	2	5	Tr	0	0.0	0.0	0.0
884	Low sodium	1 tsp	4.3	1	5	Tr	0	0.0	0.0	0.0
885	Catsup	1 cup	273	69	290	5	1	0.2	0.2	0.4
886		1 tbsp	15	69	15	Tr	Tr	Tr	Tr	Tr
887	Celery seed	1 tsp	2	6	10	Tr	1	Tr	0.3	0.1
888	Chili powder	1 tsp	2.6	8	10	Tr	Tr	0.1	0.1	0.2
	Chocolate:									
889	Bitter or baking	1 oz	28	2	145	3	15	9.0	4.9	0.5
	Semisweet, see Candy, (item 715).									
890	Cinnamon	1 tsp	2.3	10	5	Tr	Tr	Tr	Tr	Tr
891	Curry powder	1 tsp	2	10	5	Tr	Tr	([1])	([1])	([1])
892	Garlic powder	1 tsp	2.8	6	10	Tr	Tr	Tr	Tr	Tr
893	Gelatin, dry	1 envelope	7	13	25	6	Tr	Tr	Tr	Tr
894	Mustard, prepared, yellow	1 tsp or individual packet	5	80	5	Tr	Tr	Tr	0.2	Tr
	Olives, canned:									
895	Green	4 medium or 3 extra large	13	78	15	Tr	2	0.2	1.2	0.1
896	Ripe, Mission, pitted	3 small or 2 large	9	73	15	Tr	2	0.3	1.3	0.2
897	Onion powder	1 tsp	2.1	5	5	Tr	Tr	Tr	Tr	Tr
898	Oregano	1 tsp	1.5	7	5	Tr	Tr	Tr	Tr	0.1
899	Paprika	1 tsp	2.1	10	5	Tr	Tr	Tr	Tr	0.2
900	Pepper, black	1 tsp	2.1	11	5	Tr	Tr	Tr	Tr	Tr
	Pickles, cucumber:									
901	Dill, medium, whole, 3-3/4 in long, 1-1/4-in diam.	1 pickle	65	93	5	Tr	Tr	Tr	Tr	0.1
902	Fresh-pack, slices 1-1/2-in diam., 1/4 in thick	2 slices	15	79	10	Tr	Tr	Tr	Tr	Tr
903	Sweet, gherkin, small, whole, about 2-1/2 in long, 3/4-in diam.	1 pickle	15	61	20	Tr	Tr	Tr	Tr	Tr
	Popcorn. See Grain Products, (items 497-499).									
904	Relish, finely chopped, sweet	1 tbsp	15	63	20	Tr	Tr	Tr	Tr	Tr
905	Salt	1 tsp	5.5	0	0	0	0	0.0	0.0	0.0
906	Vinegar, cider	1 tbsp	15	94	Tr	Tr	0	0.0	0.0	0.0
	Yeast:									
907	Baker's, dry, active	1 pkg	7	5	20	3	Tr	Tr	0.1	Tr
908	Brewer's, dry	1 tbsp	8	5	25	3	Tr	Tr	Tr	0.0

[1]Value not determined.

Cholesterol	Carbohydrate	Calcium	Phosphorus	Iron	Potassium	Sodium	Vitamin A value (IU)	Vitamin A value (RE)	Thiamin	Riboflavin	Niacin	Ascorbic acid	Item No.
Milligrams	Grams	Milligrams	Milligrams	Milligrams	Milligrams	Milligrams	International units	Retinol equivalents	Milligrams	Milligrams	Milligrams	Milligrams	
0	1	58	87	0.0	5	329	0	0	0.00	0.00	0.0	0	881
0	1	183	45	0.0	4	290	0	0	0.00	0.00	0.0	0	882
0	1	239	359	0.0	6	312	0	0	0.00	0.00	0.0	0	883
0	1	207	314	0.0	891	Tr	0	0	0.00	0.00	0.0	0	884
0	69	60	137	2.2	991	2,845	3,820	382	0.25	0.19	4.4	41	885
0	4	3	8	0.1	54	156	210	21	0.01	0.01	0.2	2	886
0	1	35	11	0.9	28	3	Tr	Tr	0.01	0.01	0.1	Tr	887
0	1	7	8	0.4	50	26	910	91	0.01	0.02	0.2	2	888
0	8	22	109	1.9	235	1	10	1	0.01	0.07	0.4	0	889
0	2	28	1	0.9	12	1	10	1	Tr	Tr	Tr	1	890
0	1	10	7	0.6	31	1	20	2	0.01	0.01	0.1	Tr	891
0	2	2	12	0.1	31	1	0	0	0.01	Tr	Tr	Tr	892
0	0	1	0	0.0	2	6	0	0	0.00	0.00	0.0	0	893
0	Tr	4	4	0.1	7	63	0	0	Tr	0.01	Tr	Tr	894
0	Tr	8	2	0.2	7	312	40	4	Tr	Tr	Tr	0	895
0	Tr	10	2	0.2	2	68	10	1	Tr	Tr	Tr	0	896
0	2	8	7	0.1	20	1	Tr	Tr	0.01	Tr	Tr	Tr	897
0	1	24	3	0.7	25	Tr	100	10	0.01	Tr	0.1	1	898
0	1	4	7	0.5	49	1	1,270	127	0.01	0.04	0.3	1	899
0	1	9	4	0.6	26	1	Tr	Tr	Tr	0.01	Tr	0	900
0	1	17	14	0.7	130	928	70	7	Tr	0.01	Tr	4	901
0	3	5	4	0.3	30	101	20	2	Tr	Tr	Tr	1	902
0	5	2	2	0.2	30	107	10	1	Tr	Tr	Tr	1	903
0	5	3	2	0.1	30	107	20	2	Tr	Tr	0.0	1	904
0	0	14	3	Tr	Tr	2,132	0	0	0.00	0.00	0.0	0	905
0	1	1	1	0.1	15	Tr	0	0	0.00	0.00	0.0	0	906
0	3	3	90	1.1	140	4	Tr	Tr	0.16	0.38	2.6	Tr	907
0	3	[78]17	140	1.4	152	10	Tr	Tr	1.25	0.34	3.0	Tr	908

[78]Value may vary from 6 to 60 mg.

C Nutritional Analysis of Fast Foods

Dashes indicate information not provided by sources.

Complete Nutritional Values	Weight (gm.)	Calories	Protein (gm.)	Carbohydrates (gm.)	Added Sugar (gm.)	Fat (gm.)	Fat % Calories	Saturated Fat (gm.)	Cholesterol (mg.)	Sodium (mg.)	Vitamin A (% U.S. RDA)	Vitamin C (% U.S. RDA)	Iron (% U.S. RDA)	Calcium (% U.S. RDA)
ARBY'S														
Arby's Sauce	28	30	0	6	4	0	9	0	0	227	0	0	10	0
Bac 'N Cheddar Deluxe	229	532	29	35	5	33	55	8	83	1672	0	2	25	15
Bacon Platter	217	869	17	49	0	32	33	10	366	1051	8	6	20	6
Baked Potato, Broccoli & Cheddar	340	417	10	55	0	18	39	7	22	361	6	75	15	10
Baked Potato, Butter/Margarine and Sour Cream	312	463	8	53	0	25	49	12	40	203	4	55	15	10
Baked Potato, Deluxe	348	621	17	59	0	36	53	18	58	605	10	55	15	15
Baked Potato, Mushroom and Cheese	347	515	15	57	0	27	47	6	47	923	15	55	15	25
Baked Potato, Plain	241	240	6	50	0	2	7	0	0	58	0	55	15	0
Beef 'N Cheddar	198	451	25	43	5	20	40	7	52	955	4	0	20	2
Biscuit, Bacon	98	318	7	35	0	18	51	4	8	904	0	0	15	10
Biscuit, Ham	124	323	13	34	0	17	46	4	21	1169	0	0	15	10
Biscuit, Plain	82	280	6	34	0	15	48	3	0	730	0	0	15	10
Biscuit, Sausage	118	460	12	35	0	32	62	9	60	1000	0	0	20	10
Blueberry Muffin	71	200	3	34	15	6	25	2	22	269	0	0	6	4
Butterfinger Polar Swirl	329	457	12	62	40	18	36	8	28	318	4	0	2	25
Cheddar Fries	142	399	6	46	0	22	49	9	9	443	0	0	8	8
Cheese Cake	85	306	5	21	18	23	67	7	95	220	20	0	4	6
Chicken Breast Sandwich	184	489	23	48	5	26	47	4	45	1019	0	8	20	8
Chicken Cordon Bleu	216	658	31	50	5	37	50	9	65	1824	0	0	20	15
Chicken Fajita Pita	312	256	15	32	—	9	32	—	33	787	—	—	—	—
Chocolate Chip Cookie	27	130	2	17	10	4	28	2	0	95	0	0	2	0
Cinnamon Nut Danish	99	340	7	59	16	9	25	2	0	230	0	0	15	4
Coca-Cola Classic, 12 fl. oz.	358	144	0	38	27	0	0	0	0	15	0	0	0	0
Croissant, Bacon and Egg	113	389	12	30	0	26	61	14	221	582	4	0	20	4
Croissant, Ham and Cheese	119	345	16	29	0	21	54	12	90	939	0	0	15	15
Croissant, Mushroom and Cheese	148	493	13	34	0	38	69	15	116	935	0	0	15	20
Croissant, Sausage and Egg	142	519	17	29	0	39	68	19	271	632	4	0	20	6
Croissant (plain)	63	260	6	28	0	16	54	10	49	300	0	0	15	4
Croutons	14	59	2	8	0	2	34	0	1	155	0	0	2	0
Curly Fries	99	337	4	43	0	18	47	7	0	167	0	0	8	2
Egg Platter	201	460	15	45	0	24	47	7	346	591	8	6	20	6
Fish Fillet Sandwich	193	537	21	47	5	29	49	6	79	994	0	0	20	8
French Dip (roast beef sandwich)	150	345	24	34	5	12	32	6	5	678	0	0	15	2
French Dip 'N Swiss (roast beef sandwich)	178	425	30	36	5	18	39	8	87	1078	4	0	15	25
French Fries, large	142	492	4	60	0	26	48	6	0	228	0	12	12	0
French Fries, medium	114	394	3	48	0	21	48	5	0	182	0	10	10	0
French Fries, small	71	246	2	30	0	13	48	3	0	114	0	6	6	0
Grilled Chicken Barbecue	185	378	21	44	0	14	34	4	44	1059	0	0	20	10
Grilled Chicken Deluxe	228	426	21	39	0	21	45	5	44	877	0	0	20	10
Ham Platter	258	518	24	45	0	26	46	8	374	1177	8	6	20	6
Heath Polar Swirl	329	543	11	76	38	22	36	5	39	346	4	0	0	25
Horsey Sauce	14	55	0	3	0	5	82	1	1	105	0	0	0	2

Complete Nutritional Values	Weight (gm.)	Calories	Protein (gm.)	Carbohydrates (gm.)	Added Sugar (gm.)	Fat (gm.)	Fat % Calories	Saturated Fat (gm.)	Cholesterol (mg.)	Sodium (mg.)	Vitamin A (% U.S. RDA)	Vitamin C (% U.S. RDA)	Iron (% U.S. RDA)	Calcium (% U.S. RDA)
ARBY'S—*Continued*														
Hot Chocolate, 8 fl. oz.	244	110	2	23	13	1	10	1	0	120	0	0	2	6
Hot Ham 'N Cheese	162	330	23	33	5	14	38	4	45	1350	4	0	15	10
Light Roast Beef Deluxe	182	296	18	33	—	10	30	—	42	826	6	2	20	0
Light Roast Chicken Deluxe	189	253	17	33	—	5	17	—	39	874	6	2	20	0
Light Roast Turkey Deluxe	189	249	19	33	—	4	15	—	30	1172	6	2	20	0
Maple Syrup	43	120	0	29	29	0	1	0	0	52	0	0	0	0
Milk, 2% Low-fat, 8 fl. oz.	244	121	8	12	0	4	33	3	18	122	10	4	0	30
Orange Juice, 6 fl. oz.	180	82	1	20	0	0	0	0	0	2	0	119	0	0
Oreo Polar Swirl	329	482	10	66	38	20	37	10	35	521	4	0	4	25
Peanut Butter Cup Polar Swirl	329	517	14	61	54	24	42	8	34	385	4	0	0	25
Philly Beef 'N Swiss	196	498	26	37	5	26	47	6	91	1194	6	4	20	30
Potato Cakes	85	204	2	20	0	12	53	2	0	397	0	15	8	0
Roast Beef, Giant	227	530	36	41	5	27	46	10	78	908	0	0	35	6
Roast Beef, Junior	85	218	13	21	5	11	44	3	23	345	0	0	10	2
Roast Beef, Regular	147	353	22	32	5	15	38	7	39	588	0	0	20	4
Roast Beef, Super	246	529	33	46	5	28	48	8	47	798	6	2	25	6
Roast Chicken Club	234	513	31	40	5	29	51	5	75	1423	0	0	20	15
Roast Chicken Deluxe	208	373	17	37	5	19	47	3	2	913	0	0	20	4
Salad Dressing, Blue Cheese, 2 fl. oz.	57	295	2	2	8	31	95	6	50	489	2	0	2	6
Salad Dressing, Buttermilk Ranch, 2 fl. oz.	57	349	0	2	8	38	99	6	6	471	0	0	0	0
Salad Dressing, Honey French, 2 fl. oz.	65	322	0	22	20	27	75	4	0	486	8	2	10	0
Salad Dressing, Thousand Island, 2 fl. oz.	62	298	0	10	8	29	88	4	24	493	2	2	4	0
Salad Dressing, Weight Watchers Creamy French, 1 fl. oz.	30	29	—	—	—	3	93	—	—	—	—	—	—	—
Salad Dressing, Weight Watchers Creamy Italian, 1 fl. oz.	30	29	—	—	—	3	93	—	—	—	—	—	—	—
Salad, Chef	383	217	20	11	0	11	44	—	172	706	40	40	15	10
Salad, Garden	295	109	7	10	0	5	43	—	12	134	35	35	10	10
Salad, Roast Chicken	383	172	15	12	0	7	35	—	45	562	—	—	—	—
Salad, Side	150	25	2	4	0	0	0	0	0	30	20	6	4	4
Sausage Platter	238	640	21	46	0	41	58	13	406	861	8	6	20	8
Shake, Chocolate	340	451	10	76	48	12	23	3	36	341	6	0	4	25
Shake, Jamocha	326	368	9	59	33	10	26	2	35	262	6	0	0	25
Shake, Vanilla	312	330	10	46	28	11	31	4	32	281	6	0	0	30
Snickers Polar Swirl	329	511	12	73	35	19	33	7	33	351	6	0	0	25
Soup, Beef with Vegetables and Barley, 6 fl. oz.	244	96	5	14	0	3	26	1	10	996	30	8	8	2
Soup, Boston Clam Chowder, 6 fl. oz.	244	207	10	18	0	11	46	4	28	1157	10	6	10	20
Soup, Cream of Broccoli, 6 fl. oz.	244	180	8	19	0	8	40	5	3	1113	10	15	4	30
Soup, French Onion, 6 fl. oz.	244	67	2	7	0	3	42	0	0	1248	2	4	4	2
Soup, Lumberjack Mixed Vegetable, 6 fl. oz.	244	89	2	13	0	4	36	2	4	1075	50	15	6	2
Soup, Old Fashioned Chicken Noodle, 6 fl. oz.	244	99	6	15	1	2	16	0	25	929	20	0	8	0
Soup, Pilgrim's Corn Chowder, 6 fl. oz.	244	193	10	18	1	11	49	4	28	1157	35	6	4	15
Soup, Split Pea with Ham, 6 fl. oz.	244	200	8	21	1	10	43	5	30	1029	30	2	12	2
Soup, Tomato Florentine, 6 fl. oz.	244	84	3	15	0	1	16	1	2	910	20	20	8	4
Soup, Wisconsin Cheese, 6 fl. oz.	244	287	9	19	0	19	59	8	31	1129	4	4	4	35
Sub Deluxe	226	482	24	38	5	26	49	5	50	1530	0	4	20	15
Toastix	99	420	8	43	0	25	54	5	20	440	0	0	15	0
Turkey Deluxe	221	399	27	35	5	20	46	4	39	1047	6	8	15	8
Turnover, Apple	85	303	4	27	13	18	54	7	0	178	2	2	4	0
Turnover, Blueberry	85	320	3	32	8	19	53	6	0	240	0	10	4	0

Complete Nutritional Values	Weight (gm.)	Calories	Protein (gm.)	Carbohydrates (gm.)	Added Sugar (gm.)	Fat (gm.)	Fat % Calories	Saturated Fat (gm.)	Cholesterol (mg.)	Sodium (mg.)	Vitamin A (% U.S. RDA)	Vitamin C (% U.S. RDA)	Iron (% U.S. RDA)	Calcium (% U.S. RDA)
ARBY'S MEALS														
Blueberry Muffin, Orange Juice	251	282	4	54	15	6	18	2	22	271	0	119	6	4
Toastix with Maple Syrup, Orange Juice, Coffee	566	625	9	92	29	25	36	5	20	497	0	119	15	0
Sausage Biscuit, Potato Cakes, Hot Chocolate	447	774	16	78	13	45	52	12	60	1517	0	15	30	16
Light Roast Chicken Deluxe, Garden Salad, Orange Juice	664	444	25	63	0	10	20	—	51	1010	41	156	30	10
French Dip, Baked Potato (plain), Orange Juice	571	667	31	104	5	14	19	6	5	738	0	174	30	2
Plain Baked Potato, Chef Salad with Light Italian Dressing, Orange Juice	795	555	28	77	3	14	23	5	115	1890	30	184	23	15
Grilled Chicken Barbecue, Side Salad, 2% Low-fat Milk	579	524	31	61	0	19	32	7	62	1211	30	10	24	44
Turkey Deluxe, Tomato Florentine Soup, Plain Baked Potato	706	723	36	100	5	24	29	5	41	2015	26	83	38	12
Regular Roast Beef, Potato Cakes, Side Salad with Light Italian Dressing	444	605	26	59	8	28	42	10	39	2125	20	21	32	8
Giant Roast Beef, Large Fries, Coca-Cola Classic	727	1166	41	139	32	54	41	17	78	1151	0	12	47	6
Chicken Cordon Bleu, Curly Fries, Jamocha Shake, Cherry Turnover	726	1643	50	178	49	83	45	24	100	2453	6	8	32	42
BURGER KING														
Apple Pie	125	311	3	44	16	14	41	4	4	412	0	8	7	0
BK Broiler Chicken Sandwich	154	267	22	28	5	8	27	2	45	728	4	6	14	5
BK Broiler Sauce	11	37	0	1	0	4	97	1	5	74	0	0	0	0
Bacon Bits, 1 packet	3	16	1	0	0	1	56	0	5	0	0	0	0	0
Bacon Double Cheeseburger	160	515	32	26	5	31	54	14	105	748	8	0	21	18
Bacon Double Cheeseburger Deluxe	195	592	33	28	5	39	59	16	111	804	12	5	21	18
Bull's Eye Barbecue Sauce	14	22	0	5	0	0	0	0	0	47	0	0	0	0
Burger Buddies	129	349	18	31	0	17	44	7	52	717	9	8	19	11
Burger King A.M. Express Dip	28	84	0	21	0	0	0	0	0	18	0	0	0	0
Cheese, Processed American	25	92	5	1	0	7	68	5	25	312	8	0	0	14
Cheeseburger	121	318	17	28	5	15	42	7	50	661	7	5	15	11
Cheeseburger Deluxe	151	390	18	29	5	23	53	8	56	652	10	9	15	11
Chicken Sandwich (fried)	229	685	26	56	5	40	53	8	82	1417	3	0	19	8
Chicken Tenders, 6 pieces	90	236	16	14	0	13	50	3	46	541	0	0	4	0
Coke, Kids Club, 10 fl. oz.	300	120	0	32	32	0	0	0	0	—	0	0	0	0
Coke, large (27 fl. oz.)	810	324	0	86	86	0	0	0	0	—	0	0	0	0
Coke, medium (18 fl. oz.)	540	216	0	57	57	0	0	0	0	—	0	0	0	0
Coke, small (13 fl. oz.)	390	156	0	41	41	0	0	0	0	—	0	0	0	0
Cream Cheese	28	98	2	1	0	10	92	5	28	86	7	0	0	2
Croissan'wich with Bacon, Egg and Cheese	118	361	15	19	5	24	60	8	227	719	10	0	10	14
Croissan'wich with Egg and Cheese	110	315	13	19	5	20	57	7	222	607	10	0	10	14
Croissan'wich with Ham, Egg and Cheese	144	346	19	19	5	21	55	7	241	962	10	0	11	15
Croissan'wich with Sausage, Egg and Cheese	159	534	21	22	6	40	67	13	268	985	10	0	16	15
Croissant (plain)	41	180	4	18	5	10	50	2	4	285	0	0	6	3
Croutons, 1 packet	7	31	1	5	0	1	29	—	0	90	0	0	0	0
Diet Coke, medium (18 fl. oz.)	540	1	0	0	0	0	0	0	0	—	0	0	0	0
Dipping Sauce, Barbecue	28	36	0	9	8	0	0	0	0	397	3	4	0	0
Dipping Sauce, Honey	28	91	0	23	23	0	0	0	0	12	0	0	0	0
Dipping Sauce, Ranch	28	171	0	2	1	18	95	3	0	208	0	0	0	0

Complete Nutritional Values

	Weight (gm.)	Calories	Protein (gm.)	Carbohydrates (gm.)	Added Sugar (gm.)	Fat (gm.)	Fat % Calories	Saturated Fat (gm.)	Cholesterol (mg.)	Sodium (mg.)	Vitamin A (% U.S. RDA)	Vitamin C (% U.S. RDA)	Iron (% U.S. RDA)	Calcium (% U.S. RDA)
BURGER KING—*Continued*														
Dipping Sauce, Sweet & Sour	28	45	0	11	9	0	0	0	0	52	0	0	0	0
Double Cheeseburger	172	483	30	29	5	27	50	13	100	851	11	5	21	18
French Fries, medium	116	372	5	43	0	20	48	5	0	238	0	5	7	0
French Toast Sticks	141	538	10	53	2	32	54	5	80	537	0	0	16	8
Frozen Yogurt, Breyers Vanilla	65	120	2	20	9	3	23	2	10	40	2	0	0	8
Frozen Yogurt, Breyers Chocolate	65	130	3	21	9	3	21	2	10	40	2	0	0	8
Hamburger	108	272	15	28	5	11	36	4	37	505	3	5	15	4
Hamburger Deluxe	138	344	15	28	5	19	50	6	43	496	5	9	15	4
Mayonnaise, 2 tbsp.	28	194	0	2	0	21	97	4	16	142	0	0	0	0
Milk, 2% Low-fat, 8 fl. oz.	244	121	8	12	0	5	37	3	18	122	10	4	0	30
Milk, Whole, 8 fl. oz.	244	157	8	11	0	9	52	6	35	119	7	6	0	29
Mini Muffins, Blueberry	95	292	4	37	18	14	43	3	72	244	0	0	7	4
Mustard	3	2	0	0	0	0	0	0	0	34	0	0	0	0
Ocean Catch Fish Filet	194	495	20	49	5	25	45	4	57	879	0	4	14	6
Onion Rings	97	339	5	38	0	19	50	5	0	628	15	0	3	11
Orange Juice, 6 fl. oz.	183	82	1	20	0	0	0	0	0	2	3	119	0	0
Salad Dressing, Bleu Cheese, 2 fl. oz.	59	300	3	2	0	32	96	7	58	512	0	0	0	0
Salad Dressing, French, 2 fl. oz.	64	290	0	23	22	22	68	3	0	400	31	0	0	0
Salad Dressing, Olive Oil and Vinegar, 2 fl. oz.	56	310	0	2	0	33	96	5	0	214	0	0	0	0
Salad Dressing, Ranch, 2 fl. oz.	57	350	1	4	0	37	95	7	20	316	0	0	0	0
Salad Dressing, Reduced Calorie Light Italian, 2 fl. oz.	59	170	0	3	3	18	95	3	0	762	0	0	0	0
Salad Dressing, Thousand Island, 2 fl. oz.	63	290	1	15	0	26	81	5	36	403	64	0	0	0
Salad, Chef	273	178	17	7	0	9	46	4	103	568	95	25	9	16
Salad, Chunky Chicken	258	142	20	8	0	4	25	1	49	443	92	34	7	4
Salad, Garden	223	95	6	8	0	5	47	3	15	125	100	58	6	15
Salad, Side	135	25	1	5	0	0	0	0	0	27	88	20	3	3
Sausage Breakfast Buddy (test product)	84	255	11	15	0	16	56	6	127	492	5	0	10	8
Shake, Chocolate, large	410	472	13	71	49	15	29	9	45	286	10	6	6	45
Shake, Chocolate (with syrup), large	438	598	14	103	80	14	21	9	44	357	0	0	2	42
Shake, Strawberry (with syrup), large	438	569	12	99	66	14	22	8	44	319	0	2	0	43
Shake, Vanilla, regular	293	345	9	53	35	11	29	6	34	220	0	0	0	32
Shake, Vanilla, large	410	483	13	74	49	15	28	9	47	308	0	0	0	44
Snickers Ice Cream Bar	57	220	5	20	—	14	57	7	15	65	2	0	2	6
Sprite, medium (18 fl. oz.)	540	216	0	54	54	0	0	0	0	—	0	0	0	0
Tartar Sauce	28	134	0	2	0	14	94	2	20	202	0	0	0	0
Tater Tenders	71	213	2	25	0	12	51	3	0	318	12	9	2	0
Whopper	270	614	27	45	5	36	53	12	90	865	11	20	27	8
Whopper with Cheese	294	706	32	47	5	44	56	16	115	1177	19	20	27	22
Whopper, Double	351	844	46	45	5	53	57	19	169	933	11	20	40	9
Whopper, Double, with Cheese	375	935	51	47	5	61	59	24	194	1245	19	20	40	24
BURGER KING MEALS														
Croissant (plain), Orange Juice, 2% Low-fat Milk	468	383	13	50	5	15	35	4	22	409	13	123	6	33
French Toast Sticks, Burger King A.M. Express Dip, 2% Low-fat Milk, Orange Juice	596	825	19	106	2	37	40	8	98	679	13	123	16	38
Croissan'wich with Sausage, Egg and Cheese, 2% Low-fat Milk	403	655	29	34	6	45	62	16	286	1107	20	4	16	45
BK Broiler Chicken Sandwich, Side Salad (no dressing), Orange Juice	472	374	24	53	5	8	19	2	45	757	95	145	17	8

226

Complete Nutritional Values	Weight (gm.)	Calories	Protein (gm.)	Carbohydrates (gm.)	Added Sugar (gm.)	Fat (gm.)	Fat % Calories	Saturated Fat (gm.)	Cholesterol (mg.)	Sodium (mg.)	Vitamin A (% U.S. RDA)	Vitamin C (% U.S. RDA)	Iron (% U.S. RDA)	Calcium (% U.S. RDA)
BURGER KING MEALS–*Continued*														
Chicken Tenders, 6 Pieces, BBQ Dipping Sauce, Side Salad with Reduced Calorie Light Italian Dressing	312	467	17	31	11	31	60	6	46	1727	91	24	7	3
Chunky Chicken Salad with Thousand Island Dressing, Onion Rings, Diet Coke, medium	1078	772	26	61	0	49	57	11	85	1474	171	34	10	15
Whopper, Side Salad with French Dressing, Orange Juice	652	1011	29	93	27	58	52	15	90	1294	133	159	30	11
Garden Salad with Reduced Calorie Light Italian Dressing, Chicken Tenders, 6 pieces, BBQ Dipping Sauce, Vanilla Shake, large	810	1020	35	108	60	51	45	18	108	2133	103	62	10	59
Ocean Catch Fish Fillet, Side Salad with Bleu Cheese Dressing, Fries, medium, Coke, medium	1044	1408	29	156	62	77	49	16	115	1656	88	29	24	9
Double Whopper with Cheese, French Fries, medium, Strawberry Shake, large, Apple Pie	1054	2187	71	233	87	109	45	41	242	2214	19	35	54	67
DAIRY QUEEN/BRAZIER														
BBQ Beef Sandwich	128	225	12	34	5	4	16	1	20	700	8	0	20	10
Banana Split	369	510	9	93	—	11	19	8	30	250	0	0	20	30
Buster Bar	149	450	11	40	—	29	58	9	15	220	2	0	8	30
Chicken Fillet Sandwich (breaded)	191	430	24	37	5	20	42	4	55	760	0	0	10	4
Chicken Fillet Sandwich with Cheese (breaded)	205	480	27	38	5	25	47	7	70	980	8	0	10	10
Cone, Chocolate, large	213	350	8	54	24	11	28	8	30	170	10	0	6	25
Cone, Chocolate, regular	142	230	6	36	16	7	27	5	20	115	6	0	4	15
Cone, Vanilla, large	213	340	9	53	23	10	26	7	30	140	6	0	6	20
Cone, Vanilla, regular	142	230	6	36	16	7	27	5	20	95	4	0	4	15
Cone, Vanilla, small	85	140	4	22	10	4	26	3	15	60	2	0	2	10
DQ Homestyle Ultimate Burger	276	700	43	30	5	47	60	21	140	1110	20	15	40	20
DQ Sandwich	61	140	3	24	9	4	26	2	5	135	0	0	4	6
Dilly Bar	85	210	3	21	7	13	56	6	10	50	0	0	4	25
Dipped Cone, Chocolate, large	234	525	9	61	33	24	41	12	30	145	6	0	8	45
Dipped Cone, Chocolate, regular	156	330	6	40	22	16	44	8	20	100	4	0	6	30
Dipped Cone, Chocolate, small	92	190	4	25	13	10	47	5	10	60	2	0	4	20
Fish Fillet Sandwich	170	370	16	39	5	16	39	3	45	630	0	0	10	4
Fish Fillet Sandwich with Cheese	184	420	19	43	5	21	45	6	60	850	8	0	10	10
French Fries, large	128	390	5	52	—	18	42	4	0	200	0	15	8	0
French Fries, regular	99	300	4	40	—	14	42	3	0	160	0	10	6	0
French Fries, small	71	210	3	29	—	10	43	2	0	115	0	8	4	0
Grilled Chicken Fillet Sandwich	184	300	25	33	5	8	24	2	50	800	2	4	20	6
Hamburger, Double	198	460	31	29	5	25	49	12	95	630	0	0	30	4
Hamburger, Double with Cheese	226	570	37	31	5	34	54	18	120	1070	15	0	30	20
Hamburger, Single	142	310	17	29	5	13	38	6	45	580	0	0	20	4
Hamburger, Single with Cheese	156	365	20	30	5	18	44	9	60	800	8	0	20	15
Heath Blizzard, regular	404	820	16	114	55	36	40	17	60	410	8	0	10	40
Heath Blizzard, small	291	560	11	79	38	23	37	11	40	280	6	0	8	30
Heath Breeze (yogurt), regular	379	680	15	113	—	21	28	6	15	360	0	0	10	50
Heath Breeze (yogurt), small	273	450	11	78	—	12	24	3	10	230	0	0	8	40
Hot Dog	99	280	9	23	4	16	51	6	25	700	0	0	8	4
Hot Dog with Cheese	113	330	12	24	4	21	57	9	35	920	8	0	8	10
Hot Dog with Chili	127	320	11	26	4	19	53	7	30	720	0	0	8	4

Complete Nutritional Values

	Weight (gm.)	Calories	Protein (gm.)	Carbohydrates (gm.)	Added Sugar (gm.)	Fat (gm.)	Fat % Calories	Saturated Fat (gm.)	Cholesterol (mg.)	Sodium (mg.)	Vitamin A (% U.S. RDA)	Vitamin C (% U.S. RDA)	Iron (% U.S. RDA)	Calcium (% U.S. RDA)
DAIRY QUEEN/BRAZIER—*Continued*														
Hot Fudge Brownie Delight	305	710	11	102	—	29	37	14	35	340	8	0	30	30
Lettuce	14	2	0	0	0	0	0	0	0	1	0	0	0	0
Malt, Vanilla, regular	418	610	13	106	34	14	21	8	45	230	8	0	8	40
Mr. Misty Float	411	390	5	74	46	7	16	5	20	95	4	0	4	20
Mr. Misty Freeze	411	500	9	91	59	12	22	9	30	140	8	0	8	30
Mr. Misty, large	439	340	0	84	84	0	0	0	0	0	0	0	0	0
Mr. Misty, regular	330	250	0	63	63	0	0	0	0	0	0	0	0	0
Mr. Misty, small	248	190	0	48	48	0	0	0	0	0	0	0	0	0
Nutty Double Fudge	276	580	10	85	—	22	34	10	35	170	6	0	20	30
Onion Rings, regular	85	240	4	29	0	12	45	3	0	135	0	0	6	0
Peanut Buster Parfait	305	710	16	94	—	32	41	10	30	410	6	0	20	35
QC Chocolate Big Scoop	127	310	5	40	—	14	41	10	35	100	15	0	8	15
QC Vanilla Big Scoop	127	300	5	39	—	14	42	9	35	100	15	0	0	15
Salad Dressing, Reduced Calorie French, 2 oz.	57	90	0	11	—	5	50	1	0	450	15	0	0	0
Salad Dressing, Thousand Island, 2 oz.	57	225	0	10	—	21	84	3	25	570	4	4	0	0
Salad, Garden	284	200	13	7	0	59	0	7	185	240	60	35	10	25
Salad, Side	135	25	1	4	0	0	0	0	0	15	50	25	4	2
Shake, Chocolate, regular	397	540	12	94	47	14	23	8	45	290	8	0	8	40
Shake, Vanilla, large	461	600	13	101	51	16	24	10	50	260	10	0	8	45
Shake, Vanilla, regular	397	520	12	88	44	14	24	8	45	230	8	0	8	40
Strawberry Blizzard, regular	383	740	13	92	—	16	19	11	50	230	8	40	10	35
Strawberry Blizzard, small	266	500	9	64	—	12	22	8	35	160	6	25	6	25
Strawberry Breeze (yogurt), regular	354	590	12	90	—	1	2	0	5	170	0	40	10	50
Strawberry Breeze (yogurt), small	248	400	9	63	—	0	0	0	5	115	0	25	6	35
Strawberry Waffle Cone Sundae	173	350	8	56	—	12	31	5	20	220	4	10	8	15
Sundae, Chocolate, regular	177	300	6	54	34	7	21	5	20	140	4	0	6	15
Super Dog, Quarter Pound	198	590	20	41	4	38	58	16	60	1360	0	0	15	10
Tomato	14	3	0	1	0	0	0	0	0	0	2	4	0	0
Yogurt Cone, large	213	260	9	56	35	0	0	0	0	115	0	0	6	35
Yogurt Cone, regular	142	180	6	38	24	0	0	0	0	80	0	0	4	20
Yogurt Strawberry Sundae, regular	170	200	6	43	—	0	0	0	0	80	0	20	4	25
Yogurt, Cup, large	198	230	8	49	30	0	0	0	0	100	0	0	6	30
Yogurt, Cup, regular	142	170	6	35	22	0	0	0	0	70	0	0	4	25
DAIRY QUEEN MEALS														
Grilled Chicken Fillet Sandwich, Side Salad, Reduced Calorie French Dressing	376	415	26	48	5	13	28	3	50	1265	67	29	24	8
Single Hamburger with Lettuce and Tomato, French Fries, regular, Vanilla Cone, regular	411	845	27	106	21	34	36	14	65	836	6	14	30	19
Fish Fillet Sandwich, Yogurt Cone, regular, Vanilla Shake, regular	709	1070	34	165	73	30	25	11	90	940	8	0	22	64
Quarter Pound Super Dog, Yogurt Cone, regular, Vanilla Malt, regular	758	1380	39	185	62	52	34	24	105	1670	8	0	27	70
Double Hamburger with Cheese, French Fries, large, Vanilla Shake, large	815	1560	55	184	56	68	39	32	170	1530	25	15	46	65
DQ Homestyle Ultimate Burger, French Fries, large, Vanilla Shake, large	865	1690	61	183	56	61	43	35	190	1570	30	30	56	65
DOMINO'S PIZZA														
Cheese Pizza, 2 slices, 16 in. (thin-crust)	—	376	22	56	3	10	24	5	19	483	7	2	13	17

Complete Nutritional Values	Weight (gm.)	Calories	Protein (gm.)	Carbohydrates (gm.)	Added Sugar (gm.)	Fat (gm.)	Fat % Calories	Saturated Fat (gm.)	Cholesterol (mg.)	Sodium (mg.)	Vitamin A (% U.S. RDA)	Vitamin C (% U.S. RDA)	Iron (% U.S. RDA)	Calcium (% U.S. RDA)
DOMINO'S PIZZA—*Continued*														
Deluxe Pizza, 2 slices, 16 in. (thin-crust)	—	498	27	59	5	20	37	9	40	954	9	4	23	23
Double Cheese/Pepperoni, 2 slices, 16 in. (thin-crust)	—	545	32	55	4	25	42	13	48	1042	9	4	22	45
Ham, 2 slices, 16 in. (thin-crust)	—	417	23	58	3	11	24	6	26	805	4	2	19	19
Pepperoni Pizza, 2 slices, 16 in. (thin-crust)	—	460	24	56	3	17	34	8	28	825	7	2	15	19
Sausage/Mushroom Pizza, 2 slices, 16 in. (thin-crust)	—	430	24	55	3	16	33	8	28	552	8	2	17	20
Veggie Pizza, 2 slices, 16 in. (thin-crust)	—	498	31	60	4	18	33	10	36	1035	10	4	26	39
DUNKIN' DONUTS														
Apple Filled Cinnamon Donut	64	190	4	25	—	9	43	2	0	220	—	—	—	—
Apple N'Spice Muffin	100	300	6	52	—	8	24	—	25	360	—	—	—	—
Bagel, Cinnamon 'N' Raisin	87	250	8	49	—	2	7	—	0	370	0	0	15	2
Bagel, Egg	87	250	9	47	—	2	7	—	15	380	0	0	15	2
Bagel, Onion	87	230	9	46	—	1	4	—	0	480	0	0	15	2
Bagel, Plain	87	240	9	47	—	1	4	—	0	450	0	0	15	2
Banana Nut Muffin	103	310	7	49	—	10	29	—	30	410	—	—	—	—
Bavarian Filled Donut with Chocolate Frosting	79	240	5	32	—	11	41	—	0	260	—	—	—	—
Blueberry Filled Donut	67	210	4	29	—	8	34	—	—	240	—	—	—	—
Blueberry Muffin	101	280	6	46	—	8	26	—	30	340	—	—	—	—
Boston Kreme Donut	79	240	4	30	—	11	41	2	0	250	—	—	—	—
Bran Muffin with Raisins	104	310	6	51	—	9	26	—	15	560	—	—	—	—
Chocolate Chunk Cookie	43	200	3	25	—	10	45	—	30	110	—	—	—	—
Chocolate Chunk Cookie with Nuts	43	210	3	23	—	11	47	—	30	100	—	—	—	—
Chocolate Frosted Yeast Ring	55	200	4	25	—	10	45	2	0	190	—	—	—	—
Corn Muffin	96	340	7	51	—	12	32	—	40	560	—	—	—	—
Cranberry Nut Muffin	98	290	6	44	—	9	28	—	25	360	—	—	—	—
Croissant, Almond	105	420	8	38	—	27	58	—	0	280	—	—	—	—
Croissant, Chocolate	94	440	7	38	—	29	59	—	0	220	—	—	—	—
Croissant, Plain	72	310	7	27	—	19	55	—	0	240	—	—	—	—
Dunkin' Donut (plain cake with handle)	60	240	4	26	—	14	53	3	0	370	0	4	7	0
Glazed Buttermilk Ring	74	290	4	37	—	14	43	—	10	370	—	—	—	—
Glazed Chocolate Ring	71	324	3	34	—	21	58	—	2	383	—	—	—	—
Glazed Coffee Roll	81	280	5	37	—	12	39	—	0	310	—	—	—	—
Glazed French Cruller	38	140	2	16	—	8	51	—	30	130	—	—	—	—
Glazed Whole Wheat ring	81	330	4	39	—	18	49	—	5	380	—	—	—	—
Glazed Yeast Ring	55	200	4	26	—	9	41	2	0	230	—	—	—	—
Honey Dipped Cruller	69	260	4	36	—	11	38	2	0	330	—	—	—	—
Honey Dipped Yeast Ring Donut	55	200	4	26	—	9	41	2	0	230	0	4	4	0
Jelly Filled Donut	67	220	4	31	—	9	37	2	0	330	—	—	—	—
Lemon Filled Donut	79	260	4	33	—	12	42	—	0	280	—	—	—	—
Munchkin (average)	—	60	—	—	—	—	—	—	—	—	—	—	—	—
Oat Bran Muffins, plain	97	330	7	50	—	11	30	—	0	450	—	—	—	—
Oatmeal Pecan Raisin Cookie	46	200	3	28	—	9	41	—	25	100	—	—	—	—
Plain Cake Ring Donut	57	262	3	23	—	18	62	4	0	330	—	—	—	—
Powdered Cake Ring	62	270	3	28	—	16	53	3	0	340	—	—	—	—
HARDEES														
Apple Turnover	91	270	3	38	8	12	40	4	0	250	—	—	4	0
Bacon Cheeseburger	219	610	34	31	5	39	58	16	80	1030	—	—	30	20
Barbecue Sauce, 1 packet (1/2 oz.)	14	14	0	4	0	0	0	0	0	140	—	—	0	0
Big Cookie	49	250	3	31	16	13	47	4	5	240	—	—	4	0

Complete Nutritional Values	Weight (gm.)	Calories	Protein (gm.)	Carbohydrates (gm.)	Added Sugar (gm.)	Fat (gm.)	Fat % Calories	Saturated Fat (gm.)	Cholesterol (mg.)	Sodium (mg.)	Vitamin A (% U.S. RDA)	Vitamin C (% U.S. RDA)	Iron (% U.S. RDA)	Calcium (% U.S. RDA)
HARDEES—*Continued*														
Big Deluxe Burger	216	500	27	32	5	30	54	12	70	760	—	—	30	20
Big Twin	173	450	23	34	5	25	50	11	55	580	—	—	20	20
Biscuit 'N' Gravy	221	440	9	45	0	24	49	6	15	1250	—	—	10	15
Biscuit, Bacon	93	360	10	34	0	21	53	4	10	950	—	—	10	10
Biscuit, Bacon & Egg	124	410	15	35	0	24	53	5	155	990	—	—	20	15
Biscuit, Bacon, Egg & Cheese	137	460	17	35	0	28	55	8	165	1220	—	—	20	20
Biscuit, Canadian Rise 'N' Shine	161	470	22	35	0	27	52	8	180	1550	—	—	20	20
Biscuit, Chicken	146	430	17	42	0	22	46	4	45	1330	—	—	10	15
Biscuit, Cinnamon 'N' Raisin	80	320	4	37	0	17	48	5	0	510	—	—	10	10
Biscuit, Country Ham	108	350	11	35	0	18	46	3	25	1550	—	—	15	10
Biscuit, Country Ham & Egg	139	400	16	35	0	22	50	4	175	1600	—	—	20	15
Biscuit, Ham	106	320	10	34	0	16	45	2	15	1000	—	—	10	10
Biscuit, Ham & Egg	138	370	15	35	0	19	46	4	160	1050	—	—	20	15
Biscuit, Ham, Egg & Cheese	151	420	18	35	0	23	49	6	170	1270	—	—	20	20
Biscuit, Rise 'N' Shine	83	320	5	34	0	18	51	3	0	740	—	—	10	12
Biscuit, Sausage	118	440	13	34	0	28	57	7	25	1100	—	—	15	15
Biscuit, Sausage & Egg	150	490	18	35	0	31	57	8	170	1150	—	—	20	15
Biscuit, Steak	148	500	15	46	0	29	52	7	30	1320	—	—	20	15
Biscuit, Steak & Egg	179	550	20	47	0	32	52	8	175	1370	—	—	25	15
Cheeseburger	122	320	16	33	5	14	39	7	30	710	—	—	20	20
Chicken Fillet	173	370	19	44	0	13	32	2	55	1060	—	—	15	10
Chicken Stix, 6 pieces	100	210	19	13	0	9	39	2	35	680	—	—	4	2
Cool Twist Cone, chocolate	119	200	4	31	14	6	27	4	20	65	—	—	10	10
Cool Twist Cone, vanilla	119	190	5	28	14	6	28	4	15	100	—	—	0	10
Cool Twist Cone, vanilla/chocolate	119	190	4	29	14	6	28	4	20	80	—	—	10	10
Cool Twist Sundae, caramel	169	330	6	54	33	10	27	5	20	290	—	—	4	20
Cool Twist Sundae, hot fudge	168	320	7	45	33	12	34	6	25	270	—	—	6	20
Cool Twist Sundae, strawberry	166	260	5	43	33	8	28	5	15	115	—	—	4	15
Crispy Curls (fries)	85	300	4	36	0	16	48	3	0	840	—	—	8	2
Dipping Sauce, BBQ, 1 oz.	28	30	0	8	0	0	0	0	0	300	—	—	0	9
Dipping Sauce, Honey, 1/2 oz.	14	45	0	11	11	0	0	0	0	0	0	0	0	0
Dipping Sauce, Sweet 'n' Sour, 1 oz.	28	40	0	10	9	0	0	0	0	95	—	—	0	6
Dipping Sauce, Sweet Mustard, 1 oz.	28	50	0	10	9	0	0	0	0	160	—	—	0	15
Fisherman's Fillet	207	500	23	49	5	24	43	6	70	1030	—	—	20	20
French Fries, "Big Fry," 5 1/2 oz.	156	500	6	66	0	23	41	5	0	180	—	—	10	2
French Fries, large, 4 oz.	113	360	4	48	0	17	43	3	0	135	—	—	8	0
French Fries, regular, 2.5 oz.	71	230	3	30	0	11	43	2	0	85	—	—	6	0
Fried Chicken Breast	—	412	33	17	0	24	52	—	0	609	—	—	—	—
Fried Chicken Breast and Wing	—	604	44	25	0	37	55	—	165	894	—	—	—	—
Fried Chicken Leg	—	140	12	6	0	8	51	—	40	190	—	—	—	—
Fried Chicken Leg and Thigh	—	436	30	17	0	28	58	—	125	596	—	—	—	—
Fried Chicken Thigh	—	296	18	12	0	20	61	—	85	406	—	—	—	—
Fried Chicken Wing	—	192	11	9	0	13	61	—	47	285	—	—	—	—
Grilled Chicken Sandwich	192	310	24	34	5	9	26	1	60	890	—	—	15	15
Hamburger	110	270	13	33	5	10	33	4	20	490	—	—	15	10
Hash Rounds	79	230	3	24	0	14	55	3	0	560	—	—	6	0
Horseradish, 1 packet (1/4 oz.)	7	25	0	1	0	2	72	0	5	35	0	0	0	0
Hot Dog, All Beef	120	300	11	25	5	17	51	8	25	710	—	—	15	8
Hot Ham 'N' Cheese	149	330	23	32	5	12	33	5	65	1420	—	—	15	30
Margarine/Butter Blend	5	35	0	0	0	4	103	0	5	40	—	—	0	0
Mayonnaise, 1/2 oz.	14	50	0	1	1	5	90	1	5	75	0	0	0	0
Milk, 2% Low-fat, 8 fl. oz.	244	121	8	12	0	4	33	3	18	122	10	4	0	30
Muffin, Blueberry	106	400	6	51	24	19	43	4	80	320	—	—	6	4
Muffin, Oat Bran Raisin	122	440	8	62	15	18	37	3	55	350	—	—	—	8

Complete Nutritional Values	Weight (gm.)	Calories	Protein (gm.)	Carbohydrates (gm.)	Added Sugar (gm.)	Fat (gm.)	Fat % Calories	Saturated Fat (gm.)	Cholesterol (mg.)	Sodium (mg.)	Vitamin A (% U.S. RDA)	Vitamin C (% U.S. RDA)	Iron (% U.S. RDA)	Calcium (% U.S. RDA)
HARDEES—*Continued*														
Mushroom 'N' Swiss Burger	186	490	30	33	5	27	50	13	70	940	—	—	30	30
Pancakes, 3	137	280	8	56	0	2	6	1	15	890	—	—	20	6
Pancakes, 3 with 1 Sausage Patty	176	430	16	56	0	16	33	6	40	1290	—	—	20	8
Pancakes, 3 with 2 Bacon Strips	150	350	13	56	0	9	23	3	25	1110	—	—	20	6
Quarter-Pound Cheeseburger	182	500	29	34	5	29	52	14	70	1060	—	—	30	25
Real Lean Deluxe	205	340	23	35	5	13	22	—	80	650	—	—	25	10
Roast Beef Sandwich (RR)	—	350	26	37	5	11	28	—	58	732	—	—	—	—
Roast Beef Sandwich with Cheese (RR)	—	403	29	37	5	15	33	—	70	954	—	—	—	—
Roast Beef Sandwich with Cheese, large (RR)	—	427	38	31	5	17	36	—	94	1062	—	—	—	—
Roast Beef Sandwich, large (RR)	—	373	35	31	5	12	29	—	82	840	—	—	—	—
Roast Beef, Big	169	360	24	33	5	15	38	6	65	1150	—	—	30	10
Roast Beef, Regular	141	310	20	32	5	12	35	5	50	930	—	—	25	10
Salad Dressing, Blue Cheese, 2 oz.	56	210	1	10	9	18	77	3	20	790	—	—	0	23
Salad Dressing, House, 2 oz.	56	290	1	6	0	29	90	4	25	510	—	—	0	0
Salad Dressing, Reduced Calorie French, 2 oz.	56	130	1	21	17	5	35	1	0	480	—	—	0	0
Salad Dressing, Reduced Calorie Italian, 2 oz.	56	90	0	5	4	8	80	1	0	310	—	–	0	7
Salad Dressing, Thousand Island, 2 oz.	56	250	1	9	8	23	83	3	35	540	—	—	0	9
Salad, Chef	294	240	22	5	0	15	56	9	115	930	—	—	10	30
Salad, Chicken Fiesta/Grilled Chicken	298	280	26	4	5	15	48	9	145	640	—	—	10	30
Salad, Garden	241	210	14	3	0	14	60	8	105	270	—	—	6	30
Salad, Side	112	20	2	1	0	0	0	0	0	15	—	—	2	2
Shake, Chocolate	341	460	11	85	55	8	16	5	45	340	—	—	6	50
Shake, Strawberry	341	440	11	82	54	8	16	5	40	300	—	—	0	50
Shake, Vanilla	341	400	13	66	41	9	20	6	50	320	—	—	0	50
Syrup	43	120	0	31	31	0	0	0	0	25	0	0	4	0
Tartar Sauce, 2/3 oz.	19	90	0	2	0	9	90	1	10	160	—	—	0	3
Turkey Club	208	390	29	32	5	16	37	4	70	1280	—	—	15	15
Yogurt Cone (only)	5	20	1	4	—	0	0	0	0	10	—	—	0	0
Yogurt, Chocolate, Frozen, Soft Serve	113	170	6	27	—	4	21	3	10	75	—	—	8	15
Yogurt, Vanilla, Frozen, Soft Serve	113	160	6	27	—	4	23	3	10	75	—	—	4	15
Yogurt, NutraSweet Chocolate	113	120	6	22	0	0	0	0	0	75	—	—	0	20
Yogurt, NutraSweet Vanilla	113	110	5	21	0	1	8	1	0	75	—	—	2	15
HARDEE'S MEALS														
Pancakes (3) with Syrup & Margarine/ Butter Blend, Orange Juice, 2% Low-fat Milk	612	638	17	119	31	11	16	4	38	1079	13	123	24	36
Big Country Breakfast (Ham)	251	620	28	51	0	33	48	7	325	1780	—	—	30	15
Chicken Biscuit, Hash Rounds, 2% Low-fat Milk	469	781	28	78	0	41	47	10	63	2012	—	—	16	45
Big Country Breakfast (Bacon)	217	660	24	51	0	40	55	10	305	1540	—	—	30	15
Big Country Breakfast (Country Ham)	254	670	29	52	0	38	51	9	345	2870	—	—	35	15
Big Country Breakfast with Sausage, Orange Juice, 2% Low-fat Milk	701	1053	42	83	0	62	53	19	358	2104	—	—	35	50
Big Country Breakfast (Sausage)	274	850	33	51	0	57	60	16	340	1980	—		35	20
Grilled Chicken Sandwich, French Fries (regular), Orange Juice	446	622	28	84	5	20	29	3	60	977	—	—	21	15
Real Lean Deluxe, Side Salad with Reduced Calorie Italian Dressing, Orange Juice	556	530	26	60	9	21	36	—	80	975	—	—	27	19

Complete Nutritional Values

	Weight (gm.)	Calories	Protein (gm.)	Carbohydrates (gm.)	Added Sugar (gm.)	Fat (gm.)	Fat % Calories	Saturated Fat (gm.)	Cholesterol (mg.)	Sodium (mg.)	Vitamin A (% U.S. RDA)	Vitamin C (% U.S. RDA)	Iron (% U.S. RDA)	Calcium (% U.S. RDA)
HARDEE'S MEALS—*Continued*														
Hamburger, French Fries (regular), Big Cookie, Diet Coke (medium)	890	751	19	94	21	34	41	10	25	815	—	—	25	10
Regular Roast Beef Sandwich, Garden Salad with Reduced Calorie French Dressing, French Fries (regular)	509	880	38	86	22	42	43	16	155	1765	—	—	37	40
Large Roast Beef Sandwich, Crispy Curls, Vanilla Shake	426	1073	52	133	46	37	31	9	132	2000	—	—	8	52
Fisherman's Fillet Sandwich, French Fries (Big Fry), Vanilla Cool Twist Cone	482	1190	34	143	19	53	40	15	85	1310	—	—	30	32
Fried Chicken Breast and Wing, French Fries (large), Strawberry Shake	454	1404	59	155	54	62	40	8	205	1329	—	—	8	50
Bacon Cheeseburger, French Fries (Big Fry), Chocolate Shake, Apple Turnover	807	1840	54	220	68	82	40	30	125	1800	—	—	50	72
KFC														
Baked Beans	113	133	6	—	—	2	11	1	1	492	—	—	—	—
Buttermilk Biscuit	65	235	4	28	—	12	45	3	1	655	0	0	9	10
Chicken Littles Sandwich	47	169	6	14	3	10	54	2	18	331	0	0	10	2
Chocolate Pudding	93	156	2	20	—	7	43	6	2	127	0	0	3	6
Cole Slaw	91	119	2	13	0	7	50	1	5	197	6	36	0	3
Colonel's Chicken Sandwich	166	482	21	39	5	27	51	6	47	1060	0	0	7	5
Colonel's Deluxe Chicken Sandwich	187	547	25	—	0	32	53	8	64	1362	—	—	—	—
Corn on the Cob	143	176	5	32	0	3	16	0	0	0	5	4	4	0
Extra Tasty Crispy Center Breast*	135	342	33	12	0	20	52	5	114	790	0	0	5	3
Extra Tasty Crispy Drumstick	69	204	14	6	0	14	61	3	71	324	0	0	4	1
Extra Tasty Crispy Side Breast*	110	343	22	14	0	22	59	5	81	748	0	0	5	3
Extra Tasty Crispy Thigh	119	406	20	14	0	30	66	8	129	688	3	0	7	5
Extra Tasty Crispy Wing	65	254	12	9	0	19	66	4	67	422	0	0	4	2
French Fries	77	244	3	31	—	12	44	3	2	139	0	26	3	0
Hot Wings, 6 pieces	119	376	22	17	0	24	58	5	148	677	0	0	—	—
Kentucky Nuggets, 6 pieces	96	276	17	13	0	17	57	4	71	840	0	0	4	1
Mashed Potatoes and Gravy	98	71	2	12	0	2	20	0	0	339	0	0	2	2
Nugget Sauce, Barbecue	28	35	0	7	—	1	15	0	0	450	7	0	0	0
Nugget Sauce, Honey	14	49	0	12	12	0	0	0	0	0	0	0	0	0
Nugget Sauce, Mustard	28	36	1	6	—	1	23	0	0	346	0	0	0	0
Nugget Sauce, Sweet 'n Sour	28	58	0	13	—	1	9	0	0	148	0	0	0	0
Original Recipe Center Breast*	115	283	28	9	0	15	49	4	93	672	0	0	5	4
Original Recipe Drumstick	57	146	13	4	0	8	52	2	67	275	0	0	6	2
Original Recipe Side Breast*	90	267	19	11	0	16	56	4	77	735	0	0	7	7
Original Recipe Thigh	104	294	18	11	0	20	60	5	123	619	2	0	7	7
Original Recipe Wing	55	178	12	6	0	12	59	3	64	372	0	0	7	5
Parfait, Apple Shortcake	123	276	2	44	—	10	33	5	23	248	0	83	3	3
Parfait, Chocolate Creme	132	360	4	44	30	19	48	11	3	231	0	0	7	5
Parfait, Fudge Brownie	120	331	3	55	—	11	30	5	40	299	0	0	6	4
Parfait, Lemon Cream	151	513	8	74	—	20	36	9	9	232	4	8	3	22
Parfait, Strawberry Shortcake	113	230	2	36	24	9	34	5	20	162	1	30	3	3
Potato Salad	113	177	2	—	0	12	59	2	14	497	—	—	—	—
Vanilla Pudding	94	159	2	21	—	7	41	6	1	130	0	0	1	6

Complete Nutritional Values

	Weight (gm.)	Calories	Protein (gm.)	Carbohydrates (gm.)	Added Sugar (gm.)	Fat (gm.)	Fat % Calories	Saturated Fat (gm.)	Cholesterol (mg.)	Sodium (mg.)	Vitamin A (% U.S. RDA)	Vitamin C (% U.S. RDA)	Iron (% U.S. RDA)	Calcium (% U.S. RDA)
KFC MEALS														
Kentucky Nuggets (6 pieces), French Fries, Chocolate Pudding	266	676	22	64	0	37	49	13	75	1106	0	26	10	7
Original Recipe 2-Piece Dinner with Side Breast & Drumstick	401	838	41	68	0	45	48	11	150	2201	6	36	24	24
Hot Wings (6 piece), Cole Slaw, Corn on the Cob, Lemon Cream Parfait	504	1184	38	136	0	54	41	16	162	1106	15	48	7	25
Original Recipe 2-Piece Dinner with Center Breast & Thigh	473	1002	55	73	0	55	49	14	222	2482	8	36	23	26
Extra Tasty Crispy 2-Piece Dinner with Side Breast & Drumstick	433	972	44	73	0	56	52	14	158	2263	6	36	20	19
Original Recipe 3-Piece Dinner with Center Breast, Wing, & Drumstick	481	1032	62	72	0	54	48	14	230	2510	6	36	29	26
Original Recipe 3-Piece Dinner with Thigh, Side Breast, & Drumstick	505	1132	59	79	0	65	51	16	273	2820	8	36	31	31
Extra Tasty Crispy 2-Piece Dinner with Center Breast & Thigh	508	1173	62	79	0	69	53	17	249	2669	9	36	23	23
Extra Tasty Crispy 3-Piece Dinner with Center Breast, Wing, & Drumstick	523	1225	68	80	0	72	53	17	258	2727	6	36	24	21
Extra Tasty Crispy 3-Piece Dinner with Side Breast, Thigh, & Drumstick	552	1378	64	88	0	86	56	21	287	2951	9	36	27	24
MCDONALD'S														
Apple Juice, 6 fl. oz.	180	91	0	50	0	0	0	0	0	5	0	2	4	0
Apple Pie	85	260	2	30	12	15	52	4	6	240	0	20	4	0
Bacon Bits	3	15	1	0	0	1	60	1	1	95	0	0	0	0
Barbeque Sauce, 1 fl. oz.	32	50	0	12	11	1	9	0	0	340	4	4	2	0
Big Mac	215	500	25	42	5	26	47	9	100	890	6	2	20	25
Biscuit with Biscuit Spread	75	260	5	32	1	13	45	3	1	730	0	0	8	8
Biscuit with Bacon, Egg & Cheese	153	430	15	33	1	26	54	8	248	1190	10	0	15	20
Biscuit with Sausage	118	420	12	32	1	28	60	8	44	1040	0	0	10	8
Biscuit with Sausage & Egg	175	500	19	33	1	33	59	10	270	1210	6	0	20	10
Breakfast Burrito	105	280	12	21	0	17	55	6	135	580	10	10	8	10
Carrot Sticks	85	37	0	9	0	0	0	0	0	40	240	10	2	2
Celery Sticks	85	14	0	3	0	0	0	0	0	100	0	10	0	2
Cheerios, 3/4 cup	19	80	3	14	1	1	11	0	0	210	15	15	30	2
Cheeseburger	116	305	15	30	5	13	38	5	50	710	8	4	15	20
Chicken Fajitas	82	185	11	20	0	8	39	3	35	310	2	8	4	8
Chicken McNuggets, 6 pieces	113	270	20	17	0	15	50	4	56	580	0	0	6	0
Chocolaty Chip Cookies	56	330	4	42	18	16	43	5	4	280	0	0	10	2
Coca-Cola Classic,* 12 fl. oz.	360	140	0	38	38	0	0	0	0	15	0	0	0	0
Coca-Cola Classic, 32 fl. oz.	960	380	0	101	101	0	0	0	0	40	0	0	0	0
Coke, Diet, 12 fl. oz.	360	1	0	0	0	0	0	0	0	30	0	0	0	0
Croutons	11	50	1	7	0	2	36	1	0	140	0	0	0	0
Danish, Apple	115	390	6	51	30	17	39	4	25	370	0	25	8	0
Danish, Cinnamon Raisin	110	440	6	58	32	21	43	5	34	430	0	6	10	4
Danish, Iced Cheese	110	390	7	42	24	21	48	6	47	420	4	0	8	4
Danish, Raspberry	117	410	6	62	36	16	35	3	26	310	0	6	8	0
English Muffin with Margarine	58	170	5	26	0	5	26	1	0	230	2	0	8	15
Filet-O-Fish	141	370	14	38	5	18	44	4	50	930	2	0	10	15
French Fries, large	122	400	6	46	0	22	50	5	0	200	0	25	6	0
French Fries, medium	97	320	4	36	0	17	48	4	0	150	0	20	4	0
French Fries, small	68	220	3	26	0	12	49	3	0	110	0	15	2	0
Frozen Yogurt Cone, Vanilla, Low-fat	85	105	4	22	6	1	7	0	3	80	2	0	0	10

233

Complete Nutritional Values	Weight (gm.)	Calories	Protein (gm.)	Carbohydrates (gm.)	Added Sugar (gm.)	Fat (gm.)	Fat % Calories	Saturated Fat (gm.)	Cholesterol (mg.)	Sodium (mg.)	Vitamin A (% U.S. RDA)	Vitamin C (% U.S. RDA)	Iron (% U.S. RDA)	Calcium (% U.S. RDA)
MCDONALD'S—*Continued*														
Frozen Yogurt Sundae, Hot Caramel, Low-fat	174	270	7	59	30	3	9	2	13	180	6	0	0	20
Frozen Yogurt Sundae, Hot Fudge, Low-fat	169	240	7	50	29	3	12	2	6	170	4	0	2	25
Frozen Yogurt Sundae, Strawberry, Low-fat	171	210	6	49	30	1	5	1	5	95	4	2	0	20
Grapefruit Juice, 6 fl. oz.	183	80	1	19	0	0	0	0	0	0	0	100	0	0
Grilled Chicken Breast Sandwich (test product)	177	252	24	30	5	4	14	1	50	740	8	8	15	15
Hamburger	102	255	12	30	5	9	32	3	37	490	4	4	15	10
Hashbrown Potatoes	53	130	1	15	0	7	48	1	0	330	0	2	0	0
Honey, 1/2 oz.	14	45	0	12	12	0	0	0	0	0	0	0	0	0
Hot Mustard Sauce, 1 fl. oz.	30	70	0	8	8	4	46	1	5	250	0	0	0	2
Hotcakes with Margarine and Syrup	176	410	8	74	17	9	20	1	8	640	4	0	10	10
McChicken	187	415	19	39	5	20	43	4	42	770	2	4	15	15
McDonaldland Cookies	56	290	4	47	13	9	29	2	0	300	0	0	10	0
McLean Deluxe	206	320	22	35	5	10	28	4	60	670	10	10	20	15
McLean Deluxe with Cheese	219	370	24	35	5	14	34	5	75	890	15	10	20	20
McMuffin, Egg	135	280	18	28	0	11	35	4	224	710	10	0	15	25
McMuffin, Sausage	135	345	15	27	0	20	52	7	57	770	4	0	15	20
McMuffin, Sausage with Egg	159	415	21	27	0	25	54	8	256	915	10	0	20	25
McRib Sandwich	184	445	24	48	0	22	44	0	75	972	—	—	—	—
Milk Shake, Chocolate Low-fat	293	320	11	66	35	2	5	1	10	240	6	0	0	35
Milk Shake, Strawberry Low-fat	293	320	11	67	35	1	4	1	10	170	6	0	0	35
Milk Shake, Vanilla Low-fat	293	290	11	60	33	1	4	1	10	170	6	0	0	35
Milk, 1% Low-fat, 8 fl. oz.	240	110	9	12	0	2	16	2	10	130	10	4	0	30
Muffin, Fat-free Apple Bran	75	180	5	40	9	0	0	0	0	200	0	0	6	4
Muffin, Fat-free Blueberry	75	170	3	40	0	0	0	0	0	220	0	2	4	8
Orange Drink, 12 fl. oz.	360	130	0	33	33	0	0	0	0	10	0	0	0	0
Orange Juice, 6 fl. oz.	183	80	1	19	0	0	0	0	0	0	0	120	0	0
Orange Sorbet Ice, cone (4 oz.)	—	106	0	27	23	0	2	0	0	25	0	30	0	0
Orange Sorbet Ice, sundae (6 1/2 oz.), no topping	—	142	0	38	30	0	0	0	0	0	0	55	0	0
Orange Sorbet Ice/Low-fat Frozen Yogurt Twist Cone	—	104	2	25	18	1	4	0	1	50	0	15	0	6
Orange Sorbet Ice/Low-fat Frozen Yogurt Twist Sundae	—	138	3	34	23	1	3	0	2	45	0	25	0	10
Pork Sausage	48	180	8	0	0	16	82	6	48	350	0	0	4	0
Quarter Pounder	166	410	23	34	5	20	44	8	85	650	4	6	20	15
Quarter Pounder with Cheese	194	510	28	34	5	28	49	11	115	1090	15	6	20	30
Salad Dressing, Bleu Cheese, 2.5 fl. oz.	75	250	2	5	3	20	72	5	35	750	0	0	0	0
Salad Dressing, Lite Vinaigrette, 2 fl. oz.	60	48	0	8	7	2	38	0	0	240	0	0	0	0
Salad Dressing, Ranch, 2 fl. oz.	60	220	0	4	3	20	82	4	20	520	0	0	0	0
Salad Dressing, Red French Reduced-Calorie, 2 fl. oz.	60	160	0	20	18	8	45	1	0	460	0	0	0	0
Salad Dressing, Thousand Island, 2.5 fl. oz.	75	390	0	10	8	40	92	5	40	500	0	0	0	0
Salad, Chef	265	170	17	8	0	9	48	4	111	400	100	35	8	15
Salad, Chunky Chicken	255	150	25	7	0	4	24	1	78	230	170	45	6	4
Salad, Garden	189	50	4	6	0	2	36	1	65	70	90	35	8	4
Salad, Side	106	30	2	4	0	1	30	0	33	35	80	20	4	2
Sausage	43	160	7	0	0	15	84	5	43	310	0	0	4	0
Scrambled Eggs	100	140	12	1	0	10	64	3	399	290	10	0	10	6
Sprite, 12 fl. oz.	360	140	0	36	36	0	0	0	0	15	0	0	0	0
Sweet and Sour Sauce, 1 fl. oz.	32	60	0	14	12	0	3	0	0	190	6	0	0	0
Wheaties, 3/4 cup	23	90	2	19	3	1	10	0	0	220	20	20	20	2

Complete Nutritional Values	Weight (gm.)	Calories	Protein (gm.)	Carbohydrates (gm.)	Added Sugar (gm.)	Fat (gm.)	Fat % Calories	Saturated Fat (gm.)	Cholesterol (mg.)	Sodium (mg.)	Vitamin A (% U.S. RDA)	Vitamin C (% U.S. RDA)	Iron (% U.S. RDA)	Calcium (% U.S. RDA)
MCDONALD'S MEALS														
Cheerios, 1% Low-fat Milk, Orange Juice, Fat-Free Apple Bran Muffin	517	450	18	85	10	3	6	2	10	540	25	139	36	36
Hotcakes with Margarine & Syrup, Orange Juice, 1% Low-fat Milk	597	600	18	105	17	11	17	3	18	770	14	124	10	40
Cinnamon Raisin Danish, Orange Juice	293	520	8	76	32	21	36	4	34	430	0	126	10	24
Scrambled Eggs, English Muffin with Margarine, black coffee	158	310	17	27	0	15	44	4	399	520	12	0	18	21
Biscuit with Sausage & Egg, 1% Low-fat Milk, Orange Juice, Hash Brown Potatoes	651	820	30	79	1	42	46	13	280	1670	16	126	20	40
Chunky Chicken Salad, Lite Vinaigrette Dressing, Orange Juice	498	278	26	34	7	6	19	1	78	470	170	165	6	4
Happier Meal: Hamburger, Carrot Sticks, Low-fat Milk	427	402	21	51	5	11	25	5	47	660	254	18	17	42
McLean Deluxe, Side Salad, 1% Low-fat Milk	552	460	33	51	5	13	25	6	103	835	100	34	24	47
Filet-O-Fish, Side Salad, Lite Vinaigrette Dressing, Diet Coke	667	449	16	50	12	21	42	5	83	1235	82	20	14	17
Happy Meal: Hamburger, French Fries, small, Coca-Cola, 12 fl. oz.	530	620	16	94	43	22	31	7	37	585	4	19	17	10
Chef Salad, Croutons, Bacon Bits, Ranch Dressing, Diet Coke	699	456	19	19	3	32	63	9	132	1185	100	35	8	15
Hamburger, French Fries, medium, Strawberry Low-fat Frozen Yogurt Sundae, Coca-Cola Classic, 12 fl. oz.	730	925	22	153	73	27	26	7	42	750	8	26	19	30
Chicken McNuggets (6 pieces), Barbecue Sauce, French Fries, medium, Strawberry Low-fat Milk Shake	535	960	35	132	46	34	32	8	66	1240	10	24	12	35
McChicken, French Fries, medium, Coca-Cola Classic, 32 fl. oz., Low-fat Frozen Yogurt Hot Fudge Sundae	1413	1355	30	226	135	40	27	10	48	1130	6	24	21	40
Quarter Pounder, French Fries, medium, Side Salad, Blue Cheese Dressing, Low-fat Frozen Yogurt	529	1115	35	101	14	59	47	17	156	1665	86	46	28	27
Quarter Pounder with Cheese, French Fries, large, Chocolate Low-fat Milk Shake, Apple Pie	669	1490	47	176	52	67	40	21	131	1770	21	51	30	65
PIZZA HUT														
Pan Pizza, Cheese, medium, 2 slices	205	492	30	57	0	18	33	9	34	940	9	12	30	63
Pan Pizza, Pepperoni, medium, 2 slices	211	540	29	62	0	22	37	9	42	1127	10	14	35	52
Pan Pizza, Super Supreme, medium, 2 slices	257	563	33	53	0	26	42	12	55	1447	12	18	37	54
Pan Pizza, Supreme, medium, 2 slices	255	589	32	53	0	30	46	14	48	1363	12	16	28	50
Personal Pan Pizza, Supreme, whole	264	647	33	76	0	28	39	11	49	1313	12	18	37	52
Personal Pan Pizza, Pepperoni, whole	256	675	37	76	0	29	39	12	53	1335	12	17	32	73
Thin 'n Crispy Pizza, Cheese, medium, 2 slices	148	398	28	37	0	17	38	10	33	867	7	8	18	66
Thin 'n Crispy Pizza, Pepperoni, medium, 2 slices	146	413	26	36	0	20	44	11	46	986	7	10	18	45
Thin 'n Crispy Pizza, Super Supreme, medium, 2 slices	203	463	29	44	0	21	41	10	56	1336	10	14	27	46

Complete Nutritional Values	Weight (gm.)	Calories	Protein (gm.)	Carbohydrates (gm.)	Added Sugar (gm.)	Fat (gm.)	Fat % Calories	Saturated Fat (gm.)	Cholesterol (mg.)	Sodium (mg.)	Vitamin A (% U.S. RDA)	Vitamin C (% U.S. RDA)	Iron (% U.S. RDA)	Calcium (% U.S. RDA)
PIZZA HUT—*Continued*														
Thin 'n Crispy Pizza, Supreme, medium 2 slices	200	459	28	41	0	22	43	11	42	1328	10	16	33	43
Traditional Hand-Tossed Pizza, Cheese, medium, 2 slices	220	518	34	55	0	20	35	14	55	1276	10	16	30	75
Traditional Hand-Tossed Pizza, Pepperoni, medium, 2 slices	197	500	28	50	0	23	41	13	50	1267	10	12	28	44
Traditional Hand-Tossed Pizza, Super Supreme, medium, 2 slices	243	556	33	54	0	25	40	13	54	1648	11	20	38	44
Traditional Hand-Tossed Pizza, Supreme, medium, 2 slices	239	540	32	50	0	26	43	14	55	1470	11	20	45	48
TACO BELL														
Burrito Supreme with Red Sauce	255	503	20	55	0	22	39	8	33	1181	18	43	22	19
Burrito, Bean, with Red Sauce	206	447	15	63	0	14	28	2	9	1148	7	88	21	19
Burrito, Beef, with Red Sauce	206	493	25	48	0	21	38	8	57	1311	10	3	23	15
Burrito, Chicken, no Red Sauce	171	334	17	38	0	12	32	4	52	880	9	19	43	11
Burrito, combination	198	407	18	46	0	16	35	5	33	1136	9	45	19	15
Burrito, Fiesta	114	226	8	29	—	9	36	3	9	652	5	57	15	15
Chilito	156	383	18	36	0	18	42	8	47	893	17	0	14	27
Cinnamon Twists	–no data–					–no data–								
Enchirito with Red Sauce	213	382	20	31	0	20	47	9	54	1243	19	47	16	27
Green Sauce, 1 oz.	28	4	0	1	0	0	0	0	0	136	2	0	0	0
Guacamole, 3/4 oz.	21	34	0	3	0	2	53	0	0	113	2	5	1	1
Hot Taco Sauce, 1 packet (1/3 fl. oz.)	11	3	0	0	0	0	0	0	0	82	3	0	1	0
Jalapeno Peppers	100	20	1	4	0	0	0	0	0	1370	5	4	2	4
Mexican Pizza	223	575	21	40	0	37	58	11	52	1031	20	51	21	26
Meximelt, Beef	106	266	13	19	0	15	51	8	38	689	16	3	11	25
Meximelt, Chicken	107	257	14	19	0	15	53	7	48	779	10	4	20	22
Nacho Cheese	56	103	4	5	0	8	70	3	9	393	3	2	2	11
Nachos	106	346	7	37	0	18	47	6	9	399	11	3	5	19
Nachos Bellgrande	287	649	22	61	0	35	49	12	36	997	23	96	19	30
Nachos Supreme	145	367	12	41	0	27	66	5	18	471	14	50	2	26
Pico de Gallo	28	8	0	1	0	0	0	0	1	88	11	3	1	1
Pintos 'n Cheese with Red Sauce	128	190	9	19	0	9	43	4	16	642	9	86	8	16
Red Sauce, 1 oz.	28	10	0	2	0	0	0	0	0	261	5	0	0	1
Salad, Chicken	153	125	8	5	0	8	58	4	32	252	16	17	17	9
Salad Dressing, Ranch, 2 1/2 fl. oz.	74	236	2	1	0	25	95	5	35	571	5	0	3	3
Salsa, 1/3 fl. oz.	10	18	1	4	0	0	0	0	0	376	5	0	3	4
Sour Cream, 2/3 fl. oz.	21	46	1	1	0	4	78	2	0	0	3	0	0	2
Taco, hard shell, beef	78	183	10	11	0	11	54	5	32	276	7	2	6	8
Taco Bellgrande	163	335	18	18	0	23	62	11	56	472	17	9	11	18
Taco, hard shell, chicken	86	171	12	11	0	9	47	3	52	337	6	5	31	8
Taco, Fiesta (beef)	57	127	6	10	—	7	50	3	16	139	5	1	4	6
Taco, Soft, Fiesta	68	147	7	15	—	7	43	3	16	361	3	1	6	5
Taco Salad, without shell	520	484	28	22	0	31	58	14	80	680	33	124	22	29
Taco Salad, with shell	575	905	34	55	0	61	61	19	80	910	33	125	33	32
Taco Sauce, 1 packet (1/3 fl. oz.)	11	2	0	0	0	0	0	0	0	126	4	0	0	0
Taco, Soft, Beef	92	225	12	18	0	12	48	5	32	554	4	2	13	12
Taco, Soft, Chicken	107	213	14	19	0	10	42	4	52	615	4	4	35	8
Taco, Soft, Steak	100	218	14	18	0	11	45	5	14	456	3	2	16	11
Taco Supreme	92	230	11	12	0	15	59	8	32	276	11	5	6	11
Taco Supreme, Soft	124	272	13	19	0	16	53	8	32	554	9	5	13	14
Tostada, Beef, with Red Sauce	156	243	9	27	0	11	41	4	16	596	13	75	9	18
Tostada, Chicken, with Red Sauce	164	264	12	20	0	15	51	7	37	454	18	36	19	18

236

Complete Nutritional Values	Weight (gm.)	Calories	Protein (gm.)	Carbohydrates (gm.)	Added Sugar (gm.)	Fat (gm.)	Fat % Calories	Saturated Fat (gm.)	Cholesterol (mg.)	Sodium (mg.)	Vitamin A (% U.S. RDA)	Vitamin C (% U.S. RDA)	Iron (% U.S. RDA)	Calcium (% U.S. RDA)
TACO BELL—*Continued*														
Tostada, Fieta	93	167	6	17	—	7	38	2	9	324	8	45	5	11
TACO BELL MEALS														
Chicken Soft Taco, Pintos 'n Cheese														
with Red Sauce	228	400	22	37	0	19	43	8	60	1232	15	90	18	27
Taco, Bean Burrito with Red Sauce	284	630	25	74	0	25	36	7	41	1424	14	90	27	27
Kids' Fresh Meal with Beef Taco,														
Cinnamon Twist, Soft Drink, small	473	494	12	73	46	19	35	8	32	525	7	2	8	8
Enchirito with Red Sauce, Beef Meximelt	319	648	33	50	0	35	49	17	92	1932	35	50	27	52
Nachos Bellgrande, Guacamole, Cinnamon														
Twists	343	854	24	88	8	45	47	15	36	1344	25	101	22	31
Mexican Pizza, Nachos, Cinnamon Twists	364	1092	30	101	8	63	52	20	61	1664	31	54	28	45
Taco Salad with Shell and Ranch														
Dressing, Guacamole	670	1175	36	59	0	88	67	24	115	1594	40	130	37	36
WENDYS														
Alfalfa Sprouts, fresh, 1 oz.	28	8	1	0	0	0	0	0	0	0	0	4	0	0
Alfredo Sauce, 2 oz.	56	35	1	5	0	1	26	1	0	300	0	0	0	6
Applesauce, Chunky, 1 oz.	28	22	0	6	0	0	0	0	0	0	0	0	0	0
Bacon Bits, 1/2 oz.	14	40	5	0	0	2	45	1	10	400	0	2	2	0
Baked Potato, Hot Stuffed Bacon & Cheese	362	520	20	70	0	18	31	5	20	1460	10	60	25	8
Baked Potato, Hot Stuffed Broccoli &														
Cheese	350	400	8	58	0	16	36	3	0	455	14	60	15	10
Baked Potato, Hot Stuffed Cheese	318	420	8	66	0	15	32	4	10	310	10	50	20	6
Baked Potato, Hot Stuffed Chili & Cheese	403	500	15	71	0	18	32	4	25	630	15	60	28	8
Baked Potato, Hot Stuffed Sour Cream &														
Chives	323	500	8	67	0	23	41	9	25	135	50	75	20	10
Baked Potato, Plain	250	270	6	63	0	0	0	0	0	20	0	50	20	2
Bananas, 1 oz.	28	26	0	7	0	0	0	0	0	0	0	4	0	0
Big Classic	260	570	27	47	5	33	52	6	90	1085	10	20	35	15
Big Classic with Cheese	278	640	31	47	5	39	55	9	105	1345	16	20	35	27
Big Classic, Double	334	750	46	47	5	45	54	11	155	1295	10	20	55	15
Big Classic, Double, with Cheese	352	820	50	47	5	51	56	14	170	1555	16	20	55	27
Breadsticks, 2	7	30	1	5	0	1	30	0	0	30	0	0	2	2
Broccoli, fresh, 1/2 cup	43	12	1	2	0	0	0	0	0	10	6	65	2	2
Butterscotch Pudding, 1/4 cup	57	90	1	11	9	4	40	—	0	85	0	0	2	6
Cantaloupe, fresh, 2 oz.	57	20	0	5	0	0	0	0	0	5	20	30	0	0
Carrots, fresh, 1/4 cup	27	12	0	2	0	0	0	0	0	10	80	4	0	0
Cauliflower, fresh, 1/2 cup	57	14	1	3	0	0	0	0	0	10	0	70	2	2
Cheddar Cheese, shredded, 1 oz.	28	110	7	1	0	10	82	6	30	175	10	0	0	20
Cheddar Chips, 1 oz.	28	160	3	12	0	12	68	—	5	445	0	0	2	6
Cheese Sauce, 2 oz.	56	39	1	5	0	2	46	1	0	305	0	0	0	6
Cheese, Parmesan, grated, 1 oz.	28	130	12	1	0	9	62	5	20	525	6	0	0	40
Cheese, Parmesan, imitation, 1 oz.	28	80	9	4	0	3	34	3	0	410	20	0	0	50
Cheese, Shredded, Salad Bar, Imitation, 1 oz.	28	90	6	1	0	6	60	4	0	125	4	0	0	20
Cheeseburger	144	410	28	30	5	21	46	9	80	760	6	0	30	22
Cheeseburger, Double	218	590	47	30	5	33	50	14	145	970	6	0	50	22
Chicken Club Sandwich	205	506	30	42	5	25	44	5	70	930	2	15	80	10
Chicken Salad, 2 oz.	56	120	7	4	0	8	60	1	0	215	0	4	2	0
Chicken Sandwich, fried	219	430	26	41	5	19	40	3	60	725	2	8	80	10
Chili, 9 oz.	255	220	21	23	1	7	29	3	45	750	15	15	35	8
Chives, 1 oz.	28	71	6	18	0	1	13	0	0	20	195	313	30	25
Chocolate Chip Cookie	64	275	3	40	20	13	43	4	15	256	2	0	8	2

Complete Nutritional Values

	Weight (gm.)	Calories	Protein (gm.)	Carbohydrates (gm.)	Added Sugar (gm.)	Fat (gm.)	Fat % Calories	Saturated Fat (gm.)	Cholesterol (mg.)	Sodium (mg.)	Vitamin A (% U.S. RDA)	Vitamin C (% U.S. RDA)	Iron (% U.S. RDA)	Calcium (% U.S. RDA)
WENDYS—*Continued*														
Chocolate Milk, 8 fl. oz.	240	160	7	24	11	5	28	3	15	140	15	4	4	25
Chocolate Pudding, 1/4 cup	57	90	0	12	9	4	40	—	0	70	0	0	2	15
Chow Mein Noodles, 1/2 oz.	14	74	1	8	0	4	49	1	0	60	0	0	4	0
Coca-Cola, Biggie (28 fl. oz.)	840	350	0	88	88	0	0	0	0	35	0	0	0	0
Coca-Cola, large (16 fl. oz.)	480	200	0	50	50	0	0	0	0	20	0	0	0	0
Coca-Cola, medium (12 fl. oz.)	360	150	0	38	38	0	0	0	0	15	0	0	0	0
Coca-Cola, small (8 fl. oz.)	240	100	0	25	27	0	0	0	0	10	0	0	0	0
Coke, Diet, small (8 fl. oz.)	240	1	0	0	0	0	0	0	0	20	0	0	0	0
Cole Slaw, 2 oz.	57	70	0	8	0	5	64	1	5	130	4	25	0	2
Cottage Cheese, 1/2 cup	105	108	13	3	0	4	33	3	15	425	6	0	0	6
Crispy Chicken Nuggets, 6 pieces	93	280	14	12	0	20	64	4	50	600	0	0	4	4
Croutons, 1/2 oz.	14	60	2	8	0	3	45	—	—	155	0	0	4	0
Cucumber, fresh, 4 slices	14	2	0	0	0	0	0	0	0	0	0	0	0	0
Dr Pepper, small (8 fl. oz.)	240	100	0	26	26	0	0	0	0	5	0	0	0	0
Eggs, hard-cooked, 1 Tbsp.	20	30	3	0	0	2	60	1	90	25	4	0	0	0
Fettucini, 2 oz.	56	190	4	27	0	3	14	1	10	3	0	0	6	0
Fish Fillet Sandwich	170	460	18	42	5	25	49	5	55	780	2	2	15	10
Flour Tortilla, 1	37	110	3	19	0	3	25	0	—	220	0	0	2	8
French Fries, Biggie (6 oz.)	170	449	6	62	0	22	45	5	0	271	0	19	7	0
French Fries, large (4.2 oz.)	118	312	4	43	0	16	45	3	0	189	0	13	5	0
French Fries, small (3.2 oz.)	91	240	3	33	0	12	45	2	0	145	0	10	4	0
Frosty Dairy Dessert, large (14.5 oz.)	413	680	14	100	34	24	32	8	85	374	17	0	10	51
Frosty Dairy Dessert, medium (11 oz.)	316	520	10	77	26	18	32	6	65	286	13	0	9	39
Frosty Dairy Dessert, small (8.5 oz.)	243	400	8	59	20	14	32	5	50	220	10	0	6	30
Garbanzo Beans	28	46	3	8	0	1	20	0	0	5	0	0	6	0
Garlic Toast	18	70	2	9	0	3	39	1	0	65	4	0	2	2
Green Peas, frozen, 1 oz.	28	21	1	4	0	0	0	0	0	30	4	8	2	0
Green Peppers, fresh, 1/4 cup	37	10	0	2	0	0	0	0	0	0	4	60	0	0
Grilled Chicken Sandwich	175	320	24	37	5	9	25	2	60	715	2	8	20	10
Hamburger, Double	200	520	43	30	5	27	47	11	130	710	0	0	50	10
Hamburger, Single, plain	126	340	24	30	5	15	40	6	65	500	0	0	30	10
Hamburger, Single, with Everything	210	420	25	35	5	21	45	7	70	890	5	15	30	10
Honeydew Melon, 2 oz.	57	20	0	5	0	0	0	0	0	5	0	25	0	0
Honey Mustard, 1/2 oz.	14	50	0	5	—	3	54	1	5	170	0	0	0	0
Hot Chocolate, 6 fl. oz.	180	110	2	22	13	1	8	9	0	115	0	0	2	6
Jalapeño Peppers, canned, 1 Tbsp.	14	2	0	0	0	0	0	0	0	0	190	0	0	0
Jr. Bacon Cheeseburger	155	430	22	32	5	25	52	5	50	835	2	15	20	10
Jr. Cheeseburger	125	310	18	33	5	13	38	5	34	770	2	4	20	10
Jr. Hamburger	111	260	15	33	5	9	31	3	34	570	2	4	20	10
Jr. Swiss Deluxe	163	360	18	34	5	18	45	3	40	765	4	10	20	20
Lemon-Lime soft drink, small (8 fl. oz.)	240	100	0	24	24	0	0	0	0	20	0	0	0	0
Lemonade, 8 fl. oz.	240	90	0	24	40	0	0	0	0	0	0	15	2	0
Lettuce, iceberg, 1 cup	55	8	0	1	0	0	0	0	0	5	2	4	2	0
Lettuce, romaine, 1 cup	55	9	0	1	0	0	0	0	0	5	15	20	4	2
Milk, 2% Low-fat, 8 fl. oz.	240	110	8	11	0	4	33	3	20	115	10	4	0	30
Mushrooms, fresh, 1/4 cup	17	4	0	0	0	0	0	0	0	0	0	0	0	0
Olives, Black, 1 oz.	28	35	0	2	0	3	77	0	0	245	0	0	4	2
Oranges, fresh, 2 oz.	56	26	0	7	0	0	0	0	0	0	0	50	0	2
Pasta Medley, 2 oz.	56	60	2	9	0	2	30	0	0	5	6	15	4	0
Pasta Salad, 1/4 cup	57	35	2	6	0	0	0	—	0	120	0	0	2	0
Peaches, in syrup, 2 pieces, 2 oz.	57	31	0	8	0	0	0	0	0	5	2	2	0	0
Pepperoni, Sliced, 1 oz.	28	140	5	2	0	12	77	4	35	435	0	0	2	0
Picante Sauce, 2 oz.	56	18	0	4	0	0	1	0	—	5	10	30	2	0
Pineapple Chunks in natural juice, 1/2 cup	100	60	0	16	0	0	0	0	0	0	0	15	2	0

Complete Nutritional Values

	Weight (gm.)	Calories	Protein (gm.)	Carbohydrates (gm.)	Added Sugar (gm.)	Fat (gm.)	Fat % Calories	Saturated Fat (gm.)	Cholesterol (mg.)	Sodium (mg.)	Vitamin A (% U.S. RDA)	Vitamin C (% U.S. RDA)	Iron (% U.S. RDA)	Calcium (% U.S. RDA)
WENDYS—Continued														
Potato Salad, 1/4 cup	57	125	0	6	0	11	79	1	10	90	0	10	2	0
Red Onions, fresh, 3 rings	9	2	0	0	0	0	0	0	0	0	0	0	0	0
Red Peppers, Crushed, 1 oz.	28	120	5	15	0	4	30	—	0	5	200	15	15	2
Refried Beans, 2 oz.	56	70	4	10	0	3	39	1	0	215	0	0	6	2
Rotini, 2 oz.	56	90	3	15	0	2	20	0	0	0	0	0	4	0
Salad Dressing, Blue Cheese, 4 Tbsp.	60	360	0	0	0	40	100	8	40	420	0	0	0	0
Salad Dressing, Celery Seed, 4 Tbsp.	60	280	0	12	0	18	58	4	20	260	0	0	0	0
Salad Dressing, French, 4 Tbsp.	60	240	0	16	14	24	90	3	0	712	0	0	0	0
Salad Dressing, Golden Italian, 4 Tbsp.	60	180	0	12	11	16	80	2	0	1000	0	0	0	0
Salad Dressing, Hidden Valley Ranch, 4 Tbsp.	60	200	0	0	0	24	108	1	20	380	0	0	0	0
Salad Dressing, Italian Caesar, 4 Tbsp.	60	320	0	0	0	36	101	6	20	560	0	0	0	0
Salad Dressing, Reduced Calorie Bacon and Tomato, 4 Tbsp.	60	180	0	12	11	16	80	2	0	760	0	0	0	0
Salad Dressing, Reduced Calorie Italian, 4 Tbsp.	57	100	0	6	5	9	77	1	0	700	0	0	0	0
Salad Dressing, Sweet Red French, 4 tbsp.	60	280	0	20	18	24	77	3	0	500	0	0	0	0
Salad Dressing, Thousand Island, 4 Tbsp.	60	280	0	8	4	28	90	4	20	420	0	0	0	0
Salad, Chef	331	180	15	10	0	9	45	—	120	140	110	110	15	25
Salad, Garden	277	70	4	9	0	2	26	0	0	60	110	70	8	10
Salad, Taco	791	660	40	46	0	37	50	—	35	1110	80	80	35	80
Sauce for Chicken Nuggets, Barbecue, 1 oz.	28	50	0	11	0	0	0	0	0	100	6	0	4	0
Sauce for Chicken Nuggets, Honey, 1/2 oz.	14	45	0	12	12	0	0	0	0	0	0	0	0	0
Sauce for Chicken Nuggets, Sweet and Sour, 1 oz.	28	45	0	11	0	0	0	0	0	55	0	0	2	0
Sauce for Chicken Nuggets, Sweet Mustard, 1 oz.	28	50	0	9	0	1	18	0	0	140	0	0	0	0
Seafood Salad, 2 oz.	56	110	4	7	0	7	57	0	0	455	0	2	2	20
Sour Cream, 1 oz.	28	60	1	1	0	6	90	4	10	15	6	0	0	20
Sour Topping, 1 oz.	28	58	0	2	0	5	78	5	0	30	0	0	0	0
Spaghetti Meat Sauce, 2 oz.	56	60	4	8	0	2	30	1	10	315	4	4	4	0
Spaghetti Sauce, 2 oz.	56	28	0	7	0	0	1	0	0	345	0	0	0	0
Spanish Rice, 2 oz.	56	70	2	13	0	1	13	0	0	440	6	0	10	4
Strawberries, fresh, 2 oz.	56	17	0	4	0	0	0	0	0	0	0	50	0	0
Sunflower Seeds and Raisins, 1 oz.	28	140	5	6	0	10	64	7	0	5	0	0	10	2
Taco Chips, 1 1/2 oz.	40	260	4	40	0	10	35	1	0	20	0	0	4	8
Taco Meat, 2 oz.	56	110	10	4	0	7	57	2	25	300	0	0	10	4
Taco Sauce, 1 oz.	28	16	0	3	0	0	1	0	0	140	4	2	0	0
Taco Shells, 1	11	45	0	6	0	3	60	1	0	45	0	0	0	0
Tartar Sauce, 1 Tbsp.	21	120	0	0	0	14	105	2	15	115	0	0	0	0
Three Bean Salad, 1/4 cup	57	60	1	13	1	0	0	0	—	15	4	0	2	0
Tomatoes, fresh, 1 oz.	28	6	0	1	0	0	0	0	0	5	2	10	0	0
Tuna Salad, 2 oz.	56	100	8	4	0	6	54	1	0	290	0	4	2	0
Turkey Ham, 1/4 cup	28	5	0	0	0	1	26	0	15	275	0	0	4	0
Watermelon, 1/4 CUP	57	18	0	4	0	0	0	0	0	0	2	10	0	0
WENDY'S MEALS														
Salad (Romaine Lettuce, Tomatoes, Mushrooms, Cucumbers, Broccoli), 2% Low-fat Milk	397	143	9	15	0	4	25	3	20	135	33	99	6	34
Baked Potato (plain), Garden Salad with Reduced Calorie Italian Dressing, 2% Low-fat Milk	778	550	18	89	5	15	24	4	20	895	120	124	28	42

Complete Nutritional Values

	Weight (gm.)	Calories	Protein (gm.)	Carbohydrates (gm.)	Added Sugar (gm.)	Fat (gm.)	Fat % Calories	Saturated Fat (gm.)	Cholesterol (mg.)	Sodium (mg.)	Vitamin A (% U.S. RDA)	Vitamin C (% U.S. RDA)	Iron (% U.S. RDA)	Calcium (% U.S. RDA)
WENDY'S MEALS—*Continued*														
Grilled Chicken Sandwich, Baked Potato (plain), Garden Salad with Reduced Calorie Italian Dressing	713	760	34	115	10	20	23	3	60	1495	114	128	48	22
Chili (9 oz.), Garden Salad with Reduced Calorie Italian Dressing, 2% Low-fat Milk	783	500	33	49	6	22	39	7	65	1625	135	89	43	48
Kids' Meal: Jr. Hamburger, French Fries, small, Coca-Cola, small	442	600	18	91	32	21	32	6	34	725	2	14	24	10
Single Hamburger, French Fries, small, Coca-Cola, large	697	780	27	113	55	27	31	8	65	665	0	10	34	10
Baked Potato with Chili and Cheese, Chef Salad with Reduced Calorie Italian Dressing, 2% Low-fat Milk	1031	890	38	98	6	40	40	8	165	1585	135	174	43	63
Big Classic, French Fries, large, Coca-Cola, small	618	982	31	115	32	49	45	9	90	1284	10	33	40	15
Taco Salad with Hidden Valley Ranch Dressing, Baked Potato with Cheese, Coca-Cola, large	1649	1480	48	162	50	76	46	5	65	1820	90	130	55	86
Chicken Club Sandwich, French Fries, Biggie, Frosty, medium	691	1475	46	181	31	66	40	16	135	1487	15	34	96	49
Big Classic Double, with Cheese, French Fries, Biggie, Frosty, large, Chocolate Chip Cookie	999	2224	73	249	59	110	45	31	270	2456	35	39	80	80

D Food and Nutrition

Food and Nutrition Board, National Academy of Sciences—National Research Council Recommended Dietary Allowances[a], Revised 1989
Designed for the maintenance of good nutrition of practically all healthy people in the United States

| | | Weight[b] | | Height[b] | | Protein | Fat Soluble Vitamins | | | | Water-Soluble Vitamins | |
Category	Age (years) or Condition	(kg)	(lb)	(cm)	(in)	(g)	Vitamin A (μg RE)[c]	Vitamin D (μg)[d]	Vitamin E (mg α-TE)[e]	Vitamin K (μg)	Vitamin C (mg)	Thiamine (mg)
Infants	0.0–0.5	6	13	60	24	13	375	7.5	3	5	30	0.3
	0.5–1.0	9	20	71	28	14	375	10	4	10	35	0.4
Children	1–3	13	29	90	35	16	400	10	6	15	40	0.7
	4–6	20	44	112	44	24	500	10	7	20	45	0.9
	7–10	28	62	132	52	28	700	10	7	30	45	1.0
Males	11–14	45	99	157	62	45	1000	10	10	45	50	1.3
	15–18	66	145	176	69	59	1000	10	10	65	60	1.5
	19–24	72	160	177	70	58	1000	10	10	70	60	1.5
	25–50	79	174	176	70	63	1000	5	10	80	60	1.5
	51+	77	170	173	68	63	1000	5	10	80	60	1.2
Females	11–14	46	101	157	62	46	800	10	8	45	50	1.1
	15–18	55	120	163	64	44	800	10	8	55	60	1.1
	19–24	58	128	164	65	46	800	10	8	60	60	1.1
	25–50	63	138	163	64	50	800	5	8	65	60	1.1
	51+	65	143	160	63	50	800	5	8	65	60	1.0
Pregnant						60	800	10	10	65	70	1.5
Lactating	1st 6 months					65	1300	10	12	65	95	1.6
	2nd 6 months					62	1200	10	11	65	90	1.6

Recommended Dietary Allowances, © 1989, by the National Academy of Sciences, National Academy Press, Washington, D.C.
[a]The allowances, expressed as average daily intakes over time, are intended to provide for individual variations among most normal persons as they live in the United States under usual environmental stresses. Diets should be based on a variety of common foods in order to provide other nutrients for which human requirements have been less well defined. See text for detailed discussion of allowances and nutrients not tabulated.
[b]Weights and heights of Reference Adults are actual medians for the U.S. population of the designated age, as reported by NHANES II. The median weights and heights of those under 19 years of age were taken from Hamil et al., (1979) (see pages 16–17). The use of these figures does not imply that the height-to-weight ratios are ideal.

Water-Soluble Vitamins   **Minerals**

Riboflavin (mg)	Niacin (mg NE)[f]	Vitamin B_6 (mg)	Folate (μg)	Vitamin B_{12} (μg)	Calcium (mg)	Phosphorus (mg)	Magnesium (mg)	Iron (mg)	Zinc (mg)	Iodine (μg)	Selenium (μg)
0.4	5	0.3	25	0.3	400	300	40	6	5	40	10
0.5	6	0.6	35	0.5	600	500	60	10	5	50	15
0.8	9	1.0	50	0.7	800	800	80	10	10	70	20
1.1	12	1.1	75	1.0	800	800	120	10	10	90	20
1.2	13	1.4	100	1.4	800	800	170	10	10	120	30
1.5	17	1.7	150	2.0	1200	1200	270	12	15	150	40
1.8	20	2.0	200	2.0	1200	1200	400	12	15	150	50
1.7	19	2.0	200	2.0	1200	1200	350	10	15	150	70
1.7	19	2.0	200	2.0	800	800	350	10	15	150	70
1.4	15	2.0	200	2.0	800	800	350	10	15	150	70
1.3	15	1.4	150	2.0	1200	1200	280	15	12	150	45
1.3	15	1.5	180	2.0	1200	1200	300	15	12	150	50
1.3	15	1.6	180	2.0	1200	1200	280	15	12	150	55
1.3	15	1.6	180	2.0	800	800	280	15	12	150	55
1.2	13	1.6	180	2.0	800	800	280	10	12	150	55
1.6	17	2.2	400	2.2	1200	1200	320	30	15	175	65
1.8	20	2.1	280	2.6	1200	1200	355	15	19	200	75
1.7	20	2.1	260	2.6	1200	1200	340	15	16	200	75

[c]Retinol equivalents. 1 retinol equivalent = 1 μg retinol or 6 μg β-carotene. See text for calculation of vitamin A activity of diets as retinol equivalents.

[d]As cholecalciferol. 10 μg cholecalciferol = 400 IV of vitamin D.

[e]α-Tocopherol equivalents. 1 mg d-α tocopherol = 1 α-TE. See text for variation in allowances and calculation of vitamin E activity of the diet as a α-tocopherol equivalents.

[f]I NE (niacin equivalent) is equal to 1 mg of niacin or 60 mg of dietary tryptophan.